Jones's Animal Nursing

SECOND EDITION

Jones's Animal Nursing

SECOND EDITION

Edited by

R. S. PINNIGER

FOR THE BRITISH SMALL ANIMAL VETERINARY ASSOCIATION
WITH CONTRIBUTIONS FROM TWENTY AUTHORS

PERGAMON PRESS

OXFORD · NEW YORK · TORONTO
SYDNEY · BRAUNSCHWEIG

Pergamon Press Ltd., Headington Hill Hall, Oxford
Pergamon Press Inc., Maxwell House, Fairview Park, Elmsford,
New York 10523
Pergamon of Canada Ltd., 207 Queen's Quay West, Toronto 1
Pergamon Press (Aust). Pty. Ltd., 19a Boundary Street,
Rushcutters Bay, N.S.W. 2011, Australia
Vieweg & Sohn GmbH, Burgplatz 1, Braunschweig

First edition 1966

Second edition 1972

Reprinted with minor corrections 1973

Library of Congress Catalog Card No. 74–188111

Printed in Great Britain by A. Wheaton & Co., Exeter

ISBN 0 08 016839 6

Contents

2. THE PRINCIPLES OF ANIMAL MANAGEMENT, HYGIENE AND FEEDING

List of Authors

J. T. ABRAMS, MA, MSc, PhD
Department of Veterinary Clinical Studies
University of Cambridge School of Veterinary Medicine
Madingley Road
Cambridge

R. S. ANDERSON, BVMS, PhD, MRCVS
Animal Studies Department
Petfoods Limited
Melton Mowbray
Leicestershire

D. K. BLACKMORE, BSc, PhD, FRCVS
Medical Research Council
Laboratory Animals Centre
Woodmansterne Road
Carshalton
Surrey

J. E. COX, BVetMed, BSc, MRCVS
Department of Veterinary Clinical Studies
University Veterinary Field Station
Leahurst, Neston
Wirral, Cheshire

S. W. DOUGLAS, MA, MRCVS, DVR
University of Cambridge
Department of Veterinary Clinical Studies
School of Veterinary Medicine
Madingley Road
Cambridge

D. G. EARNSHAW, MA, BSc, MRCVS
237 Warringah Road
Beacon Hill
Sydney, NSW 2100
Australia

N. G. FOWLER, FRCVS, DipBact, DVR
The Veterinary Hospital
34 New Dover Road
Canterbury, Kent

CAROLINE J. FRANKLIN, RANA
Berkshire College of Agriculture
Hall Place
Burchetts Green
Nr. Maidenhead, Berkshire

S. F. J. HODGMAN, MRCVS
Lanwades Cottage
Kennett
Nr. Newmarket
Suffolk

JOAN O. JOSHUA, FRCVS
The University of Liverpool
Veterinary Hospital
Pembroke Gardens
Liverpool

ANNE R. KEELEY, RANA, AIAT
Medical Research Council
Laboratory Animals Centre
Woodmansterne Road
Carshalton
Surrey

A. R. W. PORTER, MA, Barrister-at-Law
Registrar of the Royal College of Veterinary Surgeons
32 Belgrave Square
London SW1

W. B. SINGLETON, MRCVS
14 Pont Street
Knightsbridge
London SW1

R. N. SMITH, PhD, DSc, FRCVS
Department of Veterinary Anatomy
University of Bristol
Park Row
Bristol

G. SUMNER-SMITH, BVSc, MSc, FRCVS
University of Guelph
Veterinary Teaching Hospital
Ontario Veterinary College
Guelph
Ontario, Canada

F. G. STARTUP, PhD, BSc, MRCVS
Grove Lodge Veterinary Hospital
Upper Brighton Road
Worthing
Sussex

J. STRATTON, MRCVS
Stone Cottage
Whitwell
Ventnor
Isle of Wight

G. T. WILKINSON, MVSc, MRCVS
Animal Health Trust
Small Animals Centre
Lanwades Park
Kennett
Nr. Newmarket
Suffolk

J. S. WILKINSON, BSc, PhD, MRCVS
University of Melbourne
Veterinary Clinical Centre
Werribee
Victoria 3030
Australia

C. E. WOODROW, MRCVS
Haxted Mill
Edenbridge
Kent

Preface to the Second Edition

THE wisdom of hindsight, and the advance in the status of the Registered Animal Nursing Auxiliary during the 6 years that have elapsed since the publication of the first edition of *Animal Nursing*, have necessitated a fully revised second edition, which includes six new sections and an increased number of illustrations.

The work of twenty authors has been combined to form the content of this book. Of these, two are RANAs, which in itself indicates the development that RANAs have achieved since the Royal College of Veterinary Surgeons first established the Register of Animal Nursing Auxillaries in 1961.

Two major sections have been completely rewritten by distinguished authors to adjust the approach in the light of experience in teaching ANA students: *Anatomy and Physiology* by Dr. R. N. Smith and *Medical Nursing and Some Common Diseases of Importance to the RANA* by Miss J. O. Joshua.

Other new sections are: *Nutrition of the Cat; Cage Birds; Smaller Mammals; Genetics and Animal Breeding; Obstetrical and Paediactric Nursing in the Cat* and *The Position of the RANA under the Veterinary Surgeons Act 1966*, and have been added because of their increasing relevance to small animal veterinary practice.

Some sections have an academic scope which may be thought to be beyond that required by ANA students in order to pass their examinations, because although that is the main object of this textbook it is by no means the only one. *Genetics and Animal Breeding* by J. E. Cox is a case in point. This section fills a gap in the published work in this field and is included for RANAs who wish to study the subject in greater depth.

The word RANA has been used throughout the text. In this country as well as abroad the RANA is now recognized in her own right. It is a name to be proud of and its use should be encouraged.

I am sincerely grateful to all the authors who have co-operated to produce this edition. They have willingly given of their time with little regard to material gain.

The Officers of the BSAVA and the RANA Committee, under the consecutive Chairmanships of John Leach and Olive Evans, have at all times given help and encouragement. I would especially mention Geoff Startup and Derek Tavernor, who have formed my editorial sub-committee, and have together accomplished a prodigious amount of work. To these, and to very many others who during the last 3 years have helped me greatly, I offer my gratitude. Theirs is the praise; the editorial errors and omissions are mine alone.

Bournemouth, August 1971 ROGER PINNIGER, MRCVS

Preface to the First Edition

THE establishment of a Register of Animal Nursing Auxiliaries by the Royal College of Veterinary Surgeons marked a notable advance in the development of small animal practice. The creation of this new group of people, together with the institution of examinations leading to the qualification to be entered on the Register, at once demanded a comprehensive text and reference book for both trainees and veterinary surgeons at approved training centres.

As soon as the details of the scheme and syllabus of subjects to be covered in the preliminary and final examinations became known the Council of the British Small Animal Veterinary Association directed that a book be prepared to aid students undertaking courses of tuition.

The Publications Committee of the BSAVA, in co-operation with fourteen authors, has produced *Animal Nursing* to meet this need. The book has been designed basically to cover the major subjects of the examination syllabus. The chapter structure has followed in general outline the subjects of the syllabus with modifications where these were felt to be editorially desirable.

Animal Nursing seeks to provide a background text for students undertaking the ANA course of tuition but it is emphasized that this theoretical knowledge must be supplemented with both the required practical training, and, where possible, with attendance at the classes provided by local education authorities.

Readers of this book will find that there is a certain element of duplication in some sections; this is partly due to the individual preparation of the chapters but also is planned to help emphasize some of the more important subject material of the course. In the main the dog has been used as the type animal for the description of the main anatomical and surgical fundamentals, but where species differences occur with the cat these are also described.

It is hoped that this will be the first of many editions of this work which will grow and improve as the ANA course develops and matures with the growth in small animal practice that it is designed to assist.

1966 BRUCE V. JONES, MRCVS

CHAPTER 1

Anatomy and Physiology

R. N. Smith, PhD, DSc, FRCVS

ILLUSTRATIONS BY T. WILTSHIRE

Introduction

This book is about dogs and cats. These are mammals, that is, animals that have backbones and warm blood and whose females feed their new-born young on milk produced in mammary glands (hence, the class name mammals). They also always have hair.

Most, but not all, mammals are placental; in other words, they have an arrangement called a placenta which develops in the pregnant female and from which the unborn animal gets its nourishment. Dogs and cats are placental mammals; so also, for example, are humans, bats, cattle and mice. However, these are all classified into divisions, called orders, of mammals. Humans are primates (have hands and feet); bats, having wings, belong to the chiroptera; cattle are ungulates (their feet are hooved); mice are examples of the rodentia, gnawing animals. Dogs and cats, like bears and lions, are in the order carnivora, the flesh-eaters.

Not all the animals that are brought to the surgery are mammals; for instance, birds are often presented and so sometimes are tortoises. Nevertheless, these have backbones and so, like the mammals, they belong to a section of animals called vertebrates. Some animals of great importance to the veterinary surgeon do not even have backbones. These are the invertebrates and examples of these that are rather too common are external parasites such as fleas and internal parasites such as round-worms and flat-worms.

The opening section of this book on nursing is concerned with how animals are constructed (their anatomy) and how they work (their physiology). This form and function are closely interrelated and interdependent and it is helpful to think of them together and not as separate disciplines.

Most sciences have their own language: this enables precise communication between colleagues. Sometimes a word in general everyday use is given a very exact meaning in some branch of science. At one time only Latin names were acceptable in biological nomenclature and some of these are still in current use in the original Latin form. It would be a great convenience if only one name were used for each structure. Unfortunately over the centuries that some of these sciences have been studied a variety of names has grown up and it is not a case of which is right or wrong, but which is the best term in common use. Opinions on this will vary and so some of the names used here may not be those used by the veterinary surgeon that you are assisting.

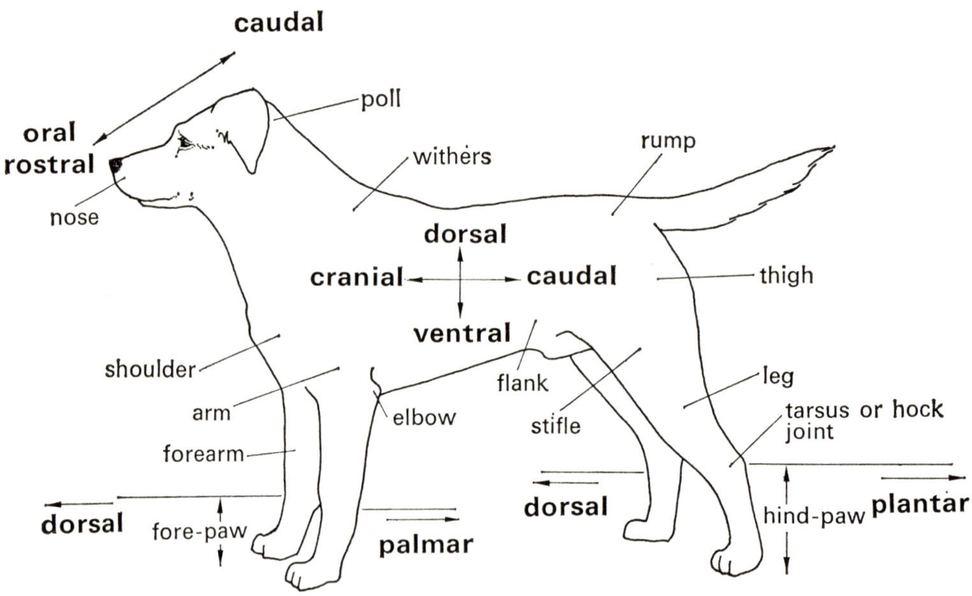

Fig. 1.1. Some points of the dog and anatomical directions: these latter are in bold type.

A series of terms is used to indicate directions with reference to parts of the body; some of these are common to all regions. *Superficial* and *deep* indicate relative distances from the surface of the body. *External* and *internal* refer to relations of depth in organs and cavities. *Medial* and *lateral* give the position nearer to and farther from the mid-line of the body.

However, many terms are used only in specific regions. When the animal is standing evenly on all four limbs with the head and tail fairly level, the surface of the head, trunk and tail nearer to the ground is *ventral:* the opposite side of the animal is *dorsal. Caudal* means that the part is nearer to the tail-end of the animal: the term is used for all the animal except the lower regions of the limbs. For this part of the forelimb the direction is *palmar* (volar is still frequently used) and for the hindlimb it is *plantar.*

The opposite to caudal is *cranial* except for the head. Here the term is *oral* (nearer the mouth) or *rostral* (towards the nose). *Anterior* and *posterior* are occasionally also used for directions in the head. For the lower parts of the limbs the *dorsal* surface is the opposite to palmar and plantar. (The conventions used for these limb regions fit best with human nomenclature and make comparison simpler.) *Distal* is another term used for the limbs and means away from the trunk; the opposite is *proximal*. These terms and some of the regions (points) of the dog are shown in Fig. 1.1.

Tissues and Systems

All the materials of which an animal is made are arranged in **tissues.** This name is taken from the French word "tissu" which means "woven" and was used by a French scientist in the eighteenth century who noticed the resemblance of the layers and structures of the body to woven material and so classified them according to their texture or "tissu".

Later work showed that these tissues, which together form the entire substance of the body, consist of three main components:

1. Cells. These are minute individual living entities.
2. Intercellular materials. These are produced by cells and as the name suggests, they are found between the cells.
3. Fluid, either bathing the cells themselves or flowing in specially formed channels between them.

A structure in which one tissue predominates and where some special function is segregated is called an **organ.** A **system** is a collection of tissues, organs, parts and structures related by position or function.

BASIC TISSUES

A tissue can be defined as a collection of cells and their products which has a common fundamental function and in which one particular type of cell predominates.

There are four basic tissues; (1) muscular, concerned with movement; (2) nervous, enabling the animal to be aware of the environment and to make any changes it needs to adapt to it; (3) epithelial, a covering tissue; (4) connective tissue which plays a general supporting role and also weaves itself through all the other tissues, connecting and binding them together.

Muscular Tissue

Muscular tissue is the one in which the property of contractility is well developed. It has a very high proportion of muscle cells, which, since they are usually long, thin and thread-like, are often called fibres. The cells are divisible into three types: skeletal, smooth and cardiac.

Skeletal muscle cells are found in muscular tissue attached to the skeleton. The cells are usually cylindrical and vary from about 1 millimetre to 5 centimetres in length although they are only about one-hundredth of a millimetre in thickness. Since skeletal muscular tissue often responds to the will of the animal, the cells may be called **voluntary** muscle cells. Skeletal muscles are formed of parallel muscle cells (fibres) held together in small bundles by connective tissue. These are collected into larger groups which are also enclosed in connective tissue, and ultimately form the muscle which is surrounded by yet more connective tissue commonly called the **muscle sheath.** Where muscles are close to one another, the muscle sheaths may thicken to form **intermuscular septa.** All the connective tissue within and around the muscles continues into the connective tissue of the structure to which the muscle is attached. Sometimes the muscle appears to attach directly but usually the connective tissue leaves the muscle as a fibrous band known as a **tendon** or as a fibrous sheet called an **aponeurosis.** Muscles vary greatly in their shapes and some are named according to the shape they have in the **human** body, although this may not be the same as in other animal bodies. Some muscles are named according to their functions and yet others according to their position in the body. When looked at under a microscope, skeletal muscle cells have regular stripes (striations) at right angles to their long axes and so this type may be called *striated muscle tissue.*

Smooth muscle cells are spindle-shaped and may be up to about half a millimetre in length although most are very much shorter. They are called "smooth" because they do not have the microscopic striations of skeletal muscle cells. Small amounts of connective tissue usually bind them together to form sheets or layers of *smooth muscle tissue.* However, they are sometimes found grouped together in small numbers, and in some parts of the body smooth muscle cells occur singly. Smooth muscle tissue is often associated with involuntary actions; that is, actions that are not usually controlled by the will of the animal. For this reason smooth muscle cells may be called **involuntary** muscle cells.

Cardiac muscle cells are confined to the heart and are involuntary in action. The cells are elongated and are the only muscle cells which frequently branch. They are held together by relatively scanty amounts of connective tissue.

Epithelial Tissue

Epithelial tissue covers the outside of the body and also lines the inner cavities and tubes: its main function is protection but in some areas it has other properties. The tissue is composed almost entirely of epithelial cells and these are fixed on to connective tissue by an intercellular substance.

It is necessary in some situations to allow absorption or filtration through the epithelial membrane (layer of cells). Obviously, it is better here to have a membrane only one cell in thickness and this is called a **simple** epithelium.

There may be cells in a simple epithelium that are specially designed to absorb material: these have a tremendous number of small processes (only recognizable under magnifications of about 40,000) on their free surface that increase the absorptive area. There may also be cells whose special function is to secrete (produce) a slippery protective fluid called **mucus.** Yet other epithelial cells may have very fine hair-like projections called **cilia** whose function is to move the mucus along over the epithelial tissue by their continuous waving action.

In some regions of the body the protective function is more important than absorption or filtration and a simple epithelium would prove to be too delicate. Here there will be several layers of cells and the tissue is called a **stratified** epithelium. Where even more protection is required and especially where the surface is dry, the outermost layers of a stratified epithelium undergo changes known as **keratinization** to become **keratin.** It is a material that is very resistant to chemical change and to bacterial invasion, as well as being fairly waterproof. This tough, resilient substance protects the underlying cells from drying out and also from other forms of damage.

There are certain areas of the body where a large amount of the epithelial secretion is required, more than could be produced by cells occupying the outermost surface. The necessary epithelial cells including, of course, the secretory type, are clustered together and push down into the connective tissue to form a **gland.** Those glands which retain a connection with the free surface and whose secretion can pass up a collecting tube or duct are called **exocrine** glands. The connective tissue in which the gland is embedded may divide it into small units or **lobules:** the gland is said to be lobulated and the connective tissue divisions are called interlobular septa. Groups of lobules may be collected by stronger connective tissue to form **lobes.** Such a gland will then be lobated and have interlobar septa.

There are some glands which do not have any connection with the free epithelial surface. Since there is no duct they may be called **ductless** glands or **endocrine** glands. They secrete very important substances called **hormones** which have special effects on the various body systems: since there is no duct, the secretion leaves the glands in one of the other fluids of the body.

Nervous Tissue

The cells of nervous tissue have the ability of responding to a stimulus by producing a wave of electrical excitation called a *nervous impulse* and of conducting the impulse rapidly over large areas of the body.

Each cell is a **neuron** and consists of a **cell body** and a number of processes. They vary tremendously in shape and in the arrangement of the processes. When the processes are thin and long (and in some cases they may be many centimetres long) their thread-like appearance gives rise to the name fibres as it does in so many other structures with this particular form.

All the processes carrying impulses *to* the cell body are called **dendrites** or **dendrons.** Only one process carries the nerve impulse away: this one is called the **axon,** and it may end by splitting into a number of branches. The nervous impulse which the axon is carrying away from its cell body may be destined immediately for an effector organ, in which case this is where the terminal branches end. It may, however, have to travel via another neuron to reach its destination. There is no continuity between successive neurons and the impulse has to pass over a junction or **synapse.** The arrangement is always one-way: the impulse leaves the axon and passes either to the cell body or to the dendrite of the next neuron, never in the reverse direction.

Connective Tissue

Connective tissue is the material that is found binding all the other tissues together, acting as a supporting medium for them and also conducting nutrition to, and waste material away from, the various cells of the body. To help perform these functions adequately, a large amount of intercellular material or **matrix** is often found in connective tissue. This is thought to be formed by some of the cells of the connective tissue and it may take one of several forms. The intercellular material may be fluid; in other cases, when it is sometimes called **ground substance,** it is gelatinous or even hard. If fibres occur in the matrix it is said to be **fibrous;** if not, then the material is considered **amorphous.** The intercellular material, its physical nature and the associated cells, together provide a variety of connective tissues depending on the proportions of each that are present. This will be decided by the function that the connective tissue has to perform: it will, however, be covered generally by the term "supporting" whether this refers to support by structure or by nutritive supplies and waste removal. The connective tissues will be described in order of increasing viscosity of their intercellular materials; that is, blood, haemopoietic tissue, loose connective tissue, dense connective tissue, cartilage, bone.

Blood (with comments on other body fluids)

Blood is a fluid connective tissue that circulates in all adult vertebrates in a continous system of tubes called **blood vessels.** It comprises about 7% of the body weight and has a supporting role for other tissues by conveying nutritive material and removing waste products. It consists of a fluid matrix called **plasma** which makes up between 55% and 70% of the blood and in this are found special blood cells called **corpuscles** and cell fragments known as **blood platelets.** The corpuscles are divided into "red blood corpuscles" (RBCs) called **erythrocytes** and "white blood corpuscles" (WBCs) called **leucocytes.** Erythrocytes have no nucleus. They are responsible for the colour of blood and in every cubic millimetre there are about 7 million. Like all the cells in the dog and cat they can only be seen under very strong magnification and in size they are about seven-thousandths of a millimetre in diameter (7 micron, or 7 μ).

The erythrocytes are concerned with the transport of gases. All the tissues of the body require a substantial supply of oxygen and they have to be relieved of the carbon dioxide which they produce. **Haemoglobin** is found in the erythrocytes and is the cause of their colour: this substance is also responsible for the carriage of oxygen.

The leucocytes are nucleated and support the body in general by taking an active part in body defence mechanisms. In the dog there are 5,000–20,000 per cubic millimetre of blood and in cats 8,000–25,000. They are colourless and are divisible into two major groups. Those that have very small granules within the cell body are called **granular** leucocytes or **granulocytes:** the others are non-granular or **agranular** leucocytes, and the most important of these are the **lymphocytes.** One of the prime functions of the leucocytes seems to be **phagocytosis,** that is, the ingestion (taking-in) and consequent removal of pieces of broken-down cells and tissues. This they do mainly outside the blood vessels, which they leave by active movement on their own account; they use the blood stream as a route to travel around the body.

If blood stops moving or if it breaks out of blood vessels which have been breached in any way it coagulates into a jelly-like mass, a phenomenon that is known as **clotting. Fibrinogen,** which is a normal constituent of circulating plasma, undergoes a physical and chemical change into **fibrin** in such circumstances. The fibrin forms into threads which become a network trapping the blood cells; in this way a clot forms. Plasma which has had the fibrinogen removed is called **serum.** When blood is taken from an animal it has to be combined with an **anti-coagulant** if it is to be kept in a fluid form; otherwise the blood settles out into the clot and the serum. It appears that blood platelets play an important role in the mechanism of blood clotting.

The gases carried by the erythrocytes have to be transported to and from the other cells of the body and yet it is unusual for the red blood corpuscles to leave the blood vessels. The gaseous exchange is achieved through the medium of **tissue fluid.** Other nutritive material and waste products also use tissue fluid as a transfer medium and the mechanism of exchange takes place through blood vessels which have walls of extreme thinness. These vessels are known as **capillaries** and their walls consist of a single layer of epithelial cells.

The capillary wall acts as a semi-permeable membrane; that is, it is permeable to some, but not all, of the constituents of blood. The part of blood that can diffuse into and out of the lumen (cavity) of the capillary is tissue fluid, the transfer medium for many of the cells' nutrients and waste products.

Outside the blood vessels, the tissue fluid bathes the cells of surrounding tissues. Much of the fluid that diffuses out of the capillary blood vessels will diffuse in again. However, not all of it takes this direct route back. Some of it diffuses through the thin walls of another system of capillary vessels which permeate the tissues to form another complex network. Once the tissue fluid has passed into the lumen of this alternative set of capillaries it is called **lymph.** These *lymph capillaries* join up to form larger *lymph vessels* and they eventually discharge their lymph into the system of blood vessels.

Haemopoietic tissue

The cells that circulate through the body wear out in a relatively short time. They must be continually replaced by new ones and the old cells must be continually removed. These two functions, replacement and removal, are both performed in one type of connective tissue. This is called haemopoietic tissue. There are two sorts of haemopoietic tissue, the main difference being the types of blood cells produced. The haemopoietic tissue producing erythrocytes and granular leucocytes is called **myeloid** tissue: that producing the agranular leucocytes is called **lymphoid (lymphatic)** tissue.

Loose connective tissue

In this form of supporting tissue the intercellular material consists of a semi-fluid gelatinous material contained in a loose meshwork of fibres. Whitish in colour, the sticky mass surrounds and supports elements of other tissues. It acts as a packing material and when it is cut and exposed to the air it often has a bubbly appearance. It is sometimes called **areolar** tissue.

The fibres of the intercellular material may be collagenous, elastic or reticular. The **collagenous** fibres are often arranged in bundles which run in all directions. Although of a soft nature they are very resistant to tensile stress, that is, to being pulled. They consist of collagen. The **elastic** fibres are not as common as the collagenous ones. They tend to run singly, to branch freely and to anastomose (join-up) to make networks. If they are present in any great number they give a yellowish tint to the tissue. **Reticular** fibres are very delicate and are common where connective tissue borders on to another tissue. One of the characteristics of loose connective tissue is that it can stretch in any direction. Fibres therefore are neither very numerous nor are they woven closely together.

The jelly-like but slightly fibrous matrix is infiltrated by several types of cellular elements such as **fibroblasts** which are usually closely associated with the collagenous fibres and are thought to play an important part in their formation, and **fat cells** which are characterized by the presence of a large drop of fat. When these occur in large numbers the nature of the connective tissue is so altered that it may be called fat or **adipose** tissue.

One of the functions of loose connective tissue is to attach the skin to underlying structures. In this way, the skin can be freely movable (it also allows the skin to be fairly readily removed from underlying tissues). In this position, the connective tissue may also be called **hypodermis;** it is sometimes called **sub-cutaneous** tissue. Both words mean "beneath the skin" and it is into this tissue that a "subcutaneous" injection is given using a "hypodermic" syringe. It is also called **superficial fascia** and it may be found arranged in definite layers.

Dense connective tissue

In this form, the proportion of fibres is very much greater than in other forms of connective tissue: it is found where great tensile strength is an advantage. Sometimes the fibres are interwoven and give the appearance of a dense mass: this is called **irregular dense** connective tissue. If the fibres are nearly parallel and tend to run in bundles or sheets they are said to form **regular dense** connective tissue.

The tissue between the epithelial layer of the skin and the superficial fascia that has just been described is irregular dense connective tissue. It is called the **dermis** and is fixed firmly on its outer surface to the epithelial **epidermis.** On its inner surface it continues into the loose connective tissue of the superficial fascia (hypodermis or subcutaneous tissue). The skeletal muscles, especially in the limbs, are often ensheathed in a tough sheet of irregular dense connective tissue. This is called the **deep fascia.** It dips down between the muscles and is continuous with the connective tissue of the intermuscular septa and the connective tissue between the muscle fibres. The deep fascia attaches in places to the skeleton; in some areas it is continuous with muscles. Irregular dense connective tissue is also found around many of the organs of the body where it is said to form a **capsule.** Sometimes the fibres in a particular part become more regularly arranged than in the remainder of the capsule. Such localized areas, which are often thicker than the surrounding connective tissue and may therefore be raised above it, are called **ligaments.**

Regular dense connective tissue is usually associated with muscles. The connective tissue fibres are nearly parallel and leave the muscle as a fibrous band known as a **tendon** or as a fibrous sheet called an **aponeurosis.**

Cartilage

Cartilage is a connective tissue which whilst being rigid can also be flexible and resilient. It is able to bear a certain amount of weight and it possesses quite considerable tensile strength.

There are relatively few cells. The intercellular material consists of a mass of fibres embedded in a gelatinous material. In some cartilage the fibres are of collagen and are not easily seen: this is called **hyaline cartilage** and the fibres are randomly arranged to form a mat. In **fibro-cartilage** there is an increase in the number of collagenous fibres and they are organised in a parallel form. Fibro-cartilage is found where it is essential that the tissue has great tensile strength. There are some areas of cartilage with a very high proportion of elastic fibres: this is called **elastic cartilage,** and, whilst still retaining the rigidity characteristic of all cartilage, this form of connective tissue is more resilient.

Perhaps the most unusual feature of cartilage is that, given a slight amount of lubrication, surfaces coated with this tissue can move and slide on one another with very little friction or wear. With the exception of such surfaces, i.e. those that move on one another, the periphery of a piece of cartilage has a less "cartilaginous" appearance than a more central zone. The collagenous fibres appear more obvious and they form a fibrous layer, the **perichondrium.** This will merge imperceptibly into cartilage.

Bone

In this form of connective tissue the matrix contains collagenous fibres and a cementing substance with a substantial proportion of chemicals such as calcium phosphate. The cells occur in microscopic cavities in this ground substance.

Mature bone is arranged in thin layers (or **lamellae**) with the collagenous fibres running in different directions in adjacent lamellae. This increases the resistance of the bone tissue to mechanical forces.

The shape and arrangement of the lamellae allow a separation into spongy (cancellous) and compact bone tissue. **Spongy** bone consists of bars and plates called **trabeculae** and these form a three-dimensional network. Each trabecula consists of a few lamellae generally arranged parallel to one another or in concentric layers. In **compact** bone most of the lamellae are arranged in cylindrical systems (**osteones** or *Haversian systems*) around narrow axial canals. The canal is called an *Haversian canal* and contains minute blood vessels and fine nerve fibres in loose connective tissue.

Bone formation is termed **ossification** or **osteogenesis;** semi-fluid ground substance already at the site of ossification condenses and undergoes a chemical change: this masks any fibres that are also present. The resulting substance is **osteoid** tissue; it becomes calcified almost immediately, and undergoes a subtle chemical change to become bone. There is a constant remodelling of bone tissue.

In the developing young animal, bone formation in some regions of the body is preceded by cartilage. When it is time for bone to be produced the cartilage becomes calcified and acts as a scaffolding. Bone is laid down on this scaffolding and the calcified cartilage is then gradually removed. *Calcified cartilage is not bone.* Bone tissue formed on a calcified cartilage scaffolding is commonly called **endochondral** bone and the process is said to be endochondral ossification. It is essential to realize that this bone tissue is formed in the same way as any other bone tissue: it is only the environment that is different. Where bone tissue is formed without the aid of a cartilage scaffold, it is said to be **intramembranous** bone and to have formed by intramembranous ossification.

SYSTEMS

The body systems are all interdependent and the fundamental purpose for which they are designed is the survival of the animal and the species. Life depends entirely on chemical reactions and many of these are so precise that they can take place in conditions that vary within only the narrowest limits. The temperature, acidity, etc., of the internal environment needs to be kept constant no matter what is happening outside the body. This is achieved by an all-pervading fluid arrangement.

The **vascular system** of heart and vessels (tubes) keeps the blood and lymph circulating through the entire animal. Tissue fluid bathes all the structures of the body and substances such as nutrients and waste products can pass between the fluid inside and outside the cells and also through the vessel walls between the tissue fluid and the blood and lymph. The vascular system ensures a constant mixing of all the fluids of the body with a resulting levelling of extreme conditions that might occur locally.

Nutrients are brought from outside the animal into the **digestive system,** a tube open at both ends. The chemical and physical extraction they undergo is **digestion,** a process helped by substances secreted (the act of producing useful material) by the cells of this system. Digestion breaks down the complex chemicals of the food into very small packages that can pass through the **intestinal wall** (part of the lining of the digestive system) and into the vascular system. This process is **absorption** and the fluid then passes the packages along to other cells where they are needed. The unwanted part of the food continues on through the digestive system and is eventually passed to the outside of the animal as **faeces** (droppings) during the act of **defaecation.** While it is travelling along the digestive system other unwanted substances are added which have passed through the wall into the lumen (cavity) of the tube. Removal of waste products from cells and from the body is called **excretion.**

The small packages of nutrient substances that have been absorbed into the blood and lymph may be used by cells without any further alteration. Sometimes special products need to be manufactured and this can only be done by cells in certain regions such as the liver. **Metabolism** is the term used to describe all the chemical reactions that go on in the body and this special manufacture is called *intermediary metabolism.*

An essential chemical in the vast majority of reactions in the animal body is the gas oxygen, and this is obtained from the air by the **respiratory system.** The air is pulled into the lungs inside the body and the oxygen passes into the blood through the extensive but very thin membrane of the lungs which terminates the respiratory system in the thorax (chest). The dissolved oxygen is carried by the ubiquitous fluid system to the cells to play its role in chemical reactions which usually end in the production of another gas, carbon dioxide. This is passed back into the blood stream and taken to the lungs where it flows back across the very thin membrane and is excreted to the outside air by the respiratory system.

There are other waste products beside carbon dioxide which result from cell metabolism and which are excreted into the blood stream. However, these are not gaseous and many are removed from the blood through the numerous small tubes within the paired kidneys. These excretory products help to form the **urine** and from the kidneys this fluid passes to the urinary bladder to be voided at intervals to the outside during the act of **urination.** This excretory arrangement forms the **urinary system** and it is very closely linked with the organs used in producing the young.

The male animal produces **sperms,** small cells carrying fundamental and chemical information from this parent and uses a tubular part (the **penis**) of the urinary system to deposit them inside the female. The potential mother produces **ova,** cells containing the contribution of the female parent to the basic chemical store of the young. Eventually the sperms meet and penetrate the ova and the resulting "fertilized" cells develop within the female. All the parts of the male and female concerned with this function of producing young constitute the **reproductive system.** Its closeness to the urinary system in the male has been outlined but there is a similar relation in the female. To get the sperms naturally into the correct place, the penis of the male has to be positioned partly in the passage of the female that is also used for voiding urine. But the male reproductive cells then pass into an adjacent tubular structure (the **uterus**) to fertilize the female germ cells and this is where the young develop. The reproductive part may also be called the **genital system** and the two closely linked arrangements are often referred to as the **urogenital system.**

But how do the male and female animals get together and how do they get around to the food they must take in? For this there is the **locomotor system.** A complex arrangement of contractile "ropes" (muscles) and fairly rigid "rods" (bones of the skeleton) is used to move the animal from place to place and in addition, this **musculo-skeletal** apparatus acts as a fairly efficient protective casing for the delicate structures forming all the other systems.

The **integumentary system** embraces all these parts of the body, keeping them together, to a certain extent insulating them from the outside and helping to keep the internal environment constant. The most extensive part of the integument is the skin and in addition to the multiple functions just outlined, it also plays an important role in excretion.

Information about the outside environment, about the position of the animal, about the relation of one part to another, about the internal environment, is all collected together by the **nervous system.** This information gathering part is the **sensory** component and its integration and evaluation takes place in the **brain** and **spinal cord.** From here instructions are sent throughout the body to deal with each situation as it arises. This part is the **motor** component and the pathways used may run side by side with those of the sensory component. The tissues forming these pathways are the **nerves** of the body and like the vessels of the vascular system, they are all-pervading.

Chemistry and Structure of the Cell

All the tissues of the body are made of chemicals and only of chemicals. These can all be purified and, if necessary, bottled and put on display. The preceding section on tissues and systems should have afforded a glimpse into the complete integration of the body, a condition requiring a fantastic interplay of delicate chemical reactions that together constitute life. However, cells are not just small compartments filled with a haphazard collection of dilute solutions of chemicals. They have their own individual structure and an appreciation of this is necessary as well as an insight into some of the chemical processes that take place there.

CHEMISTRY OF THE CELL

Chemical substances found only in living material were originally classified as **organic** compounds, as opposed to those found elsewhere which were grouped as **inorganic,** since it was thought that they were quite different and imbued with some wonderful extra "vital spirit". However, the chemists eventually showed that organic compounds could be isolated and synthesized in the same ways that were used for other compounds. Nevertheless, they did have one curious common factor: these organic compounds all contained carbon and to a certain extent organic chemistry can be considered the same as carbon chemistry. It is a branch of science that exists in its own right and so it is quite customary to continue discussing the chemistry of living material in organic and inorganic terms. Water is the commonest compound in the body and is itself an inorganic substance. Other inorganic compounds found in animals are often referred to as minerals (a very special use of the word) and since the remaining materials would all be destroyed by heat leaving only inorganic substances they are also said to make up the ash content of the body.

Inorganic Content of the Body

The body consists of 60–80% water and the other inorganic substances include calcium, phosphorus, magnesium, sodium, potassium, chlorine, iron and copper. Some others such as iodine and manganese exist in such small amounts that they are called trace elements. None of these exist as the purified element: one no more finds pure chlorine than one does a piece of metallic copper. The chemicals are found in a special combining form called an *ion;* calcium ions, magnesium ions, chloride ions, phosphate ions, etc.

Water. No living cell can exist without water and intracellular water (inside the cell) represents about 50% of body weight. Extracellular water (outside the cell) is found in tissue fluid (15% body weight) and blood plasma (5%). There is a constant interchange of water between these fluid compartments but there is quite a difference in the concentration of water in different tissues. It makes up about three-quarters of muscles and about one-quarter of bone; there is very little water in fat tissue.

Since water is a very good solvent it can act as a transport medium for a multitude of chemicals. It also plays a vital role in temperature regulation for not only can it be moved around to dissipate heat but also its evaporation from body surfaces including the mouth and the respiratory tract can have an extremely useful cooling effect. There is a high content of water in the lubricants of the joints and of the surface of the eye.

It is not convenient for an animal to store water in bulk and, since there is a continual loss through the urinary and digestive systems as well as through the lungs and skin, there must be continual replacement. Water enters the body as a liquid, in the food, and it is also formed there as a result of chemical reactions. An excessive intake is usually balanced by an increased urine output. When water is short and the amount of urine is low, the excretion through the lungs and skin may exceed urine output. Illness can cause a serious loss of fluid especially when it is accompanied by vomiting and diarrhoea. Severe bleeding (haemorrhage) can also lower the fluid level of the body.

Calcium, phosphorus, magnesium. The greater part of the mineral content of the body consists of these elements and most of it is found in the bones and teeth. The calcium level is higher than that of phosphorus and it seems that the more of one that is present the less there is of the other. A correct balance between them seems essential for the well-being of the animal. They are necessary for satisfactory nerve function and contractibility of muscle, a deficiency leading to muscular spasms and eventually paralysis and unconsciousness. An inadequacy can also result in bone conditions such as rickets. Calcium ions also play an important role in the blood-clotting mechanism. These chemicals are of exceptional importance in the pregnant animal that is having to supply them to the developing young and also in the mother supplying milk (which contains these elements) for suckling. In both cases the parent can suffer severe illnesses through even a temporary deficiency.

Sodium, potassium, chlorine. Potassium is found mainly within the cell, but sodium and chlorine ions (usually in the form of sodium chloride) are major constituents of extracellular fluid. These chemicals appear to be very important in regulating fluid balance, especially in maintaining that between the inside and outside of individual cells. They are also essential for nerve conduction and muscle contraction.

Iron and copper. These are probably distributed in all tissues but the best known site of iron is in the blood where about two-thirds of it occurs. It is part of haemoglobin, the pigment found in red blood cells, where it is essential for the transport of oxygen. Copper seems to be needed for the proper use of iron in haemoglobin formation. When the red blood cells break down, the iron is salvaged and passes to the liver, spleen and bone marrow. From here the haemopoietic tissues reissue it as newly constituted haemoglobin.

Organic Content of the Body

The organic compounds can be grouped into two classes: simple and complex substances. Those that are absorbed into the cell are relatively simple ones, amino acids, fatty acids, and sugars; but they are derived from more complex food substances, proteins, lipids and carbohydrates respectively. Not only are they derived from these but they are then used by the cell as building bricks to produce other complex substances, the proteins of muscle, skin and hair, the lipids which make up the layers of subcutaneous fat, the carbohydrates that are stored in liver and muscle.

These are, of course, complicated chemical reactions and ones that can only take place in carefully controlled conditions. This has been mentioned earlier and some of the methods for achieving this equilibrium have been discussed. Not only must the conditions be ideal, but nearly every chemical reaction in the body needs the presence of one of a group of substances called **enzymes.** These are protein compounds that assist and accelerate organic chemical reactions. They are very specific substances and will usually only be of use in one particular reaction. Since each cell performs many different reactions there must be a great number of enzymes, probably at least 200, in any one cell. It is these substances that play a decisive role in the conditions under which the reaction will take place since enzymes are very easily inactivated.

Amino acids and proteins. Each amino acid always contain nitrogen, carbon, hydrogen and oxygen and some contain sulphur and iodine. When two join together they form a **peptide.** Many amino acids joined together form a **polypeptide** and when there are several hundred they form a protein. This joining together of simple organic substances to make the complex ones is called **polymerization.**

Proteins can be grouped into two classes: structural proteins (such as the keratin found in epithelium and collagen in connective tissue) are tough substances, resistant to acids, alkalis and quite high temperatures; and functional proteins such as those associated with cellular chemical reactions, enzymes and hormones.

Fatty acids and lipids. Fatty acids are made up of carbon, hydrogen and oxygen and result from the breakdown of lipids, one example of which is fat. Fatty acids are the main forms in which fat is transported in the blood from one part of the body to another. They are involved in many of the cellular chemical reactions as well as being used as building bricks in the formation of lipids such as phospholipids and steroids, as well as fats. Phospholipids are involved in the structure of the cell membranes, including those found inside the cell as well as the enveloping one. They also act as insulators around nerves. Probably the major steroid in the body is cholesterol and in addition to playing a role in membrane function it is linked chemically with some of the acids used in digestion and with some hormones (and incidentally also with some important drugs and poisons). Fats are used as food stores: when excess food is available it may be converted to fats and be laid down subcutaneously and in other fat depots. Here they may also act as insulators against heat loss and when they surround delicate organs they will also act as protection.

Sugars and carbohydrates. Sugars also consist of carbon, hydrogen and oxygen but the oxygen forms a higher proportion than in fatty acids. Glucose is an example of the sugars (here the term is being used in a chemical sense) and forms an important source of energy for the animal. When hundreds of the simple forms of sugars like glucose are linked together they form carbohydrates (also known as polysaccharides) The simple ones dissolve easily in water, but not the more complex ones such as glycogen (sometimes called animal starch). This is the form in which animals store carbohydrates and it is found mainly in the liver and muscles. Sugars are also used in the formation of two complex acids of tremendous significance in cell chemistry and inheritance: ribonucleic acid (abbreviated as RNA) and desoxyribonucleic acid (DNA).

Chemical Reactions of the Body

n the description of the systems many actions were described that involve a lot of work. Fluids are being forced around the body, muscles are contracting, materials are brought from one group of cells to another, organized and joined together into complex organic substances. These survive for only a short while, longer than a few days is an exception even for apparently stable tissues like bone and cartilage. From these few examples of work, it can be appreciated that a lot of energy must be available.

Energy cannot be created or destroyed: it can be moved around and can also change its form, for instance heat energy can be converted to electrical energy and, as with an electric fire, electrical energy into heat energy. Energy can be locked up in a compound during synthesis and is then termed *potential energy:* this will be released when the compound is broken down. Some chemical reactions need energy whereas others release it.

When carbon (coal) is made to burn, a little heat energy has to be supplied at first. As soon as it is really burning it is undergoing a chemical reaction whereby it is combining with oxygen and this releases a tremendous amount of energy as heat. The resulting compound is carbon dioxide and the reaction can be written as follows:

$$\text{carbon} + \text{oxygen} \xrightarrow[\text{results in}]{} \text{carbon dioxide} + \text{energy.}$$

Energy in this type of reaction is measured in units called **calories** and if 1000 calories of energy were released it could be written as

$$\text{carbon} + \text{oxygen} \rightarrow \text{carbon dioxide} + 1000 \text{ calories of energy.}$$

If we wanted to turn the carbon dioxide back into carbon and oxygen, 1000 calories of energy would have to be supplied (assuming the same amounts of chemicals were being used):

$$\text{carbon dioxide} + 1000 \text{ calories of energy} \rightarrow \text{carbon} + \text{oxygen.}$$

The same sort of procedures occur in the cell: one group of reactions release energy and this is then either stored in another compound to be called upon later or it is used immediately in another cellular chemical reaction. This may result, for instance, in a nerve impulse or a muscle twitch or the synthesis of a complex substance. Generally speaking, chemical reactions in the body which result in complex substances being broken down into simpler components usually release energy: these are called **catabolic** reactions. Building-up reactions require energy and are **anabolic** reactions. The results of all the catabolic and anabolic reactions taking place at the same time will be the total metabolism of the animal.

The body constantly loses energy to the outside environment: the rate at which the resting animal produces heat is its *basal metabolism* or *basal metabolic rate.* When an animal is fed there is an increase in the production of heat and in cold weather this may warm the body. The contraction of muscles produces heat energy as a result of the chemical reactions involved. If in so doing mechanical work results, such as moving part of the body, then this will absorb some of the energy, and the remainder appears as heat. This can be an important method of heat production: animals exposed to cold undergo rapid muscular contractions, more commonly called shivering, to achieve these results.

It is wasteful to use these chemical reactions to keep an animal warm when other methods are less expensive. An alternative is to reduce heat loss from the body and this is achieved by the insulation effect of hair and of subcutaneous fat. Clipping and starvation will reverse these particular mechanisms and it must be remembered that new-born animals do not have the full advantage of these protective devices. To enable these to conserve their energy it may be necessary to supply the young with warmth as well as ensuring a satisfactory diet that will release energy for internal chemical reactions.

However, although heat production by muscular contractions may be a useful technique for the animal in a cool environment it may be an embarrassment at other times, when the exercise is prolonged or the outside temperature high. At such times there must be an efficient system that allows heat to be removed, otherwise the body temperature would rise continuously and an increase in muscular activity could lead to death. About three-quarters of the heat lost by the body can be removed as dry heat from the surface if the outside temperature is lower than that of the animal. If this cannot operate then it must be lost by evaporation of water from the integument (perspiring, sweating) and from the surfaces of the mouth (panting) and respiratory system. Evaporation is a very efficient method of heat removal and even at ordinary temperatures a quarter of all the heat lost from the resting animal goes this way.

When heat loss is balanced by heat production the temperature should remain constant and this is necessary for so many of the chemical reactions of the body. The temperature of an animal varies in different parts of the body and the veterinary surgeon usually checks it at the rectum.

For the dog and cat, the average reading here is about 38·6°C (101·5°F), but there is quite a variation between animals and the conditions under which the animal is examined can also affect the reading.

There are delicate mechanisms predominantly under nervous control that regulate heat production and loss, acting somewhat like a thermostat, so that the normal temperature is maintained. When an animal suffers from a fever, the "thermostat system" appears to be disturbed, so that it operates at a higher temperature. That is, although heat is being produced by all possible means such as increasing energy releasing reactions like shivering (in this case called a chill) and the temperature rises, the heat loss mechanisms are not brought into play. At a certain point in the illness the "thermostat" is corrected, the heat-losing mechanism is switched on but the temperature is high. Evaporation processes come into play as is shown by profuse sweating. This is the "crisis" of the fever and the body temperature should then begin to return to normal and the illness recede. If the chemical reactions of the animal diminish, as happens just prior to death, the body temperature then falls below normal.

Since energy is always leaving the animal and some is locked up in various ways, a constant supply is essential. Plants are able to use the energy from the sun to unite carbon dioxide and water to form sugars and carbohydrates. Animals are unable to do this and so they obtain their energy indirectly from the sun by eating the plants as food: indeed some animals go farther and achieve an energy balance by eating animals that have eaten plants. The foodstuff is broken down into simpler substances with the aid of enzymes during digestion and the resulting mixture of amino acids, fatty acids, fats and sugars is dissolved through the intestinal wall and eventually reaches the blood stream from where it can reach the individual cells. Here the chemicals combine with oxygen, a reaction which is energy-yielding. The principal source of energy is the oxidation (combination with oxygen) of glucose which results in the formation of carbon dioxide and water as well and this metabolism can occur in all the cells of the body. (The oxygen–carbon dioxide link has already been mentioned in the reference to the respiratory system.) If the glucose oxidation occurred in one reaction there would be so much energy released locally that the cell would probably not be able to withstand the heat. Instead, it goes through about thirty steps, using a large number of different enzymes, each yielding a small amount of energy: the total given up will still be the same as that resulting from the one large reaction. The released energy may be used immediately but in many cases it is stored in a special substance which can be broken down later and perhaps in another place to yield its energy content.

If there is more glucose available than is needed immediately as an energy source, the liver and muscle cells convert the excess to the carbohydrate glycogen by polymerizing 200–300 glucose units, and this is stored locally. These cells can also break the glycogen down to its component glucose units again when necessary and use these for energy production. When the glycogen reserve is full, the liver cells use the surplus glucose to make fat and this is deposited in various sites throughout the body.

When the glucose is in short supply and the glycogen has also been depleted, fats and fatty acids will need to be called upon as a source of energy and when these are low even the amino acids will be broken down. All this occurs mainly in the liver which can convert these compounds into glucose; this can then be dispatched to provide energy for less versatile cells.

During starvation or illness when carbohydrates are low, fat is transferred from the various depots to the liver ready for its processing and causes the condition of "fatty liver". When a large amount of fat is being metabolized, some of the breakdown products, called **ketones** or ketone bodies, accumulate in the liver and blood stream and are slowly excreted in the urine. Since they are poisonous, this condition of "ketosis" is very serious.

When all else fails and the cells still need energy, amino acids have to be broken down. This also produces a problem since these compounds contain nitrogen. There is always a limited amount of amino acid breakdown occurring and the nitrogen is excreted by being incorporated by the liver cells in the harmless compound **urea** which passes via the blood stream through the kidneys and out of the body in the urine. The amount of nitrogen absorbed from the food through the wall of the digestive system equals that passed out in the urine so that the body maintains a *nitrogen balance*. When starvation dictates that amino acids shall be used, there is no nitrogen entering the body but it is being excreted in increasing amounts due to their breakdown. The amount finally increases rapidly, followed by death.

In addition to this breakdown of complex compounds, cells must have the capacity to synthesize them. The formation of glycogen by liver and muscle cells has already been mentioned and this is how most of the carbohydrate reserve of animals exists. Lipids can be synthesized by all cells, some for their own particular use, others for export to separate tissues. Some lipids are produced in specific areas: for instance, liver cells are of major importance in cholesterol formation although other tissues can perform the process.

All cells synthesize protein, some continuously, others for only a part of their life cycle. It is an important function of cells, since even after the maximum size has been achieved, the proteins are still being broken down and then reformed. This is where the complex acids RNA and DNA play such a significant role.

There are about twenty different amino acids, and proteins consist of hundreds of these linked together in an individual sequence for each protein. Any change in the order produces a different material and so synthesis can be a complex undertaking. One form of RNA, soluble RNA, is responsible for the gathering together of the individual amino acids and passing them to the other form, insoluble "ribosomal" RNA. It is here that they are arranged in correct sequence, polymerized and released as protein. Each type of soluble RNA will be responsible for only one amino acid and each ribosomal RNA will only produce one type of protein. The formation of the RNA itself is automatically controlled by DNA.

STRUCTURE OF THE CELL

Most animal cells are very small, from one-hundredth to one-tenth of a millimetre (10–100 μ) in diameter. It is the number of cells that mainly decides the size of the animal: small animals have fewer cells not necessarily smaller ones. Although some of the structures in the cells can be seen by using light microscopes, it is only by using the electron microscopes with magnifications of up to many hundreds of thousands that detail connected with the work of the cell can be appreciated.

If the cells are free they are usually spherical or oval but when they are packed into tissues their shape becomes distorted due to pressure of other cells or because of their own growth and multiplication. When the cells are studied through microscopes it is usually necessary to kill and dye them with various stains to see the small structures: it is difficult to reconcile their dead appearance with their dynamic activity in life. The material of which cells are made is called **protoplasm** and even by using light microscopes it can be seen that nearly all cells consist of two main compartments enclosed within a **cell membrane** (Fig. 1.2). One compartment, the **nucleus,** consists of **nucleoplasm** and is embedded in the remainder of the cell which forms the other compartment and is called the **cytoplasm.**

Cytoplasm

The electron microscope has shown that this living jelly is not a substance in the ordinary sense but a highly structured organization. Within the cytoplasm organized units of living substance called **organelles** have important specific functions; these are probably always present and include mitochondria, the Golgi apparatus, endoplasmic reticulum, ribosomes, lysosomes and centrioles. **Inclusions** are accumulations of cell products often of a temporary nature such as protein, carbohydrates, lipids, pigment, crystals, and secretory droplets.

The cytoplasm is fluid or semi-fluid and physically and chemically it is in a state of flux. Its constitution will vary with age and metabolic state and cells will have different and characteristic variants.

Cell membrane. This is a thin limiting skin for the whole cell and it acts as a barrier between the cytoplasm and the surrounding materials. It has a variable and selective permeability, allowing only certain substances into and out of the cell. In some cells numerous finger-like processes may project: they increase the surface area and are called **microvilli.**

Cytoplasmic organelles. **Mitochondria:** the number of these small organelles varies with the state of the cell from a few hundred to a few thousand. They contain a very

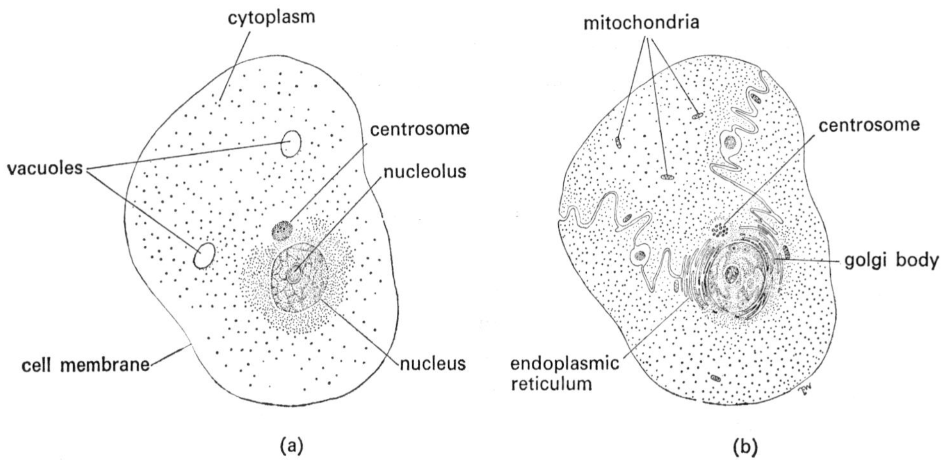

Fig. 1.2. Diagrammatic representation of a highly magnified cell: (a) as seen with a light microscope (b) when viewed by an electron microscope.

large number of enzymes responsible for releasing a vast amount of energy as well as for various synthetic pathways. They are sometimes called "mobile power plants".

The Golgi apparatus: this complex had been seen under the light microscope and is named after the man who first described it using that technique. Higher magnifications show that it consists of parallel flattened small bags. It seems certain that it plays a role in secretion in glandular cells, but it is found in nearly all cells and its function in non-glandular cells is uncertain.

Endoplasmic reticulum: this is a network of membranous tubular cavities filled by fluid. In some areas the surface of the reticulum is smooth but in others it is covered by small particles called **ribosomes** composed mainly of RNA, and these areas are described as rough-coated. The ribosomes attached to the membranes are thought to be concerned with the formation of protein that is secreted from the cell. The function of the smooth-coated reticulum is not known although lipid metabolism has been suggested.

Ribosomes: in addition to those attached to the reticulum there are numerous ribosomes found free in the cytoplasm. It is thought that the RNA in these is responsible for synthesizing protein to be used within that cell.

Lysosomes: these are membranous compartments containing enzymes that help break down the complex organic compounds. Some cells can absorb into their cytoplasm matter that is not wanted, that is perhaps even injurious to the body: this is *foreign* matter and can be taken in, for example, during phagocytosis. Once absorbed, this matter becomes surrounded by lysosomes that discharge their enzymes so that it is broken down for removal. Another use occurs when the cell is damaged: the lysosomes then release their enzymes to clear up the resulting cell debris.

Centrioles: small bodies found near the nucleus play an important role in reproduction of the cell and these centrioles will be referred to again later. Their surrounding cytoplasm is usually condensed and may be called the **centrosome** or **centrosphere.**

Cytoplasmic inclusions. Dark brown to black granules are found in cells called **melanocytes**: the granules are **melanin** and these cells occur in pigmented areas of the body. A golden-brown pigment called **haemosiderin** may be found in cells connected with haemoglobin breakdown. Other pigments, carbohydrates, lipids and protein can also be found as cell inclusions.

Other cytoplasmic contents. Many of the inorganic substances of the body are found in the cytoplasm in addition to a vast range of enzymes. Water is the commonest compound and in this the dissolved chemicals can react as necessary, either in the fluid or on the surface of the membranous organelles.

Nucleus

Nearly all cells have one nucleus and some have more than one. Metabolism is restricted and growth is impossible in cells without a nucleus. When present it is the control centre of the cell and contains large quantities of DNA. This governs the activities of the cytoplasm as well as being the material controlling heredity from parents to the young. The DNA compounds are the **genes** and are found combined with structural proteins to form **chromatin.** The DNA controls the formation of RNA and this spreads throughout the cell controlling the formation of the many proteins produced in a cell. There is also a discrete collection of RNA within the nucleus forming a **nucleolus** (there may be more than one). The nucleus is separated from the cytoplasm by a distinct nuclear membrane, but this is thought to be perforated by several small openings.

Reproduction of the Cell

There seems to be a certain size to which cells grow and this may be determined by the amount of DNA in the nucleus. In many cases the cell then doubles all its contents and divides evenly. The resulting two cells continue independently and themselves increase in size. This method of reproducing is called **mitosis** (Fig. 1.3) and growth and reproduction may be continuous in some tissues: the cells lining the surface of the intestine are one example. Other cells, such as those found in some muscle tissue, only reproduce occasionally during the life of the animal and yet others which are highly specialized such as neurons may never reproduce. Mitosis is a phase in the life of a cell and the time between the mitotic events is called the **interphase.** Although all the dynamic processes are fully active during this period, the cell is sometimes (mistakenly) said to be "resting".

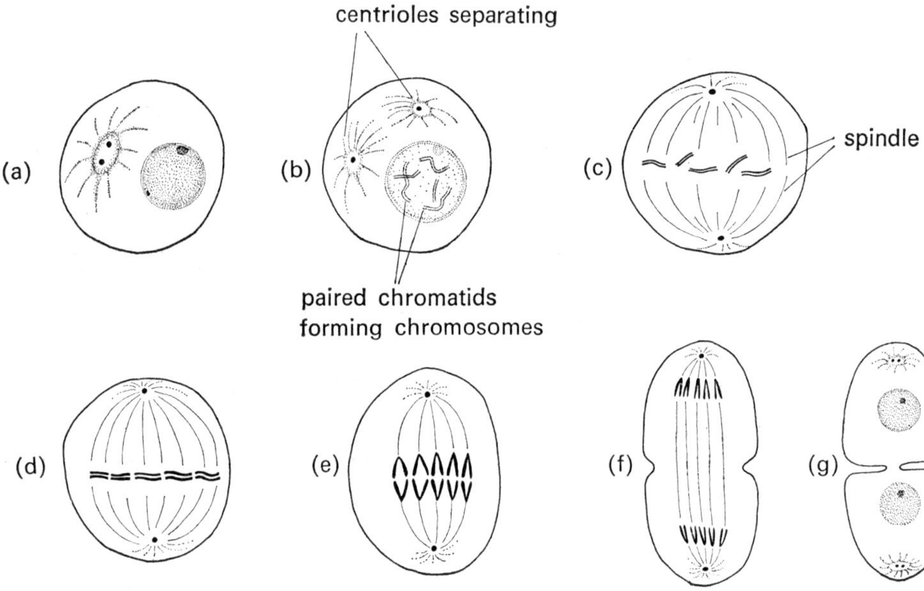

Fig. 1.3. Mitotic reproduction of a cell. See text for full explanation.

Towards the end of interphase, that is just prior to mitosis, each DNA complex (each gene) within the nucleus produces an exact copy of itself. The centrioles begin to separate and pass to opposite ends of the cell, but remain connected by a set of fibres called the **spindle** (Fig. 1.3 a, b, c). The nucleolus disappears and the chromatin of the nucleus condenses into visible threads called **chromosomes** (Fig. 1.3 b). These can be seen to be already doubled, that is, each chromosome consists of two threads lying side by side, each of which is called a **chromatid.** The nuclear membrane disappears and the chromosomes arrange themselves across the middle of the cell, half-way between the centrioles and closely applied to the spindle fibres (Fig. 1.3 c). The chromosomes separate into their component chromatids which then migrate towards opposite centrioles (Fig. 1.3 d, e, f). A nuclear membrane grows around each separated group of chromatids which can now be called chromosomes

(Fig. 1.3 g). They appear to thin out and then become invisible. The remainder of the cell becomes encircled by a furrow which deepens and eventually separates the original cell into halves. It is thought that all the other structures of the cell undergo a simultaneous duplication to supply each resulting cell with the necessary components.

Skeletal System

Part One

The hard structures that support and protect the soft tissues form the **skeleton.** They can be taken to be organs in which bone tissue and/or cartilage tissue are predominant. For convenience, one often uses the term skeletal system to include also the joints, that is the tissues which connect such organs.

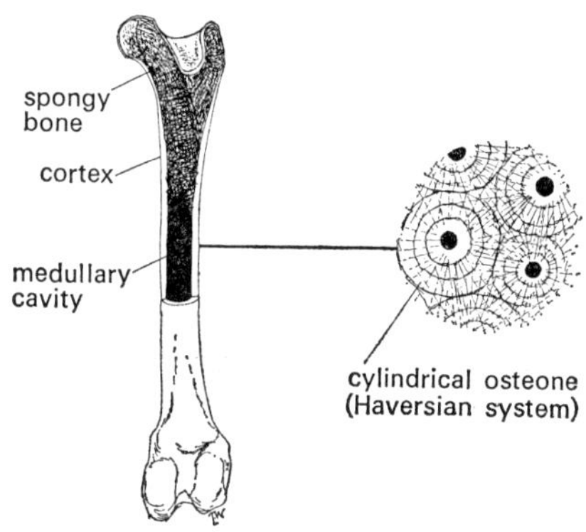

Fig. 1.4. A long bone, partly sectioned. The enlargement in the circle represents the microscopic appearance of compact bone.

BONES

A bone is an organ and includes several tissues (Fig. 1.4). The bone tissue itself is usually arranged in the compact form on the outer surface and this varies tremendously in thickness, depending on the part of the bone and its function. The layer of compact bone is often referred to as the **cortex;** inside this there is usually some spongy (cancellous) bone and there may also be a space called the **medullary cavity.**

This space and also those between the trabeculae of the spongy bone are filled with connective tissue known as **marrow.** In some bones this is very fatty and is called **yellow marrow.** In others, and also sometimes in the same bones that one finds yellow (fatty) marrow, there is **red marrow.** This is myeloid (haemopoietic) tissue, the connective tissue responsible for producing erythrocytes and granular leucocytes. In the very young animal all the marrow in all the bones is the red (myeloid) variety. Gradually fat cells replace the myeloid tissue and yellow marrow becomes substituted in many of the spaces.

Blood vessels will be intimately connected with the marrow, especially when it is the red variety and if they use one definite place to pass through the compact bone this is called the **nutrient foramen.** Do not be misled into thinking that this is the point of entry of the only vessel that is responsible for the nutrition of the bone; it receives supplies from many other vessels over its surface. Fine nerves will also be found associated with the inside of a bone.

The outer surface of a bone is covered by a layer of dense connective tissue, the **periosteum.** The deeper part of the periosteum in intimate contact with the surface of the bone can help in bone-tissue formation. The outermost part of the periosteum is more fibrous than the deeper layer and has a protective function. Fibres of the periosteum continue into the bone tissue itself and may make it extremely difficult to separate the periosteum.

There are a few regions where periosteum does not cover the bone. If one bone is in contact with another, and especially if there is movement between the bones, the contiguous areas are usually covered instead by a layer of cartilage. Sometimes, however, and especially if there is little or no movement, the uniting medium is dense connective tissue. Various structures attach to bones and nearly always the actual uniting medium is dense connective tissue. Its fibres are continuous with those of the periosteum and they may also run into the bone tissue itself.

Bones are sometimes classified according to their shape. This is not an all-embracing classification and also it is difficult to be certain to which class some bones belong.

Long bones. These bones are found in the limbs and are rather like cylinders. The ends or **extremities** are often expanded and are usually filled with spongy bone. The part of the bone between the extremities is the **shaft**, and this encloses a medullary cavity.

Short bones. These are many sided and have similar dimensions in length, breadth and height. Short bones consist of the outer compact bone enclosing spongy bone, and do not have medullary cavities.

Flat bones. Flat bones consist of two layers of compact bone, usually very close together and separated by a small amount of spongy bone. Some of the bones of the head are flat bones and in these the spongy bone is also called the **diploë**.

Irregular bones. These do not fit any of the above classes. They are found in the midline of the body and like short bones, they consist of outer compact bone enclosing spongy bone. Their shape, as the name suggests, is irregular.

Development of Bones

There is only one way in which bone tissue forms, but there are two ways in which a bone as an organ may develop. Direct formation within the connective tissue is intramembranous ossification; onto and gradually replacing a cartilage predecessor (which goes through a calcified stage) is endochondral ossification.

Some bones have one centre where ossification begins and the bone tissue is gradually added over the surface of the centre until the final shape is attained. In others, there may be two or more centres and the bone tissue around each gradually merges and obliterates the original connecting material, whether it is dense connective tissue or cartilage. Often where centres of ossification are separated, the intervening tissue continues to reproduce itself. The distance between the original centres increases but the intervening tissue is being constantly replaced by bone tissue. This is an important method whereby bones grow, usually in length. The rate of bone deposition is ultimately faster than the rate of reproduction of the intervening tissue which gradually decreases in thickness. Eventually the entire intervening tissue may be replaced by bone which is then continuous between the adjacent original centres: they are then said to have **fused.**

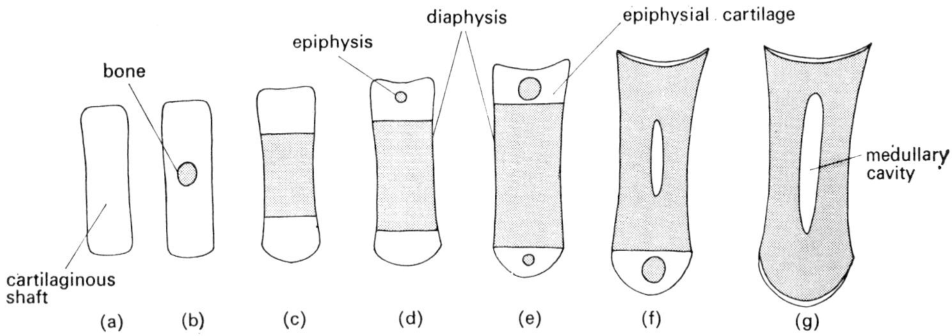

Fig. 1.5. Development and growth of a long bone. See text for full explanation.

This method of growth is especially important in long bones and also in some of the irregular bones (Fig. 1.5). The cartilaginous shaft of the very young bone is first replaced by bone tissue (Fig. 1.5 b, c). A centre of ossification then forms in one extremity, sometimes in both extremities, of the cartilaginous remainder of the bone (Fig. 1.5 d, e). Such a centre of ossification is called an **epiphysis.** The part between the epiphyses, that is, the shaft of a growing bone, is called the **diaphysis.** Between the diaphysis and each epiphysis there will be a plate of cartilage called the **epiphysial cartilage** or epiphysial plate; since this is the region where longitudinal growth is being caused it may be called the growth plate. As long as the cartilage cells in the epiphysial cartilage continue to multiply, the bone will grow in length. When they cease, bone will gradually replace the cartilaginous epiphysial plate and fusion will occur (Fig. 1.5 f, g). This takes place in different bones and even in different parts of the same bone at different times; in other words, growth does not cease at the same time in all parts of the skeleton. There is quite a variation between different species; there is an appreciable difference between animals of the same species and even between litter-mates. After fusion is complete there appears to be a condensation of bone tissue at the site of the epiphysial cartilage; this is called the **epiphysial line.**

CARTILAGES

Many parts of the skeleton develop first as cartilage and this tissue is then replaced by bone. However, some parts remain as cartilage throughout the life of the animal. Sometimes, as the animal ages, the cartilage may become calcified: calcified cartilage is not bone.

JOINTS

When two or more pieces of bone or cartilage are connected this is a joint. **Arthrosis** is another word for joint. The Latin word for an arthrosis is *articulatio*: therefore we often refer to an arthrosis as an **articulation** and things relating to an arthrosis as **articular.** For instance, those surfaces of a bone that can actually appose in the articulation are the *articular surfaces.* We have, then, three words that can be used for the connection of bones and/or cartilages; joint, arthrosis, articulation.

Joints have been classified in many different ways but the system which is receiving international recognition is that dependent on the tissue connecting the bones or cartilages of the joint. The classes are then **fibrous, cartilaginous** and **synovial** joints.

Fibrous joints. The connecting medium is dense connective tissue. Many of the bones of the head are connected to each other in this way and here such joints are called **sutures.** Usually there is very little movement between the bones and/or cartilages of these joints and they are sometimes known as *synarthroses.*

Cartilaginous joints. The connecting medium is cartilage and such a joint between corresponding bones on opposite sides of the body is a **symphysis.**

Those cartilaginous joints that show little or no movement are sometimes also called synarthroses: if there is a reasonable amount of movement the joint may be called an *amphiarthrosis.*

In both fibrous and cartilaginous joints, bone may eventually replace the dense connective tissue and the cartilage and unite the whole mass into a continuum of bone. Such an arrangement is a *synostosis.*

Synovial joints (Fig. 1.6). When these joints are cut, a small amount of fluid leaks out: this is called **synovia** or synovial fluid.

The articular surfaces in a synovial joint are always cartilage: even if the joint is basically between two bones, the contacting surfaces are covered by a layer of cartilage. The articular cartilages are never covered by perichondrium and they are only separated by the thin layer of synovia. The periphery of the articular cartilages are connected by a dense connective tissue membrane, which, since it is responsible for the production of synovia, is called the **synovial membrane.** The membrane does not usually hold the surfaces tightly together but often pouches outward from the **articular cavity.** (Although the term cavity is used, there is actually no empty space in a joint. Only if the joint is damaged is it possible to separate the surfaces.) The synovial membrane may also merge with the periosteum of the bone supporting the articular cartilages. Dense connective tissue forms another layer outside the synovial membrane; as it is usually very fibrous it is called the **fibrous membrane.** The two membranes are closely interconnected and together form the **articular** (or **joint**) **capsule.** Fibrous thickenings strengthen parts of the joint capsule: these are **ligaments** and usually run between the bones of the joint. The articular capsule attaches to the periosteum of the bones, or the perichondrium of the cartilages: so also will the ligaments and they will gain additional attachment by inserting into the bones or cartilages themselves.

Synovial joints are usually able to move more freely than fibrous or cartilaginous joints. They are sometimes called *diarthrodial joints.* In some situations in the skeleton the main joint is divided by an **articular disc** (or **articular meniscus**) of cartilage.

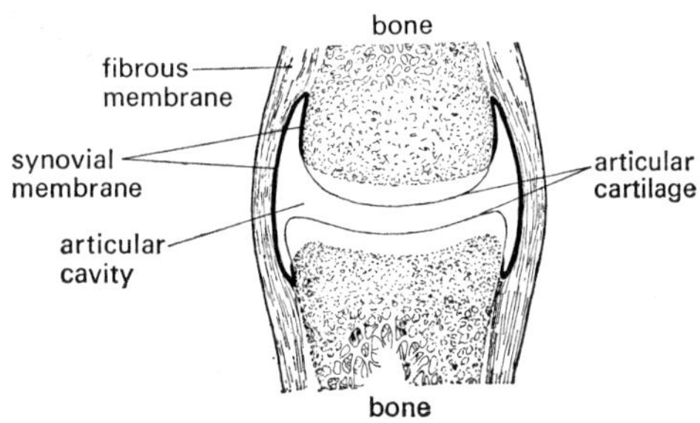

Fig. 1.6. Section of a synovial joint between two bones. Normally there is no space between the articular cartilages.

This may be connected all around its periphery to the joint capsule and one has then, in effect, two articular cavities, within the one main joint. In some the connection to the joint capsule is not complete and the articular cavities are in free communication.

Movements in Joints

The changes in position between the bones of a joint can be complex. The movements are generally approximately classified into four types but any change in position is usually the result of a combination of these. When one articular surface slides over another this is a **gliding** movement. Altering the angle between two pieces of a joint is an **angular** movement: decreasing the angle is **flexion**, increasing the angle until the components are in a straight line is **extension. Rotation** takes place when one bone rotates around its longitudinal axis. In **circumduction**, one end of the bone is involved in the articulation, the other describes a circle or a segment of one.

Skeletal System

Part Two

GENERAL ARRANGEMENT OF THE BONES AND JOINTS

The skeleton may be divided into two major parts, axial and appendicular.

Axial skeleton: as the name suggests this part of the skeleton forms a straight line from end to end of the body. It includes the bones of the head (the skull), the bones of the vertebral column (the vertebrae) and the other bones of the thorax (the ribs and sternum).

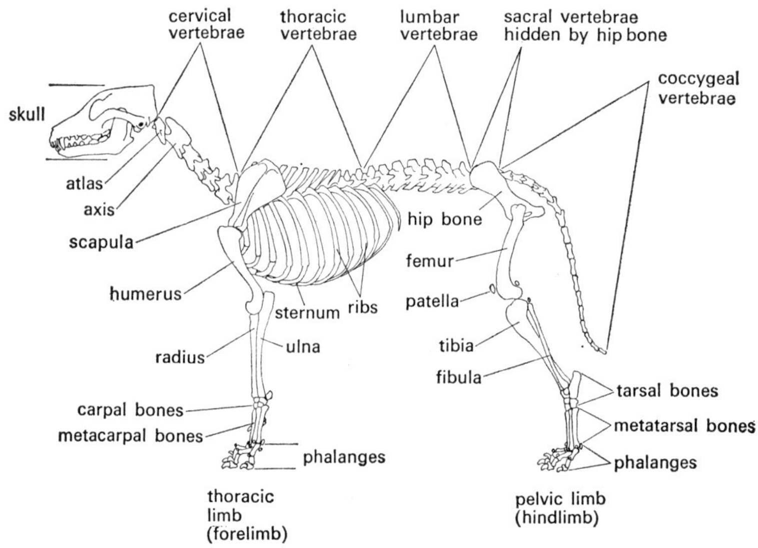

Fig. 1.7. Half skeleton of dog.

Appendicular skeleton: this is the part of the skeleton in the limbs—those parts of the body that are attached or appended to the trunk. Each limb is made up as follows.

Thoracic Limb

Thoracic (pectoral) **girdle:** a scapula is present and in the cat and dog the remnants of a clavicle.

Arm: contains the humerus.

Forearm: radius and ulna.

Fore paw: this part is the equivalent of the human hand and consists of three subdivisions. (a) Several carpal bones forming the carpus (sometimes called the wrist even in the dog). (b) A few metacarpal bones forming the metacarpus. (c) Digits: these correspond to the human fingers. The main digits each consist of a proximal phalanx, a middle phalanx and a distal phalanx.

Pelvic Limb

Pelvic girdle: this consists of three bones, the ilium, the ischium, the pubis. In the adult these three are fused together and are then called the hip (coxal) bone. (During development, a fourth bone, the acetabular bone, is also involved.) The left and right hip bones meet in the ventral midline forming a symphysis.

Thigh: contains the femur.

Leg: tibia and fibula.

Hind paw: this part is the equivalent of the human foot and consists of three subdivisions. (a) Several tarsal bones forming the tarsus. (b) A few metatarsal bones forming the metatarsus. (c) Digits: these correspond to the human toes. The main digits each consist of a proximal phalanx, a middle phalanx and a distal phalanx.

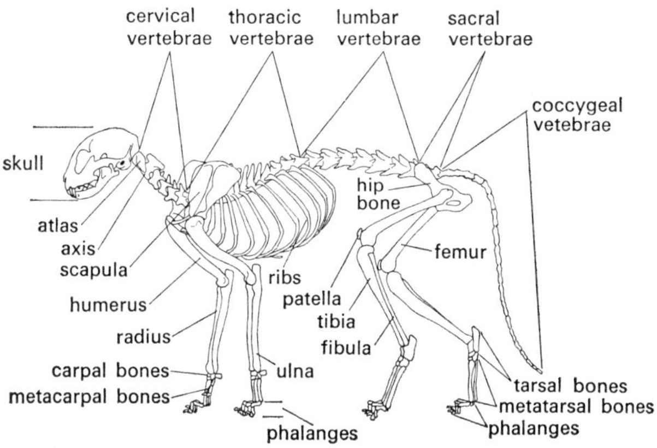

Fig. 1.8. Skeleton of cat.

THE AXIAL SKELETON

Skull (Figs. 1.9, 1.10, 1.11)

Part of the skull resembles a box, with two joined tubes attached to one end. The box is the cranium, the tubes the nasal chambers. The mandibles (the bones of the lower jaw) and the hyoid apparatus are suspended from the cranium.

Cranium. The floor of the box can be considered to consist of two bones one behind the other in the midline of the head: the **occipital** and the **sphenoidal** bones. The latter is the nearer to the nose.

The base of the occipital bone forms the floor of one end of the box. The actual end of the box consists mainly of a large hole (the **foramen magnum**) and the occipital bone forms a frame all round this hole.

An apparently solid pyramid of bone, forming part of the **temporal** bone is wedged into the space between the side parts of the occipital bone and the caudal part of the sides of the sphenoid. The organs of balance and of hearing it contains need the protection of the thick bony tissue. On its outer surface is the external acoustic meatus, the opening to which the (external) ear is attached.

Each side of the sphenoid is continued nearer the nose by a **frontal** bone and these form not only the walls in this region, but also part of the roof of the cranium.

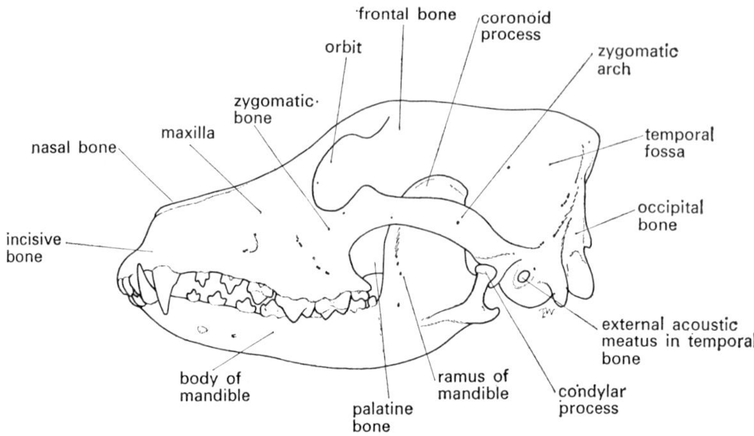

Fig. 1.9. Average dog skull.

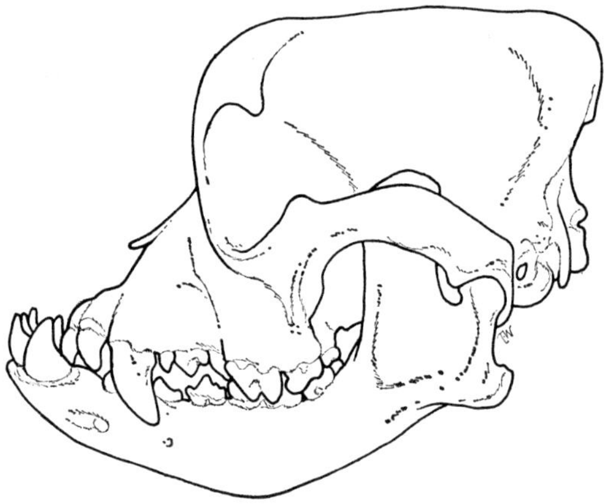

Fig. 1.10. Skull of short-nosed breed, such as Bulldog.

The box is now nearly complete; at one end the occipital bone frames the foramen magnum. At the opposite end there is a flat plate of bone with two areas where there are a large number of very small holes. This gives the bone the appearance of a sieve and it is called the **ethmoid** bone.

The space inside the box or cranium is the **cranial cavity** and in life it houses the brain. This part of the central nervous system will have nerve fibres flowing to and from it and will need a good blood supply and drainage. There are many holes, or foramina, in the boundaries of the cranial cavity for their passage. The brain is continuous with the other part of the central nervous system, the spinal cord, through the foramen magnum.

Nasal chambers. These have been described as two joined tubes and their common wall is the **nasal septum.** Much of this structure remains cartilaginous throughout life. It attaches to the midline of the ethmoid and its ventral border is strengthened by a grooved bar of bone. The floor and lateral wall of each tube are formed by three L-shaped bones; the **incisive** bone (sometimes called the pre-maxilla), the **maxilla** and the **palatine** bone. These bones are in line, with the palatine bone being nearest the cranium.

Teeth are found in the incisive and maxillary bones. The roof of each nasal chamber consists of the **nasal** bone.

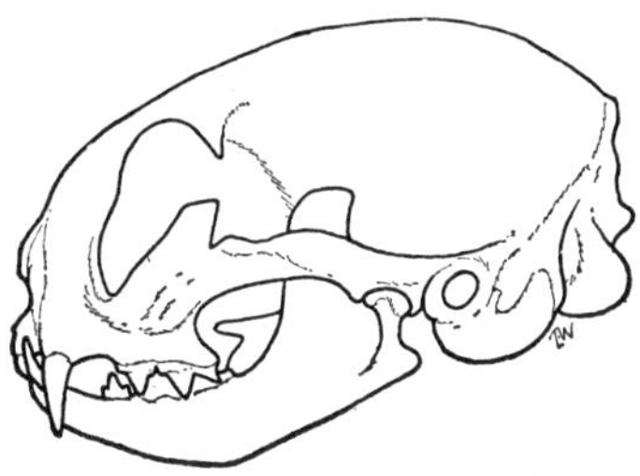

Fig. 1.11. Cat skull.

All the bones of the nasal chambers are flat bones and are interconnected by sutures. The chambers are open-ended and slightly curved; they are far from being empty spaces. Attached to the ethmoid bone and to the lateral walls and roof of each nasal chamber there is a number of thin scrolls of delicate bone: these are the **turbinates.**

Two other small bones lie on either side of the skull, near the nasal chambers and the cranium, but forming an integral part of neither. The **lacrimal** bone is between the frontal bone, the palatine bone and the maxilla. The **zygomatic** bone (sometimes called malar or jugal bone) is bounded by the lacrimal bone and the maxilla and has a projection which joins with a similar spike from the temporal bone to form the *zygomatic arch.* In the dog and cat there is a ligament connecting this arch and the frontal bone. The connection divides the space into two parts: the region nearer the nose is the **orbit**, the other part is the **temporal fossa.** The orbit houses the eye and its related structures, usually embedded in fat. Strong jaw muscles attach at one end to the walls of the temporal fossa and at the other end to the process of the mandible which projects into this region.

Mandibles. The bone of the lower jaw consists of right and left mandibles. They are joined only at the "chin". The articulating surfaces between them are rough and the projections and depressions of one side fit snugly into those of the other. They are bound together by fibrocartilage into a symphysis. Each mandible has a horizontal part, the **body**, and a vertical part, the **ramus.** Teeth are fixed in the body. The ramus has two strong processes: one, the **coronoid** process is normally in the temporal fossa and forms a point of attachment for the very strong muscle which helps to close the jaw; the other, the **condylar** process is caudal to the coronoid process and forms a synovial joint with the articular surface of the temporal bone. This temporo-mandibular joint is one that has a complete meniscus dividing the cavity into two parts; it forms the pivot for jaw movement. (Some people consider the entire lower jaw is one bone, the mandible, consisting of right and left halves. There are reasons for both points of view.)

Hyoid apparatus. There are several parts of this, which collectively are also called the **hyoid** bone. It resembles a trapeze and each of its limbs is attached by a cartilaginous joint to the petrous part of the temporal bone. The tongue and the larynx are suspended by attachments to the bar of the trapeze.

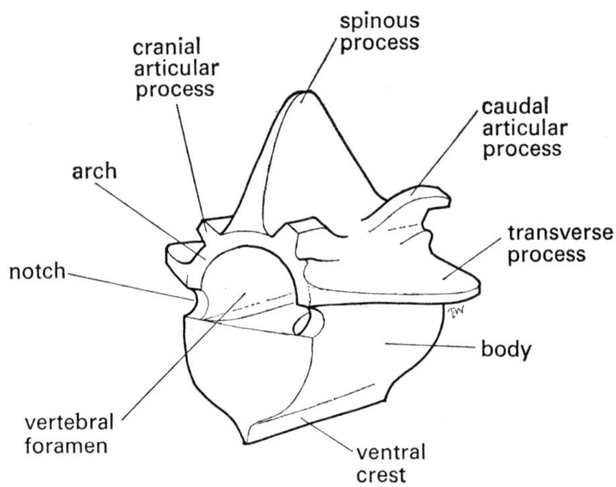

Fig. 1.12. Model of a basic vertebra.

Vertebral Column

This is the collection of bones, the **vertebrae,** in the midline of the body, stretching from the skull to the end of the tail. The bones are classified as irregular and are divided into regions according to the part of the body in which they are found. **Cervical** in the neck, **thoracic** in the chest, **lumbar** in the loins, **sacral** in the croup, **coccygeal** in the tail. The bones in each region have characteristics similar to one another but different from those of other regions. Nevertheless, a basic plan can be recognized for all vertebrae.

Basic vertebra

The **body** of the vertebra (Fig. 1.12) is somewhat cylindrical; its ventral surface sometimes bears a single midline **ventral crest.** The dorsal surface is flattened and forms the floor of the **vertebral foramen.** The **arch** of the vertebra arises from either side of the body and completes the vertebral foramen. The vertebral foramina of a series of connected vertebrae together form the **vertebral canal** which houses the spinal cord and many blood vessels in their surrounding fat. Small **notches** in the cranial and caudal borders of the arch meet in adjacent vertebrae to form **intervertebral foramina**, through which nerves and blood vessels pass. The **spinous process** rises dorsally from the middle of the arch; it varies in shape and direction in the different vertebrae. There are a pair of **articular processes** on the cranial edge, and a pair on the caudal edge, of the arch. The articular processes of adjacent vertebrae form synovial joints. The **transverse processes** are paired pieces of bone that project laterally from the junction of the body and the arch. The interior of a vertebra consists of the closely arranged trabeculae of spongy bone surrounded by red marrow.

In addition to the pair of **intervertebral synovial joints** between the articular processes of adjacent vertebrae, there are cartilaginous joints between their bodies. The intervening fibrocartilage which is very firmly attached to the vertebral bodies forms the **intervertebral disc.** This consists of a very fibrous periphery, the **anulus fibrosus** and a softer more amorphous central part, the **nucleus pulposus.** There are also short ligaments running between two or three adjacent vertebrae and longer ligaments running between two or three regions of vertebrae.

Regional differences

Cervical vertebrae. There are seven in all domestic mammals and the first two are very modified.

The first cervical vertebra is called the **atlas** (Fig. 1.13a), and seems to consist only of a pair of large flattened transverse processes (sometimes called the *wings*) joined dorsally and ventrally to enclose a large vertebral foramen. The vertebra forms a pair of large synovial joints with articular surfaces of the occipital bone of the skull, supporting the head and allowing it to nod up and down. (This supporting function is the reason for its name; Atlas was the mythical giant who supported the world on his shoulders.) The second cervical vertebra is the **axis** (Fig. 1.13b); it has a long body with a cranially-projecting process, the **dens.** There are only synovial joints between the first and the second cervical vertebrae and these are so arranged that the head and first cervical vertebra pivot around the dens of the second cervical vertebra.

Thoracic vertebrae. There are usually thirteen to fourteen thoracic vertebrae in the dog and cat. They are characterized by tall spinous processes and also articular depressions or fovea on each side of the cranial and caudal surfaces of the body. Since the function of the depressions of adjacent vertebrae is to clasp and make a synovial joint with the head of a rib they are called **costal fovea.** ("Costal" is an adjective used in phrases referring to a rib.) In addition, the transverse process also makes a synovial joint with the rib, this time with its tuberculum.

Lumbar vertebrae. There are six or seven lumbar vertebrae and these have large flat laterally projecting transverse processes.

Sacral vertebrae. The dog and cat usually have three. The bodies and the arches fuse together to form one mass which is often called the **sacrum.** This is a wedge-shaped bone with lateral parts that form a firm **sacro-iliac** joint (usually cartilaginous) with the ilium of the pelvic girdle.

Coccygeal vertebrae. The number of these will vary tremendously depending on the length of the tail. They decrease in size and become more regular so that the terminal few are like small rods of bone. A dog which has had its tail amputated is said to be *docked.* Rarely is this necessary for the well-being of the animal: it is more commonly done to subserve owners' ideas of fashion.

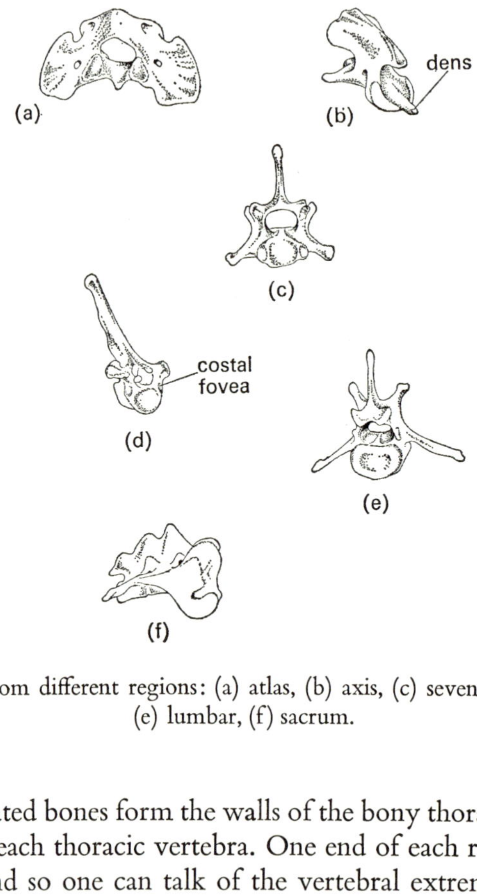

Fig. 1.13. Vertebrae from different regions: (a) atlas, (b) axis, (c) seventh cervical, (d) thoracic, (e) lumbar, (f) sacrum.

Ribs. These elongated bones form the walls of the bony thorax (Fig. 1.14). There is one pair of ribs for each thoracic vertebra. One end of each rib articulates with the vertebral column and so one can talk of the vertebral extremity. This has a **head** which for most ribs forms a synovial joint with the costal fovea of adjacent vertebrae. The head is on the end of a **neck** and adjacent to this is the **tuberculum** which forms a synovial joint with the transverse process of the thoracic vertebra. The other extremity of the rib articulates with the sternum. This sternal extremity is cartilaginous and although strictly the whole organ from the vertebral column to the sternum is a rib it is common to consider the bony part to be the rib and talk of the remainder as the **costal cartilage.**

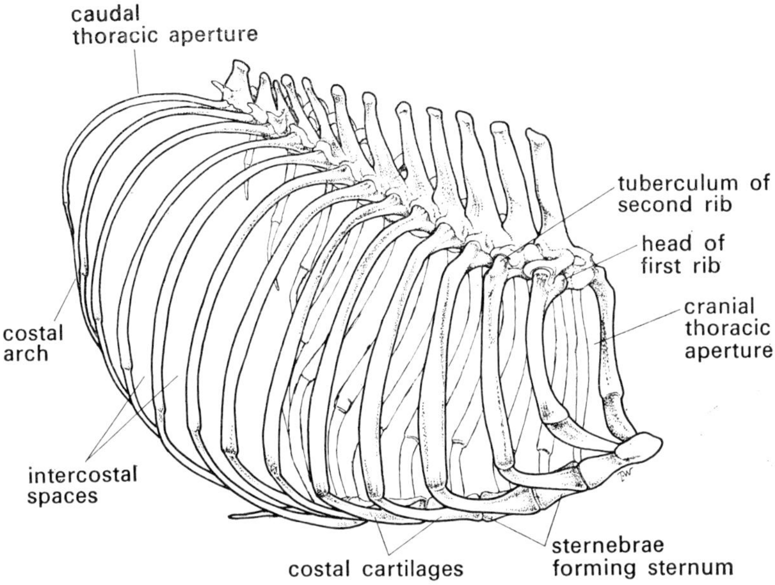

Fig. 1.14. The thorax.

Not all the ribs articulate directly with the sternum; those that do are called **true** (sternal) ribs; the others, more caudal, are **false** or asternal. The costal cartilages of the false ribs overlap and are attached to each other and so indirectly to the sternum. The line of the last rib and these overlapping cartilages forms the **costal arch.** There is no medullary cavity in a rib. The interior is filled with spongy bone packed with red marrow.

Sternum. The sternum completes the thorax ventrally. It is an axial structure, composed of a line of bones or **sternebrae,** which mostly articulate with each other by a series of cartilaginous joints. Internally they resemble vertebrae. The costal cartilages form synovial joints with the sternum.

Thoracic cavity (Fig. 1.14)

The thorax consists of the thoracic vertebrae dorsally, the sternum ventrally and the ribs and costal cartilages laterally. The gaps between adjacent ribs are **intercostal spaces.** The **cranial thoracic aperture** (the inlet) is formed by the first thoracic vertebra, the first pair of ribs and the sternum. The **caudal thoracic aperture** (the outlet) is formed by the last thoracic vertebra, the costal arch (including the last pair of ribs) and the sternum. As the cranial thoracic aperture is much smaller than the caudal thoracic aperture the **thoracic cavity** is irregularly conical in shape with the dorsal wall much longer than the ventral.

THE APPENDICULAR SKELETON

The Thoracic Limb

There is no bony connection between the thoracic limb and the trunk. The attachment is solely by muscles. These run between the scapula and humerus of the limb, and the head, neck and thorax of the trunk. During movement the scapula moves slightly over the wall of the thorax and pivots round an area rather than any specific point.

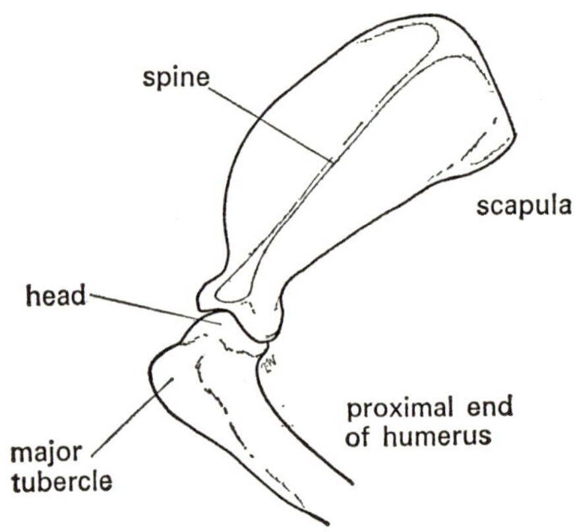

Fig. 1.15. Shoulder joint.

Scapula. This is a flat bone which is closely applied to the thorax. Its outer (lateral) surface is divided into two areas by a well-marked **spine** (Fig. 1.15). The end which forms a synovial joint (the shoulder joint) with the humerus is expanded into the **glenoid cavity.**

Clavicle. The cat has only a thin sliver of bone and the clavicle is also vestigial in the dog. In both species it lies buried in a muscle running between the forelimb and the head and neck, over the point of the shoulder.

Humerus. The proximal extremity of this long bone has a convex articular **head** which is part of the shoulder joint. This synovial joint has no well-marked ligaments. It is normally kept in place by the surrounding muscles and although it allows movements in all directions, they are chiefly flexion and extension. The *point of the shoulder* is formed by a process of bone, the **major tubercle**, which lies craniolateral to the articular head. The distal extremity is transversely cylindrical forming the **condyle** of the humerus: this forms part of the synovial **elbow joint.**

Radius. A long bone that articulates proximally with the humerus in the elbow joint (Fig. 1.16) and distally with the carpus. It is the more medial of the two forearm bones.

Ulna. The proximal end is the **olecranon**, which forms the *point of the elbow* and on its cranial edge the bone has a semi-circular **trochlear notch** (Fig. 1.16). Into this fits the condyle of the humerus, to help with the radius in forming the elbow joint. The ulna of the dog and cat is closely applied to the radius, but it is able to rotate around this bone, being attached to it by muscle tissue. The elbow joint is formed by the condyle of the humerus fitting into the trochlea of the ulna and being supported by the proximal end of the radius. There are very strong ligaments on the lateral and medial sides of the joint and these, together with the shapes of the bones, restrict movement to flexion and extension.

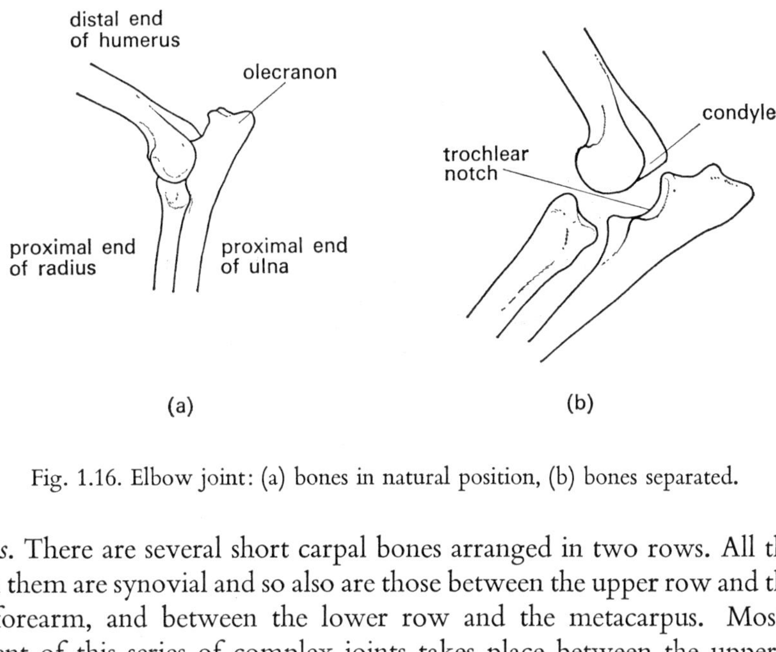

Fig. 1.16. Elbow joint: (a) bones in natural position, (b) bones separated.

Carpus. There are several short carpal bones arranged in two rows. All the joints between them are synovial and so also are those between the upper row and the bones of the forearm, and between the lower row and the metacarpus. Most of the movement of this series of complex joints takes place between the upper row of carpal bones and the forearm bones; some takes place between the proximal and distal rows. Mostly it is flexion and extension, but a small amount of lateral movement is possible. Some rotation can also take place and enables an animal to turn the paw so that it can lick the undersurface. This movement of the distal part of the limb is *supination.*

Metacarpus. In the typical mammal there are five metacarpal bones which are numbered one to five, the most medial being the first. The dog and cat are near to the typical but even here the first metacarpal bone is very reduced.

The proximal end of each metacarpal bone is flattened and forms a synovial joint with the lower row of carpal bones. There is however little movement at this joint. The distal end of each metacarpal bone is transversely cylindrical and forms the

trochlea. Its articular surface has a ridge and the synovial joint between this bone and the proximal phalanx of the digit has strong lateral ligaments. Only flexion and extension are possible. Each main metacarpal has a pair of very small sesamoid bones at the distal end on the palmar surface. They are included in the articulation between the metacarpal and phalangeal bone.

Digits. For every complete metacarpal bone there is a complete set of three phalangeal bones, a proximal, a middle and a distal (Fig. 1.28). The proximal phalanx has a concave **fovea** at the proximal extremity and a convex **trochlea** at the distal extremity. The middle phalanx resembles the proximal, except that it is a shorter

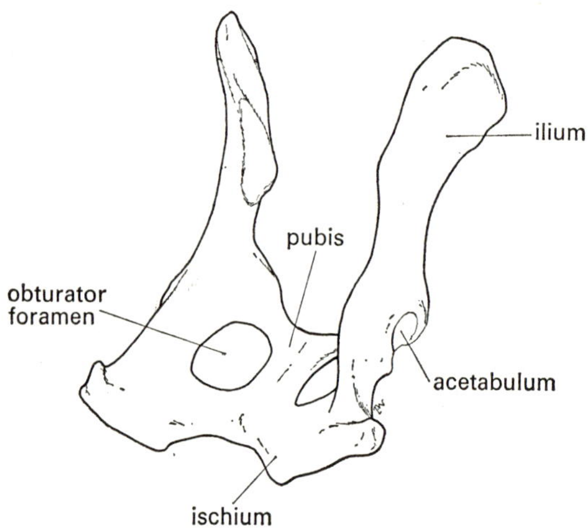

Fig. 1.17. The hip bones of a dog.

bone. The distal phalanx conforms roughly to the shape of the claw which covers it in life.

The development of the phalanges for the subsidiary metacarpal bones is variable. However, the dog and cat usually have a *dewclaw* related to the first digit.

The joints between proximal and middle, and middle and distal phalanges are synovial and are called the toe joints. All have strong lateral ligaments and are only able to flex and extend.

The Pelvic Limb

The bony pelvis is composed of the pair of hip (coxal) bones joined at the midline symphysis, the sacrum and the first few coccygeal bones.

Hip bone. Each consists of the **ilium**, the **ischium** and the **pubis** (Fig. 1.17). These are all flat bones and they meet together in an articular cavity, the **acetabulum**, into which fits the head of the femur to form the **hip joint**. The centre of the acetabulum has no articular cartilage and is called the **acetabular fossa.**

Most of the ilium is vertical and it forms a mainly cartilaginous joint with the lateral parts of the sacrum. The floor of the pelvis is formed on each side by the pubis cranially and the ischium caudally. The floor is incomplete and has a large hole on each side of the midline; this is the **obturator foramen.** The ischium also forms a part of the low side-walls of the pelvis caudal to the acetabulum. The ilium, pubis and ischium fuse together quite early in life and the right and left sides also often fuse together. There is a ligament of dense connective tissue between the sacrum and the ischium (**sacro-tuberal ligament**).

The ventral part of the body of the sacrum, the medial surface of the iliac bones, and the dorsal aspect of the pubic bones form a ring which is the **cranial pelvic aperture** (pelvic inlet). The **caudal pelvic aperture** (pelvic outlet) is formed dorsally by the ventral part of the caudal end of the sacrum, laterally by the sacro-tuberal ligaments and ventrally by the dorsal aspect of the ischial bones.

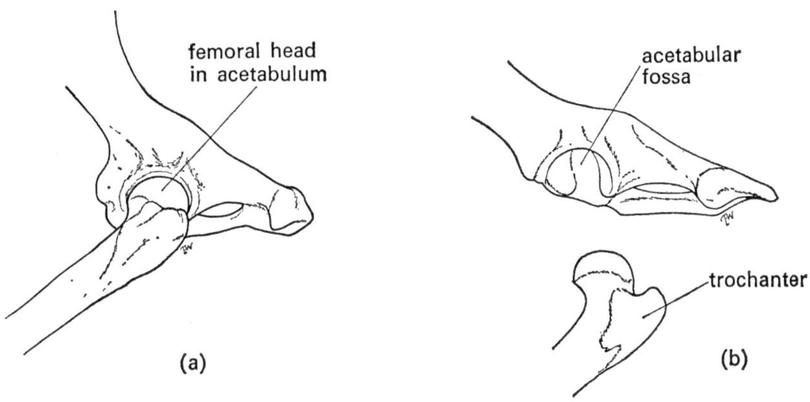

Fig. 1.18. The hip joint: (a) bones in natural position, (b) bones separated.

Femur. This long bone has proximally a rounded **head** which fits into the acetabulum to form the **hip joint** (Fig. 1.18). Like all synovial joints this has a joint capsule: it runs between the rim of the acetabulum and the neck of the bone joining the head to the rest of the femur. There is also a ligament of the head of the femur (sometimes called the teres or the round ligament) which runs from a firm attachment on the rounded articular head of the femur to the non-articular acetabular fossa. It is too long to hold the femoral head in the socket in the normal animal. The muscles surrounding the hip joint are mainly responsible for this. Although it would appear that this arrangement allows a wide range of movement, the hip joint usually only flexes and extends. There are roughened processes for muscular attachment near the head which are called **trochanters.** At the distal end, a pair of articular **condyles** take part in the formation of the **stifle** (knee) joint (Fig. 1.19). Just proximal to the condyles and merging with them the **trochlea** of the femur forms a gutter for the **patella** (knee-cap). This is a **sesamoid** bone; that is, a bone formed in a muscle or its tendon to assist its passage over another piece of bone. There are also sesamoid bones in the muscles on the side of the femur opposite to the patella. However, these are very much smaller.

Tibia and fibula. It is convenient to deal with these two leg bones together. The tibia is the main bone and is medial to the fibula. In the dog and cat the fibula is a complete bone but is much finer than the tibia.

The proximal end of the tibia is flattened and helps form the stifle joint with the femur. There are a pair of fibro-cartilaginous **menisci** between the femoral condyles and the articular surface of the tibia. There are also a pair of strong **cruciate** ligaments which help to stabilize this synovial joint. One is attached cranially between the

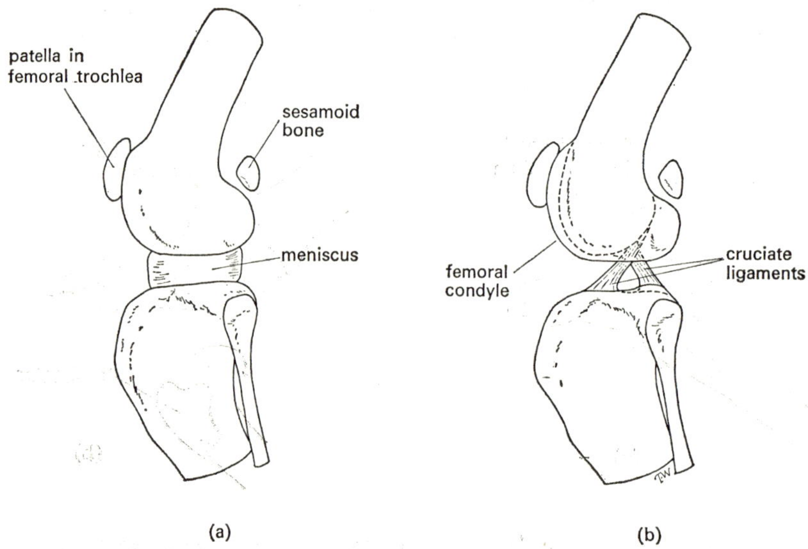

Fig. 1.19. Stifle joint: (a) with menisci in position, (b) menisci removed to show cruciate ligaments.

femoral condyles and caudally on to the head of the tibia: the other is attached opposite to this and so they cross (hence the name, which means crossing).

The distal end of the tibia forms a synovial joint with one of the tarsal bones. To conform to this the tibia has a pair of rather deep articular grooves, separated by a ridge.

Tarsus. There are several tarsal bones. They all form parts of synovial joints but the one in which there is most movement is that between the **talus** (astragalus) and the tibia. This tarsal bone has a **trochlea** which conforms very well indeed to the distal end of the tibia. The **calcaneus** (os calcis) is closely associated with the talus; it has a distinct process for muscle attachment which forms the *point of the hock.* The talus and the calcaneus can be considered to form the proximal row of tarsal bones. The distal row resembles those in the corresponding position in the carpus, forming a fairly level row to articulate with the proximal end of the metatarsal bones and being quite firmly attached to them. One tarsal bone is found between the proximal and the distal rows: this is the **central** tarsal bone. It is also known as the scaphoid bone and seems prone to fracture in the racing greyhound.

The whole region of the distal end of the tibia, the tarsus and the proximal end of the metatarsus is called the **hock joint**: but since nearly all the movement (predominantly flexion and extension) takes place between the tibia and the talus this part of the joint is sometimes said to be the "true hock joint".

Metatarsus and digits. The bones of the remainder of the hind paw are sufficiently similar to those of the corresponding region of the thoracic limb, that separate descriptions are unnecessary.

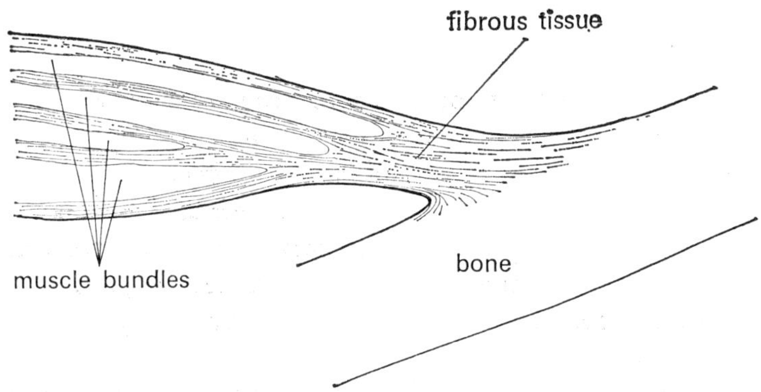

Fig. 1.20. The attachment of a muscle to a bone. Notice that it is the fibrous tissue which forms the attachment and that this runs into the bone.

Skeletal Muscles

The structure of a skeletal muscle has been outlined with the connective tissue binding the cells into bundles and the bundles into muscles enclosed in a muscle sheath. This interweaving connective tissue continues the line of the muscle fibres as a rope-like tendon or a sheet-like aponeurosis. It is this fibrous connective tissue that forms the attachment of a skeletal muscle to another structure; the muscle cells themselves do not come into direct contact with the organs (Fig. 1.20). However, there may sometimes be little fibrous tissue and then one talks of a "fleshy", as opposed to a "tendinous", attachment. The point of attachment which moves least when the muscle contracts is often termed the **origin**: the opposite end is the **insertion.** This is not entirely satisfactory and in the limbs, for instance, the more proximal end is usually called the origin. For muscles between the trunk and the limbs the more medial insertion is often termed the origin. With some muscles the term **belly** is used for the swollen part; the tapered origin is then the **head.**

One tends to think of skeletal muscles as only causing movements at a joint. However, in addition to this important function, they may have many other uses, as the following examples will show. Complete limbs are moved; softer structures, such as the eyeball and the outer part of the ear, are reorientated; the skin is twitched; apertures, such as that between the eyelids, may be closed by circular **sphincter** muscles; the entire mass of abdominal organs is supported by the muscular body wall.

It is as well to realize, also, that a muscle may be called upon to perform more than one function. Perhaps this is best illustrated by the fact that, although so far the emphasis has been on movement, one of the most important duties of a muscle is to keep a structure still. For instance, a limb is kept rigid, and so an animal is supported, by muscles on opposite sides of the limb-joints exerting forces which balance each other. No movement as such, but a necessary use of skeletal muscles.

Muscle Contraction

Contraction is controlled by motor nerve impulses passing from the central nervous system through the hundreds of nerve fibres that enter the muscle belly. After entry, each nerve fibre splits up and innervates very small bundles of muscle fibres distributed throughout the muscle. If the muscle is used for delicate movements the number of muscle fibres supplied by each nerve fibre may be very small, perhaps only about ten: for gross movement many more muscle fibres, 200 or more, may be innervated by each fibre. All the muscle fibres innervated by a single nerve fibre form a **motor unit.**

When a muscle fibre contracts it does so to its maximum: it cannot contract partly. At the same time all the muscle fibres in that unit will contract, but since they are spread throughout the muscle, innervation of only one unit will result in an overall weak contraction. Stimulation of all the motor units in a muscle will result in maximum contraction. Grading of the contraction is achieved by varying the number of motor units innervated at any one time.

If the ends of a muscle are brought closer together when it is stimulated the contraction is said to be **isotonic** and this is common during movement. Sometimes a muscle is tensed but not shortened: this often happens whilst standing and the contraction is **isometric.**

Muscles are usually in a slight state of tension: this is called **muscle tone** and is accomplished by a few nerve impulses continually leaving the central nervous system. Any additional stimulus will provoke a more rapid reaction. The rate of nerve impulses, and hence muscle tone, is increased during fear and anxiety. The animal becomes apprehensive ("jumpy" or "nervy") and may react violently to any additional stimulus. The rate of tonic impulses is reduced during sleep and muscles become more relaxed.

The more a muscle is used, the more it increases in size and strength: when the nerve supply is destroyed, however, the muscle fibres degenerate and the muscle withers and atrophies.

The complex chemical reactions of muscle contraction demand a ready source of energy and also a plentiful supply of free calcium ions. The reactions are quite inefficient and only about a quarter of the energy goes into mechanical work; the remaining three-quarters appear as heat, an occurrence that can be very embarrassing to the animal during prolonged or intense muscle activity.

Muscles of the Head

These can be intrinsic (muscles within the head region altering the position of parts of the head) or extrinsic (muscles altering the entire head in relation to the rest of the body).

The lower jaw pivots at the temporo-mandibular joint. There are very strong intrinsic muscles for closing the jaws; the one in the temporal fossa has been mentioned in the description of the skull and there are others between the upper jaw and the bodies of the mandibles. It is important that the jaws can be closed strongly and held tightly shut: they can be opened by relaxation of the "jaw-closing" muscles, but there are some relatively weak ones that can help by contraction.

There are several intrinsic muscles that adjust the lips, nostrils, eyelids and ears: these are sometimes grouped as "muscles of expression". Special eye muscles within the orbit control the eyeball and muscles between the mandibles merge into the tongue.

Extrinsic muscles attach to the occipital bone and to the vertebral column dorsal to the transverse processes. These will tend to tilt the head dorsally, with the point of fulcrum being the synovial joint between the occipital bone and the atlas. Muscles running ventral to the transverse processes and to the sternum will depress the head. There are also laterally placed muscles. All the extrinsic muscles of the head harmonise to provide it with a wide range of movement.

Muscles of the Trunk

These can be grouped into three: vertebral (spinal) muscles, the diaphragm, abdominal muscles.

Vertebral muscles. These attach to the vertebrae, ribs and ilium. Sometimes the end attachments are only one or two vertebrae apart, sometimes many vertebrae separate them. There is a lot of intermingling between the bundles that form this group, making it difficult to isolate specific muscles. However, those that run between adjacent ribs form an important part of the thoracic wall and are called intercostal muscles.

Vertebral muscles lying dorsal to the transverse processes are called **epaxial**, those lying ventral are **hypaxial.** The cervical vertebral column can be said to be ventrally concave, the thoraco-lumbar region dorsally concave. The epaxial muscles will increase the ventral concavity of the cervical region and decrease the dorsal concavity of the thoraco-lumbar region. By combination of actions the trunk can also be curved laterally to the left or right. The muscles attaching to the thorax may be used during respiration.

Diaphragm. This is a very important skeletal muscle and is found near the mid-point of the trunk. Its attachment to the ventral surfaces of the bodies of the lumbar vertebrae is by a pair of thickened muscle bundles called **crura** (singular **crus**). These run cranially and at the last thoracic vertebra spread out as a sheet stretching over the entire caudal thoracic aperture (thoracic outlet). It attaches all round its periphery to the ribs; dorsally, just cranial to the costal arch and ventrally, to the caudal end of the sternum. In this way the thoracic cavity is separated off from the remainder of the trunk; the cavity thus formed caudal to the diaphragm is the *abdominal cavity*. The diaphragm does not run the shortest distance between these attachments: in the midline it bulges cranially, to take the shape of a dome. It does have a few foramina for the passage of structures between the thoracic and the abdominal cavities. In life the central part of the diaphragm is continually moving to vary the size of the thoracic cavity and so plays a major part in respiratory movements.

Abdominal muscles. There are several muscles concerned in forming the abdominal wall on each side of the body. They have to be strong and well arranged to support the contents of this cavity. The muscle fibres extend for about half the length of the muscle which is continued by a strong fibrous aponeurosis; this meets its fellow of the opposite side ventrally in the midline stretching cranially from the sternum and caudally reaching to the pubis.

The left and right aponeuroses of most of the abdominal muscles meet at the midline and here the fibrous tissue is fused to form a strong seam which extends from the sternum to the pelvis and is called the **linea alba** (white line). The attachment to the pubis is called the **prepubic tendon.** The aponeuroses do intermingle to a certain extent other than at the midline.

The supportive action of these abdominal muscles has been mentioned. In addition, they have the important function in the dog and cat of increasing the dorsal concavity of the thoraco-lumbar part of the vertebral column by drawing sternum and pubis closer together: this is part of their method of locomotion.

Muscles of the Limbs

These can also be divided into extrinsic and intrinsic muscles. The extrinsic ones run between the trunk and the limbs, the intrinsic ones between the bones of the appendicular skeleton of each limb.

Extrinsic limb muscles. In the description of the skeletal system it was mentioned that the forelimb pivoted in the region of the scapula. The hindlimb pivots at the hip joint. If the lower part of a limb is drawn cranially it is said to be **protracted** (Fig. 1.21) and the protractor muscles attach on the trunk cranial to the limb and on the limb ventral to the pivot. Alternatively they can be attached on the limb dorsal to the pivot and on the trunk caudal to the limb. **Retraction** is the action of drawing the lower part of the limb caudally and the attachments of retractor muscles will be opposite to the protractors. Retraction and protraction are very important actions in

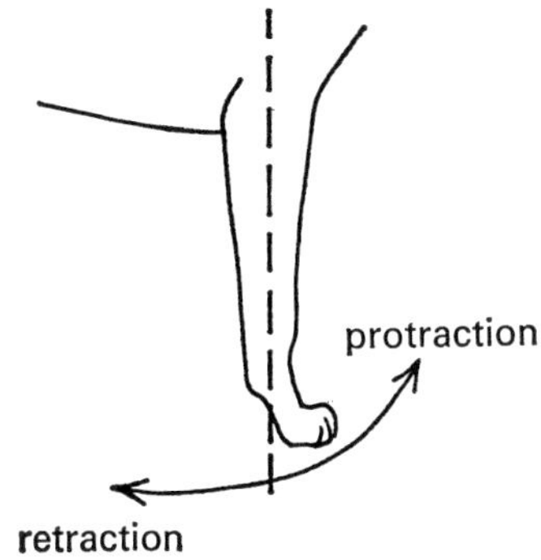

Fig. 1.21. Protraction and retraction of a forelimb.

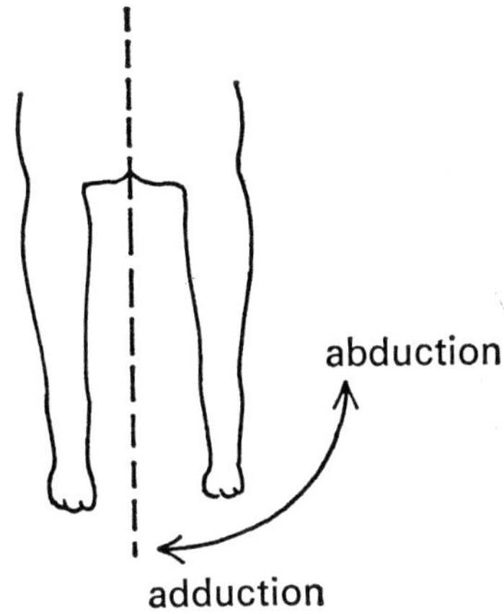

Fig. 1.22. Abduction and adduction of a forelimb.

locomotion (movement from place to place) and muscles acting about the pivot points of the entire limbs are very strong. Fortunately they are rarely damaged and consequently receive rather less attention than some of the intrinsic limb muscles.

If the entire lower limb is brought nearer to the midline it is said to be **adducted** (Fig. 1.22). Adductor muscles are attached to the trunk and to the limb ventral to the pivot point. **Abductor** muscles have the opposite effect and have their attachment dorsal to the pivots.

There is a considerable overlap of action of these extrinsic muscles. Several can both protract and adduct, for instance, and contraction of separate parts of one muscle may cause both protraction and retraction at different times.

Intrinsic limb muscles. These cause the flexion and extension of the limb joints described in the skeletal system. Some of the muscles affect one joint, only being attached to its two components, whereas others, whose attachments are further apart, may have an effect on each joint over which they pass.

It is more important to know the action of the muscles than their names and the convention that is applied to intrinsic muscles is shown in the accompanying diagram (Fig. 1.23). When the bones are brought together as shown, the joints are considered to flex. The opposite action is extension. In describing the action of a muscle it should refer to the effect at each joint it controls. It is possible for the same muscle to flex one joint and extend another: a good example is the muscle attached to the proximal end of the tibia and to the distal phalanges. On contraction this could flex the hock but it can extend the toe joints. It is not essential that these two actions

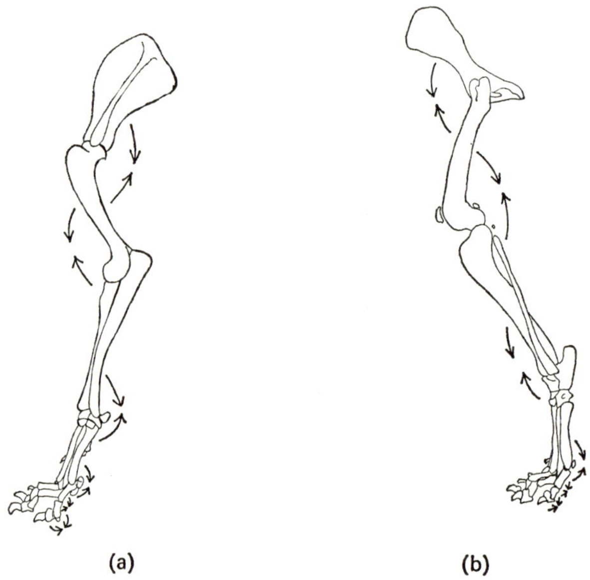

Fig. 1.23. When the bones are brought together as indicated in the diagram, each joint is said to flex: (a) forelimb, (b) hindlimb.

should occur. Opposing muscles can ensure that one joint is kept still while the other is moved.

Because of their attachments, the protractor and retractor muscles of the forelimb can extend and flex the shoulder joint and similarly those of the hindlimb can affect the hip joint.

Muscle of the Skin

The skin over various parts of the bodies of domestic mammals can be made to move or twitch. This is achieved by contractions of the **cutaneous muscle**, a thin layer that is widely distributed in the superficial fascia. It is only attached to the skeleton in a few places and the connective tissue between the muscle cells is continuous with that of the dermis and hypodermis.

SPECIAL ARRANGEMENTS

A whole variety of muscles has now been described, some with short fibrous attachments, others with vast aponeuroses. Sometimes the muscle takes origin from two or more sites: likewise there may be more than one insertion, the end of the tendon being split. Some of the limb muscles have very long tendons, the muscle belly being near the proximal end of the limb and the insertion being at the distal end.

Long tendons running beside bones are sometimes covered with fascia which is attached to the bone: the tendon may be in a groove in the bone. Such an arrangement of dense fibrous tissue is a **vaginal** ligament (sometimes called an anular ligament).

Several muscles, especially those with long tendons, have special modifications where they pass over prominences, whether this is in the normal position of the bones or as a result of movement at a joint. The bony prominence itself has usually a cartilage covering and the tendon may thicken and itself contain cartilage. In some muscles a

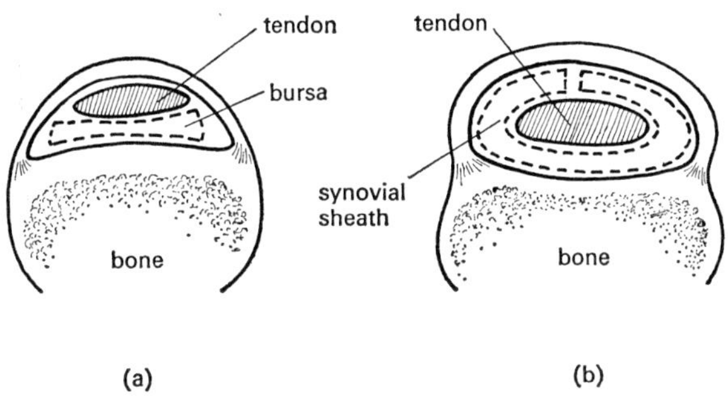

Fig. 1.24. (a) A bursa between bone and a tendon; (b) a synovial sheath wrapping round a tendon.

small bone may develop at the point of contact, especially where there is a slight change of direction. Such a structure is a **sesamoid** bone and it may form in the fleshy part of the muscle or in the tendon. The part of the sesamoid that faces the prominence is covered with cartilage (in keeping with the arrangement that moving parts of a bone are covered with cartilage) and the apposing surfaces form part of a synovial joint. All the sesamoid bones are closely related to joints between larger limb bones and the joint cavity between the sesamoid bone and the bony prominence is in free communication with the joint cavity of the major limb bones. The synovial membrane is continuous around the periphery of the articular surfaces of the main bones and of the sesamoid bones.

In some joints the synovial membrane also pouches out to lie between tendons and the extremities of bones. These extensions of the cavity are called **bursal elongations.**

Similar to these, and often, but not always, separate from a joint cavity, structures called **bursae** lie between tendons and the bone (Fig. 1.24). The lining of the bursa secretes the small amount of synovial fluid and the effect is that of a fluid-containing cushion minimizing pressure and friction. These functions may be useful in situations other than between tendons and bones; for instance, bursae are also found between the skin and bony prominences at sites where pressure and friction occur. The loose connective tissue in these regions becomes more open in texture and eventually a sac is formed, with the local cells capable of producing the small amount of synovial fluid that is required to form the cushion. Sometimes abnormal or excessive pressure and friction cause the formation of a bursa in an unusual place: this is called an *adventitial bursa.*

If one imagines the bursa to wrap all round the tendon, the structure so produced is a **synovial sheath** (Fig. 1.24), and several of these occur at the carpal and tarsal joints.

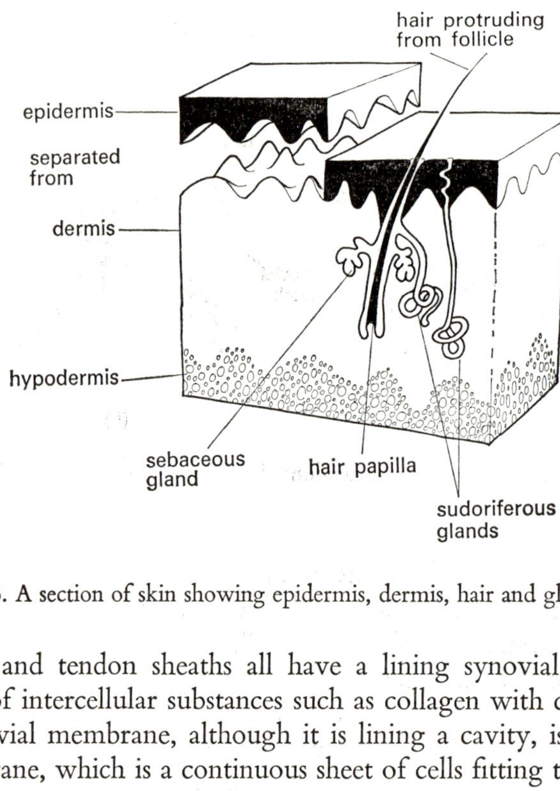

Fig. 1.25. A section of skin showing epidermis, dermis, hair and glands.

Joints, bursae and tendon sheaths all have a lining synovial membrane. This consists mainly of intercellular substances such as collagen with cells in among the fibres. The synovial membrane, although it is lining a cavity, is not therefore an epithelial membrane, which is a continuous sheet of cells fitting tightly together.

The Integument

The integument is the covering of the body. In addition to protecting the animal mechanically, it is a sensory structure, conveying information on pain, touch and pressure as well as about the temperature of the environment. Since epithelium is the tissue that forms a covering layer, the outermost part of the integument consists of epithelial cells. There are several layers of these constituting the **epidermis**; over most of the body this is quite elastic and forms part of the **skin**. The surface cells of the epidermis of the skin die and become dry and hard. As these superficial cells have a very high content of the protein *keratin*, they are said to be *keratinized* or *cornified*. There are some regions of the body where extra protection is needed and here there is a vast increase in the amount of keratin. In this way claws are formed to protect the ends of digits (horns, used as weapons, are produced in the same way). These may be described as *modified epidermal structures*; the fundamental difference between these and skin is the increase in proportion and amount of keratinization.

The epidermis, whether it is relatively lightly keratinized as in the skin, or heavily keratinized as in a claw, is avascular (has no blood supply). It is firmly attached to the

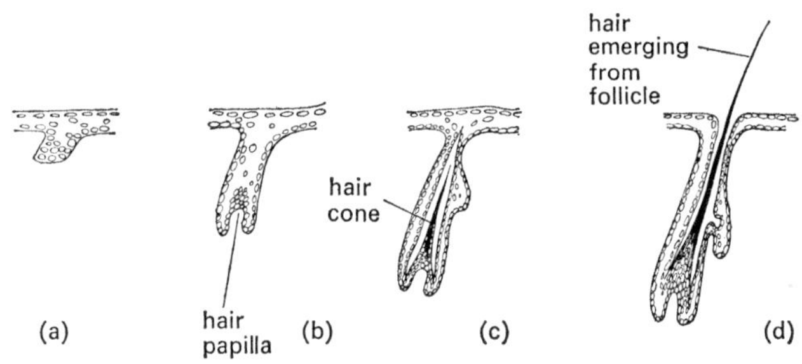

Fig. 1.26. Formation of a hair.

underlying **dermis** (Fig. 1.25) which consists of irregular dense connective tissue carrying blood vessels and nerve fibres. The **hypodermis** is deep to the dermis; it may also be called the subcutis and is actually the superficial fascia formed of loose connective tissue.

The epidermis and dermis together constitute the skin. In addition to the functions already mentioned, the skin, often helped by an underlying layer of fat, plays an important role in temperature control by acting as a blanket to conserve heat.

Epidermis

The epidermis of the skin consists of two main layers. The deeper layer is very closely attached to the dermis. By the active reproduction of its cells, more layers are formed which are gradually pushed towards the surface. The more superficial cells contain an increasing proportion of keratin and constitute the *cornified layer*.

The surface adjacent to the dermis is pitted and furrowed, with dermis fitting into all the holes and undulations that this forms. In addition to this irregular surface some epidermal structures such as hairs and glands project much further into the dermis.

Hairs

Hairs are epidermal structures formed by the epidermis thickening and extending down into the dermis (Fig. 1.26a). The deeper end flows over a knob of dermis which is then called the **hair papilla** (Fig. 1.26b). The epithelial cells immediately over the papilla produce a central **hair cone** which eventually forms the hair (Fig. 1.26c). The cells around the point of the cone disintegrate and make a canal which the growing hair uses to reach the surface of the skin. The canal opens onto the surface and can then be called the **hair follicle** (Fig. 1.26d). The deeper layer of the epidermis continues to produce the hair shaft while the hair grows. When this ceases that particular hair dies in its follicle. At any time after this it may fall from the skin, that is, it may be *shed*. The deep epidermal cells may by then be producing another hair as a replacement.

Small numbers of hairs group together to share common openings on the surface of the hairy skin of dogs. One hair in the bundle is larger and stiffer than the others and is called a **cover** or **guard** hair: the smaller, softer hairs in the bundle are **under** hairs. The number of hairs in the bundle varies with the type of hair coat.

Hairs are most common on the dorsal and lateral sides of the dog and cat but there are few inside the flanks, on the abdomen, or under the tail. There are no hairs around the nostrils nor on the foot pads but long sensory hairs (**vibrissae**) are found for instance on the sides of the nose and above the eyelids.

The hair coat is thicker in the winter than in the summer which is when some of it is normally shed: however, in house pets there is a tendency for shedding to occur throughout the year. It does not grow very quickly in the summer, but when the cool weather begins the rate increases. During active growth, about a millimetre of hair shaft is produced each week by the hair follicle. The layer of air trapped by the hair assists the insulating properties of the skin to control heat loss from the body.

Cutaneous glands

Some of the epithelial cells of the wall of the hair follicle proliferate and form glandular masses which surround the follicle and open into it (Fig. 1.25). These masses are **sebaceous** glands and their secretion, called **sebum**, keeps the skin and hair pliable and is also a protection against both drying and moisture. **Sudoriferous** or **sweat** glands may also open into the hair follicle, developing from the epithelium between the sebaceous glands and the surface of the integument. Glands may fail to function adequately during illness and malnutrition: the hair coat then becomes dull and dry. Sebum and sweat also contain some of the excretory waste of the body. The glands of some regions produce odoriferous substances which may be influential in reproductive behaviour.

There is an opening on either side of the anus, where the terminal end of the digestive tube joins the skin, which leads into an **anal sac** (also called **para-anal sinus**). These paired cavities vary from about the size of a pea in cats and small dogs up to as large as a walnut in bigger animals. The secretory glands lining these pockets of integument produce an unpleasant smelling sticky liquid which is stored in the sacs and intermittently evacuated. The openings may occasionally become blocked and the animal will show symptoms of irritation and annoyance.

Mammary glands (Fig. 1.27). These are another group of modified cutaneous glands and their function is to produce milk. There are usually eight to twelve arranged as pairs on either side of the midline, extending from about the fourth rib to the region of the pubis. They are most obvious in the female, especially towards the end of pregnancy and during and after suckling. Rudimentary structures are present in the male.

Each gland is provided with a conical teat (nipple) bearing several openings, ranging in number between about eight and sixteen. The secretory epithelium of the gland is embedded in a mass of connective tissue which varies in its nature with the age and condition of the animal. The secretions collect in dilatations called **gland sinuses**; these are drained by **teat sinuses** occupying most of the teat. Nearer the apex of the teat, the sinuses narrow to become **teat canals** that open as the **teat orifices**.

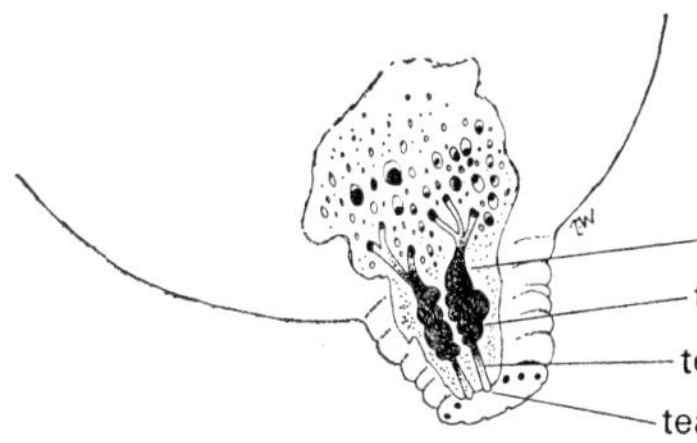

Fig. 1.27. Section of a mammary gland.

The production of milk is **lactation** and this is usually associated with the nursing of the young progeny. During pregnancy the glandular material increases in amount and size and the first milk associated with each pregnancy is called **colostrum**. This contains many substances that are vital to the new-born: after a few days the proportion of proteins, lactose (milk sugar), minerals and small fat globules changes and then stays fairly constant for the rest of the lactation.

Dermis

This may be called *corium* and is a dense feltwork of connective tissue fibres with blood vessels and nerves freely scattered in its substance. The dermis is continuous throughout the body, whether it is deep to the skin or to modified epidermal structures. Hair follicles and glands form downgrowths into its substance and the dermis forms ridges, bumps and papillae into the under-surface of the epidermis. There are many smooth muscle cells in the dermis, especially related to the hair follicles: these can alter the slope of the hair relative to the skin surface.

Hypodermis

This is very variable in amount, being virtually absent in some situations. It may merge imperceptibly into the dermis. It is the superficial fascia and consists of loose connective (areolar) tissue often arranged in sheets. Fat infiltrates between these to form the subcutaneous layer that can be such a useful insulating blanket, protection and energy store, but which when present in excess not only inconveniences the animal but also the surgeon who has to incise through these layers at an operation site.

MODIFIED INTEGUMENT OF THE FOOT

The foot consists of four toes, each of which has a **claw** and a (digital) **footpad**; there is in addition a metacarpal or metatarsal pad. (The **paw**, as opposed to the foot, includes, in the forelimb, the carpus, metacarpus, phalanges and the associated sesamoid bones. The paw of the hindlimb is composed of corresponding hindlimb bones.) The metacarpal (or metatarsal) and phalanges medial to these four toes are not

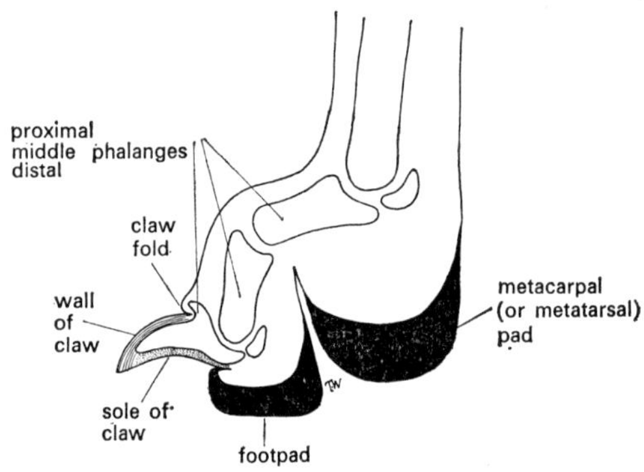

Fig. 1.28. Section of a toe of a dog.

well developed and are known as **dewclaws.** They may be completely absent: this is commonly so in the hindlimbs, especially in cats. Dewclaws do not reach the ground and may cause more trouble than claws that do. They are removed from some dogs within a few days of birth.

Footpads

The keratinized, hairless epidermis of a footpad is thick and pigmented. In the dog it is arranged in conical papillae which may become worn down on hard surfaces. Those of the cat have smoother surfaces with ridges producing a branching connected pattern. Sweat glands open on to their surface.

The subcutaneous tissue helps to form **digital cushions** deep to the footpads: they consist of fibrous adipose tissue. Sweat glands are found in this layer.

The digital pads are oval and support the distal interphalangeal joints (Fig. 1.28). The metacarpal and metatarsal pads of the dog are somewhat "heart-shaped"; the apex is distal and the two lobes are unequal in area. Those of the cat are more rounded. The joints between the proximal phalanges and the metacarpus (or metatarsus) rest on them when the paw supports weight.

There is also a carpal pad situated palmar and distal to the carpal bones.

Claws (Fig. 1.2

The claw of the carnivore is the horny covering of the distal phalanx. The beaklike shape is quite characteristic; there are two **walls** that are continuous dorsally but on the ground surface the free edges embrace a soft flaky horn which forms the **sole** of the claw. The free edges of the walls may meet, thereby covering part of the sole; sometimes the part of the sole nearest the apex of the claw is visible.

The proximal end of the claw, which may also be called its base, root, or **coronary border**, fits into a groove. There it is continuous with the epidermis of hair-free skin which, as it leaves the groove to continue as the hairy skin, constitutes the **claw fold.** The ground surface of the claw is separated from its corresponding digital pad by a furrow.

The claw is produced mainly from cells in the groove housing the coronary border; as it is produced the horny covering curves over the dermis that is tightly attached to the distal phalanx.

The dermis between the bone of the distal phalanx and the horn of the claw is very vascular and great care should be taken when trimming claws to ensure that only the epidermis is cut. The extent of the dermis can be seen by shining a light through the claw, providing it is not pigmented.

The claw grows at a rapid rate, and if it is not worn off or trimmed it will sometimes continue growing in a circular fashion until the point penetrates the ground surface of the foot. Especial notice should be taken of dewclaws which are unable to be worn down in the same way as the main claws.

Body Cavities and the Visceral Systems

BODY CAVITIES (Fig. 1.29)

The **viscera** (singular, viscus) are those organs found in the body cavities, i.e. the thoracic cavity, the abdominal cavity and the pelvic cavity.

The **thoracic cavity** is bounded by the cranial thoracic aperture (first thoracic vertebra, first pair of ribs and the cranial end of the sternum), the diaphragm, the bodies of the thoracic vertebrae, the ribs (including costal cartilages), and the sternum.

The **abdominal cavity** has as its cranial boundary the diaphragm, and as its caudal limit the cranial pelvic aperture; the dorsal boundary is formed by the diaphragm and the lumbar vertebrae, and the muscles of the abdominal wall form the dorso-lateral, lateral and ventral limits.

The **pelvic cavity** has the cranial pelvic aperture (pelvic inlet) and the caudal pelvic aperture (pelvic outlet) as its cranial and caudal limits, the sacrum and the first few coccygeal vertebrae dorsally, and the pubis and the ischium of the left and right sides as the floor. The lateral boundaries are muscles and the sacro-tuberal ligament.

Tissue is attached to the inner surfaces of these body cavities to form two sacs in the thoracic cavity and one sac in the abdominal and pelvic cavities. This tissue consists of a continuous layer of epithelial cells on the inner surface of the sacs and a thin supporting layer of connective tissue on the outer surface. The epithelial cells produce a very small amount of a watery serous fluid; the epithelium and the layer of connective tissue are therefore said to form a **serous membrane** or serosa and the sacs surround *serous cavities*. The serous membrane lining the thorax is **pleura** and this surrounds two **pleural cavities**. The serous membrane in the abdomen and most of the pelvis is the **peritoneum** and this surrounds the **peritoneal cavity**.

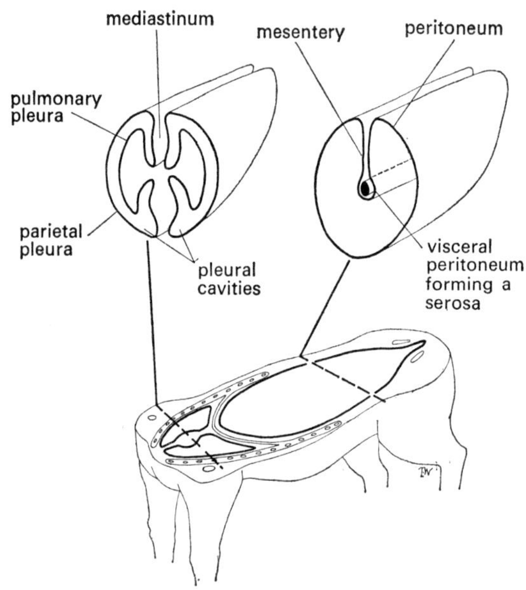

Fig. 1.29. Body cavities.

There is a left and a right pleural sac and the space between them is the **mediastinum**. Most of the organs, such as the heart, and other structures of the thoracic cavity are in the mediastinum. However, the largest viscera, the **lungs**, and one of two closely related tissues including their vascular and nerve arrangements, push laterally out of the mediastinum, taking pleura with them and reducing considerably the size of the pleural cavities. The pleura which actually covers the lungs is called **pulmonary pleura** (visceral pleura), the remaining pleura is **parietal pleura**. This is subdivided into that forming the limits of the mediastinum, **mediastinal pleura**, that covering the diaphragm, **diaphragmatic pleura**, and that lining the ribs, etc., **costal pleura**. The pleural cavity is so reduced that it is virtually non-existent and the pulmonary pleura is separated from the parietal pleura by only a thin film of *pleural fluid* produced by the pleura itself. This acts as a lubricant between the serous membranes, which will therefore be moist, shiny and slippery.

The peritoneal cavity fills the abdominal cavity and the more cranial part of the pelvic cavity. In describing a pleural cavity it was seen that the growth of the viscera laterally from the mediastinum reduced the cavity to a potential space. In the case of the peritoneal cavity a similar phenomenon can be imagined (it does not actually occur like this) but the "growth" would be downward from the *dorsal* surface of the abdominal cavity. There are many parts of several viscera involved in this "growth" and they are all coated with peritoneum which will be **visceral peritoneum.** The part closely applied to the viscus is often described as a part of that viscus; then it is called its **serosa.** The **parietal peritoneum** lines the limits of the abdominal cavity and the more cranial part of the pelvic cavity. The part of the peritoneum between the viscus and the parietal peritoneum has a variety of names depending on the viscus, e.g. **mesentery, omentum, ligament.** This part, which is very thin, consisting of a little connective tissue between the two layers of serous membrane, will carry the vessels and other structures to and from the viscus. The peritoneum-coated viscera and their attachments fill the peritoneal cavity, leaving room only for the small amount of the serous *peritoneal fluid* to act as a lubricant between the serous membranes. All the surfaces are normally moist, shiny and slippery.

It should be emphasized in completing these comments on the pleural and peritoneal cavities that only fluid is to be found within the cavities themselves and that this acts as a lubricant between the serous membranes which are constantly apposed to each other.

VISCERAL SYSTEMS

There are three visceral systems: **respiratory**, **digestive** and **urogenital.** Not every organ of these three systems is within one of the three body cavities, but since the major part of each of these systems is truly visceral they are included in this group. Conversely, because an organ is in a body cavity (and hence it is a viscus) it is not necessarily part of a visceral system.

The systems consist primarily of tubes contained within the body which eventually open to the outside. In the case of the digestive system the tube opens to the outside at both ends. In the respiratory and urogenital systems only one end of each system opens to the outside. These tubes have a continuous lining of epithelium which is usually very thin. One of the methods of protecting this membrane is by lubrication with mucus, produced either by glands or by individual cells. The epithelium of the tubes of the visceral system is therefore called **mucous membrane** or mucosa. (Note that the noun is spelt **mucus** and the adjective **muc*o*us.**)

Respiratory System

Respiration is the gaseous exchange between a living structure and its environment. Oxygen is necessary for the chemical reactions essential to animal life and carbon dioxide is an end-product. In discussing blood, it was mentioned that this tissue is capable of carrying these gases. The transfer of the oxygen from blood to all the cells of the body and of carbon dioxide from these cells to the blood is called *tissue (or internal) respiration*. The transfer of the gases between the external environment and the blood is called *external respiration* and in mammals this takes place in the lungs. The structure of these organs and of the passageways from the outside to the site of external respiration will be considered in this description of the respiratory system. It will include the nasal cavities, the pharynx, the larynx, the trachea, the bronchi and the lungs (Fig. 1.30). Occasionally the mouth is used as an additional air-way during mouth breathing and panting. The thorax, pleural cavities, diaphragm and other muscles, such as those of the abdominal wall, which can affect the size of the thoracic cavity are also essential parts of the respiratory system.

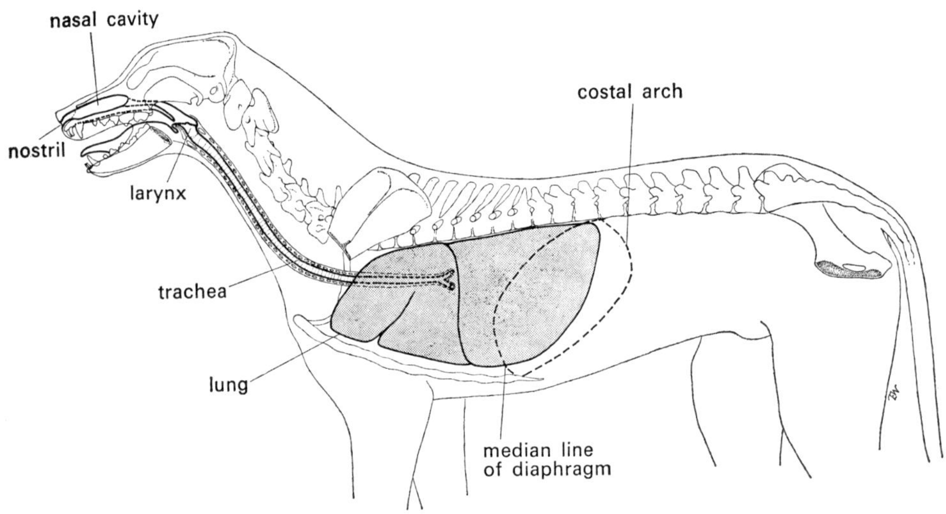

Fig. 1.30. Respiratory system.

Some regions of the respiratory system are used for other functions in addition to the passage of gases: for instance, parts of the nasal cavities play a role in the sensation of smell, the larynx helps in the production of sound and part of the lining of the respiratory system is effective in heat and water loss. In the section on the visceral system the respiratory system was described as a tube within the body that had an opening to the outside at one end only. This tube has a continuous lining called a mucous membrane, the epithelial cells of which vary with the region.

Nasal Cavities (Fig. 1.31)

The nasal chambers, and the turbinates they contain, are lined with **nasal mucous membrane** to form the **nasal cavities.** The continuation with the epithelium of the skin takes place at the **nostrils.** The animal is able to increase and decrease the size of these apertures. The openings are strengthened by cartilage and are surrounded by a zone of hairless skin, the **muzzle.**

The scrolls of bone in the nasal chambers are covered by a very vascular mucous membrane, that is, one rich in blood vessels, many of which are wide-bored and have thin walls. Near the cranial cavity, i.e. in the depth or fundus of the nasal cavity, the epithelium over the tubinates has a special arrangement to register the sensation of smell and convey the information to the brain. This part of the mucous membrane is the **olfactory region**: the remainder is the **respiratory region** and most of the mucous membrane bears minute hair-like projections called **cilia** which are constantly in wave-like motion. The mucous membrane moistens, warms and cleans the incoming air. Any small particles are trapped in the mucus which is continuously

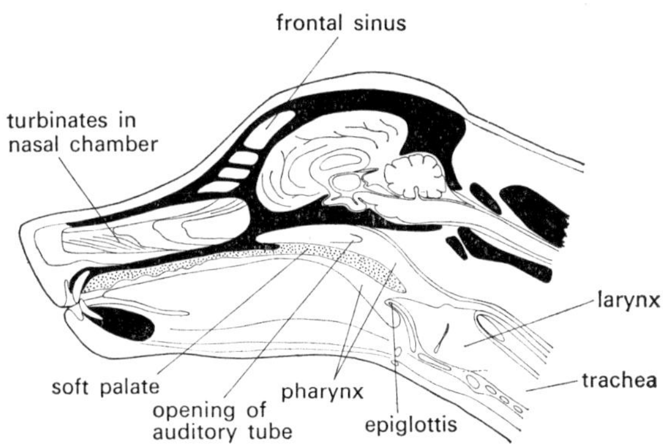

Fig. 1.31. Median section of a dog's head. Solid black represents bone.

produced by the membrane. This secretion, together with any trapped material, is wafted by the cilia into the throat and then swallowed.

The mucous membrane forms a lateral pouch called a **maxillary sinus** in the spongy interior of the maxillary bone. The epithelium of the cavity differs from that in the nasal chamber.

More of these outpouchings of the nasal mucous membrane take place between the turbinates. Here the bone that is invaded is the frontal bone and so **frontal sinuses** are formed.

All these sinuses retain their connections with the nasal cavities and all are lined by a continuation of the nasal mucous membrane. The outpouchings are collectively known as **paranasal sinuses.**

The nasal cavities are continued into the single midline **pharynx** through paired openings.

Pharynx (Fig. 1.31)

This chamber is common to the ıespiratory and the digestive systems. Both systems have entrances to it but these are separated by a musculo-membranous partition, the **soft palate**, into a dorsal **nasal part** and a ventral **oral part**. At times of respiratory distress, the mouth is used for an additional opening, and the oral part of the pharynx then becomes an air-way.

In the dorsal region of the nasal part of the pharynx, there are paired openings into the **auditory** (Eustachian) **tubes.** The tube of each side connects the middle-ear cavity with the pharynx and its lining is continuous with that of the pharynx.

The opening into the larynx is in the floor of the pharynx and just caudal and slightly more dorsal is the opening into the **oesophagus**, the continuation of the digestive system.

The wall of the pharynx is muscular and its lining is continuous with that of all the tubes which enter and leave it.

Larynx (Fig. 1.31)

The **larynx** is a complex valvular mechanism of interconnected cartilages, muscles, fibrous tissue and mucous membrane, whose function is to stop the entry of material other than gases into the more distal part of the respiratory system; if any food touches the pharynx the larynx immediately closes. The larynx also controls the flow of these gases, as well as producing sounds. It lies in the midline between the rami of the mandibles.

There are fundamentally three single, and one pair of cartilages. The single midline **epiglottis** is the most rostral cartilage and it points toward the soft palate. Caudal to the epiglottis are a pair of **vocal ligaments.** Since each vocal ligament is attached dorsally to cartilages which are slightly separated and yet ventrally they attach to a midline structure their arrangement will represent the two limbs of a V, one limb on either side of the midline.

The continuous action of the cartilages swings these two limbs alternately nearer to and further from the midline. The mucous membrane lining the cavity of the larynx covers the vocal ligaments and the combined ligament and mucous membrane forms the **vocal fold.** The space bounded by the folds and the mucous-membrane-covered cartilages to which they are attached is the **glottis.** Movement of the cartilages controls the size of the glottis and therefore regulates the flow of gases. Forced passage of gases through the glottis causes the vocal folds to vibrate and so produce a sound. This is modulated by the size of the glottis and the tension of the folds and further modified by the resonance effects of the remainder of the head region.

Trachea

The **trachea** is a permanently open tube attached to the laryngeal cartilages. It lies on the ventral aspect of the neck and passes through the cranial thoracic aperture into the mediastinum of the cranial half of the thorax. Here it ends by splitting at the **bifurcation** into right and left **bronchi** (Fig. 1.33).

The tube is kept open by a series of incomplete **tracheal cartilages**, which vary in shape but resemble a C. The open part of the cartilage is dorsal; this means that the part nearer the skin is always the solid part of the cartilage. They are connected into a tube by fibrous tissue with which smooth muscle cells are associated. The ciliated mucous membrane is continuous with that of the larynx and the bronchi and is attached to the inner surface of the cartilages.

Bronchi and Terminal Air Passages (Fig. 1.32)

The bronchi that leave the trachea branch continually in such a manner that the very apt descriptive name of bronchial tree is given to the arrangement (Fig. 1.33). The successive branches decrease in size and the smaller tubes are called **bronchioles.**

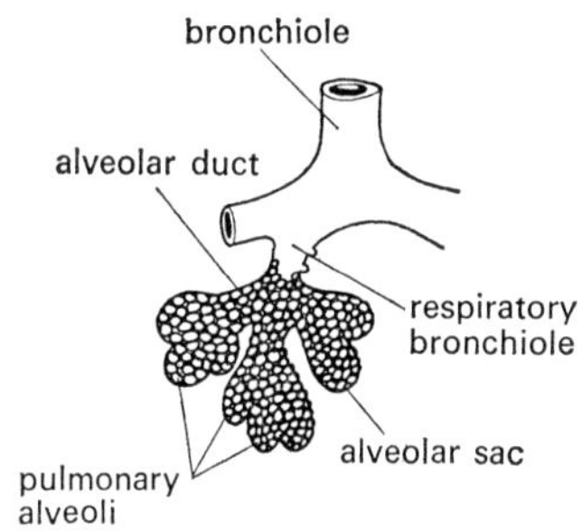

Fig. 1.32. Terminal air passages.

Although the larger tubes have a cartilage arrangement resembling that of the trachea this becomes reduced to a series of small overlapping plates and eventually the cartilage tissue ends. These tubes, which are lined by a continuation of the ciliated mucous membrane, are of a very small diameter. Ultimately the stage of the smallest bronchioles is reached. These are called **respiratory bronchioles** and each branches into several **alveolar ducts.** Each duct ends as **alveolar sacs** which consist of a large number of **pulmonary alveoli.** The epithelium of the walls of these respiratory bronchioles and their ramifications is extremely thin and has no cilia; it is sometimes called the **pulmonary membrane.** This is the level at which gaseous exchange takes place and so these structures are covered by equally thin-walled capillaries accompanied by just a trace of connective tissue. Oxygen continually leaves the air in the alveoli, diffuses across the pulmonary membrane and passes into the blood. It is replaced in the alveoli by carbon dioxide which has left the blood by a similar mechanism. As the blood vessels are followed away from this alveolar level they get larger and have thicker walls. The amount of connective and other tissue also increases. Blood leaving the lungs in an oxygenated state circulates to capillaries permeating the body and there the oxygen passes into tissue fluid and into the cells where it is rapidly used for oxidation. Most of the oxygen has been carried in combination with haemoglobin although a small amount is dissolved in the plasma. At normal times the haemoglobin only gives up about a quarter of its oxygen to the tissues; however, at times of distress it can probably release about three times as much as this.

The collection of air passages, blood vessels and surrounding connective tissue forms the lung tissue. Only the proximal parts of the bronchi are outside the lung tissue, that is, are extra-pulmonic. All the lung tissue is enclosed in pulmonary pleura to form **lungs.**

Lungs

The right and left lungs fill nearly all the thoracic cavity. They are not very similar to one another in shape and the right one is larger than the left. The bronchi and the

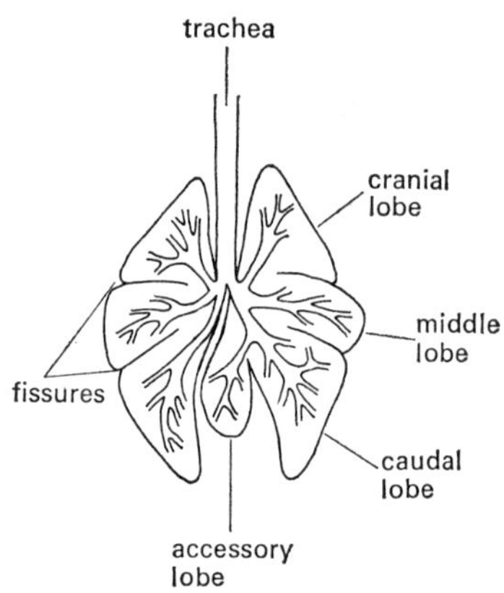

Fig. 1.33. Diagram to show bronchial tree within the lobes of the lungs.

blood vessels, nerves, etc., associated with a lung, enter it at its **root.** The lung tissue in dogs and cats is completely divided by fissures into a group of **lobes** (Fig. 1.33). A cranial (apical), middle (cardiac) and caudal (diaphragmatic) lobe can be seen in both lungs. The right lung has, in addition, an accessory (intermediate) lobe which lies between the two lungs.

BREATHING

This is accomplished by alternately enlarging and contracting the thorax. The diaphragm and some of the trunk muscles enlarge the thorax by their contractions. During quiet respiration the thorax may reduce in size by virtue of the elasticity of the tissues and the relaxation of muscles. Contraction of abdominal muscles can force the contents of that cavity against the diaphragm and so help reduce the size of the thorax. The lungs slide freely in the pleural cavity and follow the excursions of the thorax. As the lungs enlarge during inspiration air is pulled into the alveoli; as they reduce in expiration air is forced out. The muscles of respiration are not used to their maximum during quiet breathing, but have an enormous reserve that can be called upon in respiratory distress.

During quiet respiration the dog breathes 10–30 times per minute, the cat 20–30. This is called the respiratory rate.

When the lungs are distended nerve impulses are sent to a respiratory centre in the brain; this transmits information which inhibits the inspiratory muscles. A similar mechanism is used at expiration and so a rhythmic control is established. There are other nerve patterns used in a similar manner so that this vital function does not rely on only one. The rate and depth of respirations are affected by many factors, including carbon dioxide and oxygen levels in the blood.

The motor-nerve impulses leave the spinal cord in nerves at appropriate levels to reach the respiratory muscles. Some leave the cervical part of the cord and together form a **phrenic nerve** on each side which runs through the mediastinum to reach the diaphragm.

The air that passes in and out of the lungs with each respiration is the **tidal air** and the amount is the **tidal volume.** Even at the end of the most forceful expiration there is some aiı left in the lung; the amount is the **residual volume**. That which is left at the end of normal expiration is the **functional residual capacity** and this is the air that allows gaseous diffusion between breaths. A lot of the air drawn in at each inspiration is exhaled again before it reaches the alveoli; this amount is called the **dead space** and is the same as the volume of the respiratory passages from nostrils to alveoli.

In the pathological condition **pneumonia** the alveoli fill with fluid and their walls become inflamed and "waterlogged" by excess fluid. This will obviously severely restrict gaseous exchange. Another pathological state can occur if the thorax is punctured or opened in any way. Air can then enter the pleural cavity and the lungs will collapse away from the wall; this is **pneumothorax.** It may be caused intentionally during thoracic operations, and at the end the anaesthetist will ensure that the lungs are restored to their normal size, and the air expelled from the pleural cavity.

Digestive System

The normal animal requires material to incorporate into its own body to help replace worn-out tissues. The breakdown of these substances can also provide the energy required to carry on life processes. The material is *food* and the function of breaking it down and altering it to make it available for absorption into the body is *digestion* and is carried out by the **digestive system.** *Absorption* is the transference of foodstuffs from the digestive system into the blood and lymph; these carry it eventually to tissues for storage or immediate use.

In the natural state dogs and cats obtain most of their food from animal, as opposed to plant, sources; that is, they are carnivorous. As pets this is certainly not so. The food must supply water, proteins, carbohydrates, lipids and inorganic compounds. It must also provide a group of chemicals called **vitamins**. These are essential in minute traces in the food since the animal is probably incapable of manufacturing them itself. It appears that many of the vitamins form parts of enzyme systems. Diseases can occur in their absence but the average well-balanced diet probably contains an adequate supply. Vitamins will be discussed more fully in the section on feeding. Some foods need no digestion, but in most cases quite elaborate changes have to take place before the complex and sometimes insoluble substances can be absorbed.

The digestive system is basically a tube which is open at both ends and has entering into it ducts from glands producing secretions that help in the digestive process. The food is taken in at the mouth and here secretions from salivary glands are added; the breaking-down of this mixture is helped by the teeth and the tongue. The result is carried through the pharynx to the oesophagus, a musculo-membranous tube that passes along the neck and then through the mediastinum within the thorax. The oesophagus enters the abdominal cavity through the diaphragm and there it enlarges to form the stomach, a storage organ where some digestion occurs. From here material is propelled along the small intestine, in which three consecutive parts, duodenum, jejunum and ileum, are recognized. The remainder of the tube is the large intestine and consists of the caecum, the colon, the rectum and the anal canal. It has been mentioned that salivary glands add their secretion (saliva) to the contents of the mouth. The pancreas and the liver, two other glands of the digestive system, add their secretions to the contents of the small intestine. Since these glands (salivary, pancreas, liver) are remote from the tube itself, they may be considered as *extrinsic*. Glands in the wall of the digestive tube are *intrinsic* and these, together with individual cells, also pour their secretions into the lumen of the tube. Mucus is produced along the entire length of the digestive system to act as a lubricant and to protect the inner lining. The epithelium of the mucous membrane of the tube is continuous with that of the skin at the lips and at the anus (the opening to the outside of the anal canal). The part of the digestive tube caudal to the pharynx (i.e. from the oesophagus to the anus) may be spoken of as the **alimentary canal.**

Mouth

The **mouth** is supported by the bones of the upper and lower jaws which move mainly in a vertical plane. The bones of the upper jaw form the floor of the nasal chambers and act as the roof of the **mouth cavity**, forming the **hard palate** (Fig. 1.34). The caudal end of the hard palate is continued by the musculo-membranous **soft palate.** This reaches as far as the larynx and in some of the short-headed breeds of dogs (e.g. Bulldogs) it may interfere with normal respiration. The skeleton of the lower jaw consists of the paired mandibles, joined in the midline. **Teeth** are found in the body of each mandible and in the opposing part of the bones of the upper jaw. The line of the teeth in each jaw is called a **dental arch.**

The sides of the jaws are connected by muscles covered on the outside by skin and on the inside by mucous membrane. These form the **cheeks.** The **lips** are also formed by muscle covered by outside skin and inside mucous membrane and it is along the edge of the lips that the epithelium of the skin becomes continuous with that of the mucous membrane. The upper lip has a furrow or **philtrum** dividing the right and left halves.

The entire inside of the mouth cavity is lined by mucous membrane. From the inside of the lips and cheeks it is reflected on to the bones of the upper and lower jaws where it is pierced by the teeth and attaches to the periosteum of the tooth-bearing bones. The reflections of mucous membrane are the **gums** and in the upper jaw it continues on to and attaches tightly to the bones of the hard palate. The mucous membrane of the lower jaw is continuous from the gums over the free surfaces of the tongue.

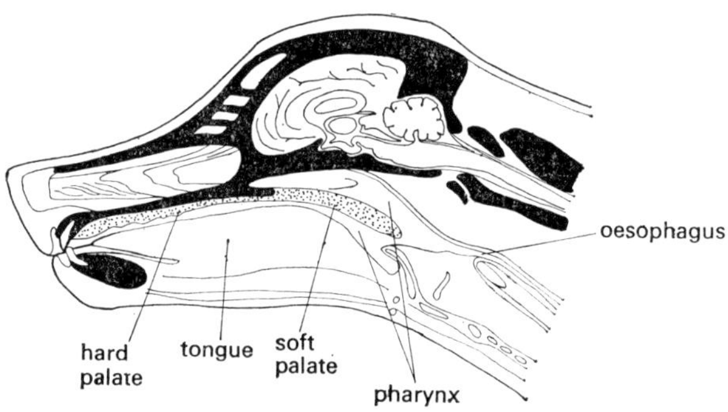

Fig. 1.34. Median section of a dog's head. Solid black represents bone.

Carnivores do not masticate food (i.e. mechanically reduce it in the mouth) very well. It is very rapidly pushed on by the tongue and cheeks into the next part of the system.

Teeth

These hard structures, embedded in the jaws, are used for grinding, tearing and crushing. The sockets in which they fit are called **alveoli.**

The centre of the tooth is the **pulp**, a soft mass of nerves, blood vessels, etc., held together in connective tissue, and this is contained in the **tooth cavity** formed by the immediately surrounding **dentine** (Fig. 1.35). This resembles bone but is much harder. The part of the tooth buried in the jaw is the **root**; some teeth may have two or even three roots. Here the dentine is covered by **cement**, a tissue that resembles bone but is softer than dentine. The part of the tooth projecting out of the jaw is the **crown.** It consists of the dentine covered by a cap of **enamel**; this is extremely hard tissue.

The surface which comes in contact with a tooth of the opposite jaw is its **masticatory surface** (grinding surface, or table).

According to their positions, four types of teeth are recognized. **Incisor** teeth are found at the opening of the mouth, and are used for tearing and cutting food. Caudal to these there is a **canine** tooth on each side in the upper and lower jaws. Continuing along the dental arch, the next teeth are the **pre-molars**. These and the yet more caudal **molars** may together be known as the *cheek teeth*, whose main function is grinding food.

The dog and cat have two consecutive sets of many of these teeth. The first set are called **deciduous** or milk teeth. Although not showing at birth (i.e. not erupted)

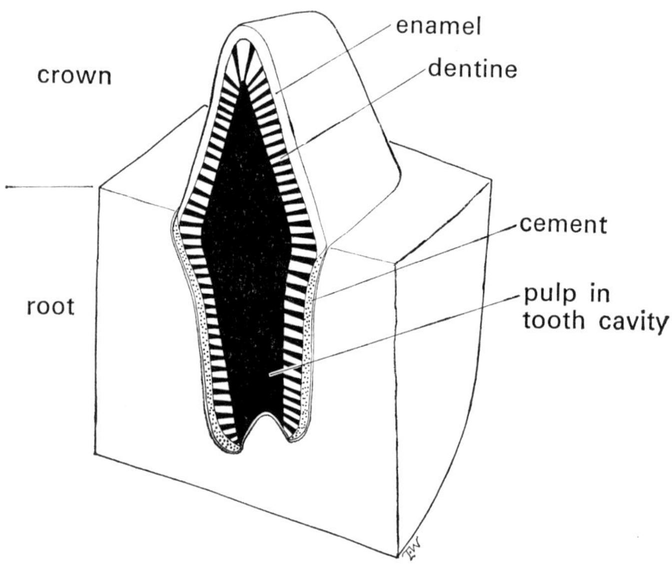

Fig. 1.35. Diagrammatic section of a tooth in an alveolus.

they are usually all functional by 1 to 2 months. In this dentition the puppy has on each side three incisors, one canine and three pre-molars in the upper jaw and the same arrangement in the lower jaw (Fig. 1.36). This information can be written as a dental formula as follows:

$$I\,\tfrac{3}{3}\quad C\,\tfrac{1}{1}\quad PM\,\tfrac{3}{3}\quad \text{(total, both sides upper and lower jaws, 28).}$$

The dental formula for the deciduous dentition of the kitten is:

$$I\,\tfrac{3}{3}\quad C\,\tfrac{1}{1}\quad PM\,\tfrac{3}{2}\quad \text{(total 26).}$$

The deciduous teeth drop out and are replaced by permanent ones. Molar teeth appear in this dentition and in the dog there is an additional pre-molar. This replacement starts at approximately four months in the dog and cat.

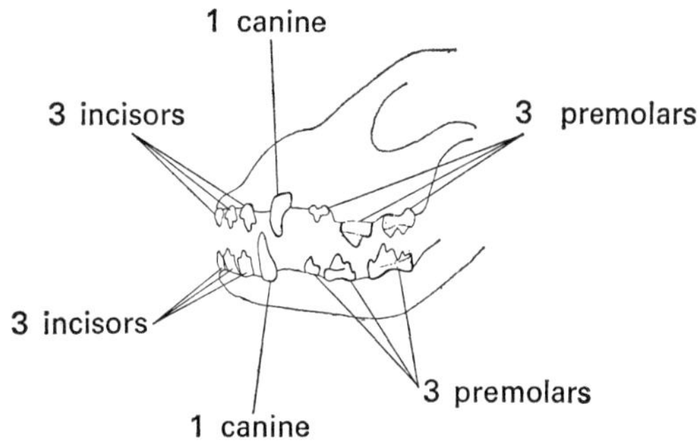

Fig. 1.36. Skull of a puppy to show deciduous teeth.

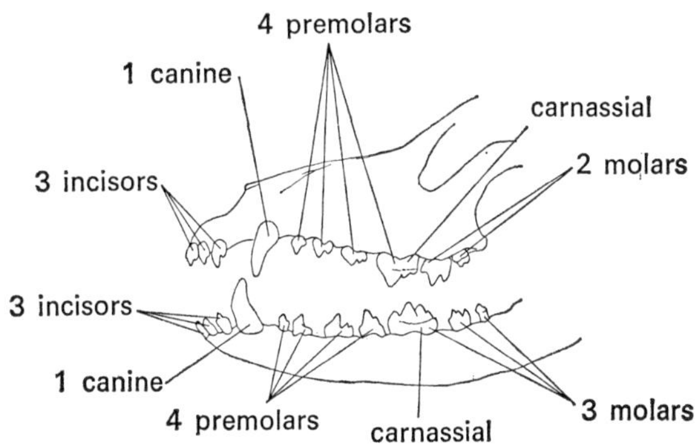

Fig. 1.37. Skull of an adult dog to show permanent dentition.

The dental formula for the permanent dentition of the dog is:

$$\mathrm{I}\,\tfrac{3}{3}\quad \mathrm{C}\,\tfrac{1}{1}\quad \mathrm{PM}\,\tfrac{4}{4}\quad \mathrm{M}\,\tfrac{2}{3}\quad \text{(total 42) (Fig. 1.37).}$$

These teeth are larger than deciduous ones. The incisors are slender with single roots. In young dogs the crowns have a central rounded projection flanked by two smaller ones. Depending on the age of the dog and the wear the teeth receive during chewing, these projections may be ground down to various levels. The canine teeth are the longest, with a curved single root almost twice as long as the cone-shaped crown. There are four pre-molar teeth in the upper and in the lower jaw. The first one is quite simple and has only one root. The masticatory surface of the other cheek teeth have two to four rounded cones called **tubercles** or **cusps.** The fourth pre-molar in the upper jaw is massive. It is called the **carnassial** tooth of the upper jaw and is especially important in cutting tough material. This tooth is very firmly fixed and, like the molars in the upper jaw, has three diverging roots. None of the lower jaw pre-molars or molars has more than two roots. The first molar is the carnassial of the lower jaw; it is about twice as large as the second and third put together. A dog will turn its head to one side in tackling hard food so that the carnassial teeth are brought into use.

The formula for the permanent dentition of the cat is:

$$I\,\tfrac{3}{3}\quad C\,\tfrac{1}{1}\quad PM\,\tfrac{3}{2}\quad M\,\tfrac{1}{1}\quad \text{(total 30) (Fig. 1.38).}$$

The incisors and canines resemble those of the dog, but are, of course, much smaller. In the upper jaw the pre-molars increase in size caudally; the third is the largest tooth in the mouth and is the only one with three roots. In the lower jaw the molar is the largest tooth. These cheek teeth resemble those of the dog in having a tuberculate (i.e. rounded cusps) arrangement of their masticatory surfaces. The significance of the number of roots lies in the difficulty they cause in tooth extraction.

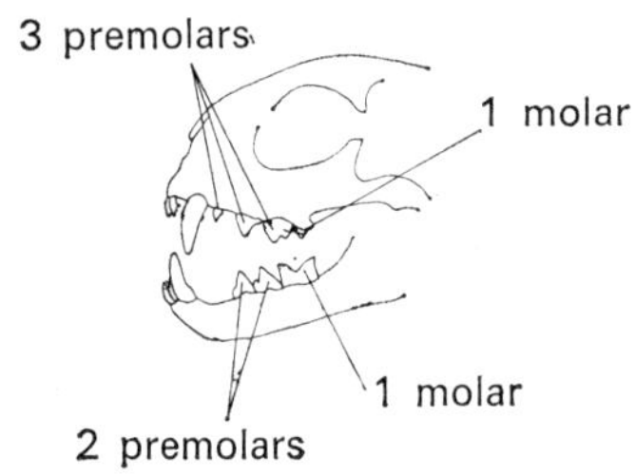

Fig. 1.38. Skull of an adult cat to show permanent dentition.

Tongue

The tongue lies on the floor of the mouth and is mainly a mass of striated muscle fibres, some of which take origin from the hyoid apparatus and from the mandibles. The caudal part is firmly attached to the local skeleton and is called the **root** of the tongue. It is continuous with the larynx and if it is necessary to pass an instrument through the glottis, pulling the tongue brings the epiglottis and other laryngeal structures nearer to the lips (Fig. 1.34). The oral end of the tongue is unattached and able to be moved over an extensive area, sometimes making quite delicate movements. It is made into a ladle-shape when the dog and cat lap up fluids. Most of the mucous membrane is arranged in a multitude of small projections called **lingual papillae**; some have **taste buds** associated with them containing special nerve endings. The papillae help the tongue to control the food during its treatment in the mouth and the rough surface they provide is also useful for grooming. The mucous membrane is well supplied with nerve fibres which convey general information as well as data about the taste of the material in the mouth. A large vein is very prominent on either side of the underneath surface of the tongue. It is especially useful for intravenous (into the vein) injections in the anaesthetized animal.

Salivary Glands

There are several paired glandular areas which produce saliva. The largest are the zygomatic, sublingual, mandibular and parotid glands and these have several ducts opening into the mouth.

The sight of food and also other signs associated with its preparation start salivary secretion. It is increased when food is in the mouth. Saliva is about 99% water and this moisture makes food easier to masticate and swallow. Since it does not stay long in the mouth, the food does not undergo any significant chemical change there.

Pharynx

This chamber is common to the digestive and respiratory systems (Fig. 1.34). The pharyngeal wall is muscular and its mucous membrane lining is continuous with that of all the tubes which enter and leave. There are many diffuse lymphoid areas in the mucous membrane of the pharynx, forming an almost complete ring round the entrances. These areas are called **tonsils**; the palatine tonsils, however, are distinct lymph nodes, one on each side of the pharynx, usually hidden in a small recess. When enlarged and inflamed as in tonsilitis, they are more obvious and can be very painful.

Food is pushed by the tongue to the back of the mouth and into the oral part of the pharynx; from here the pharyngeal muscles propel it to the oesophagus. This is *swallowing* or *deglutition* and while food is in the pharynx the glottis is closed to stop food entering the respiratory system.

Oesophagus

The oesophagus is a simple tube leading from the pharynx and in its passage along the neck it is closely related to the dorsal surface of the trachea and slightly on its left side (Fig. 1.39). In the mediastinum it is still related to the trachea as far as the bifurcation and it then continues caudally to pass into the abdominal cavity through a special foramen in the diaphragm. The mucous membrane lining the tube is surrounded by a loose submucous coat: this allows the mucosa to be arranged in many longitudinal folds that become smoothed out when the oesophagus undergoes distension.

Outside the submucosa there is a muscular coat consisting of layers of striated muscle fibres. The connective tissue that surrounds the oesophagus is usually called its **adventitial coat** and this will blend with local fascia.

Food is passed along the oesophagus by **peristalsis;** this is a circular constriction of the tube by its muscle coats which moves toward the distal end of the digestive system.

Stomach

The junction of the oesophagus and stomach is the **cardia.** The exit from the stomach into the small intestine is at the **pyloric opening** or **pylorus.** The simple tube shape is distorted by a much greater lengthening of one side (Fig. 1.39). It can adapt itself to the quantity of food and between meals it may be almost empty. Gastric digestion occurs here, and it also acts as a reservoir for the food. Nevertheless, it is not essential to life and animals that have had it removed may live apparently normally.

The glands of the mucous membrane of the stomach produce gastric juice in which are found mucus, hydrochloric acid and several enzymes used in splitting proteins and lipids. The protein-splitting enzymes need the acid environment to be able to work. Food has not normally been simplified sufficiently for absorption to occur in the stomach. The fluid or semi-fluid mixture leaving the stomach is called **chyme** (pronounced *kime*).

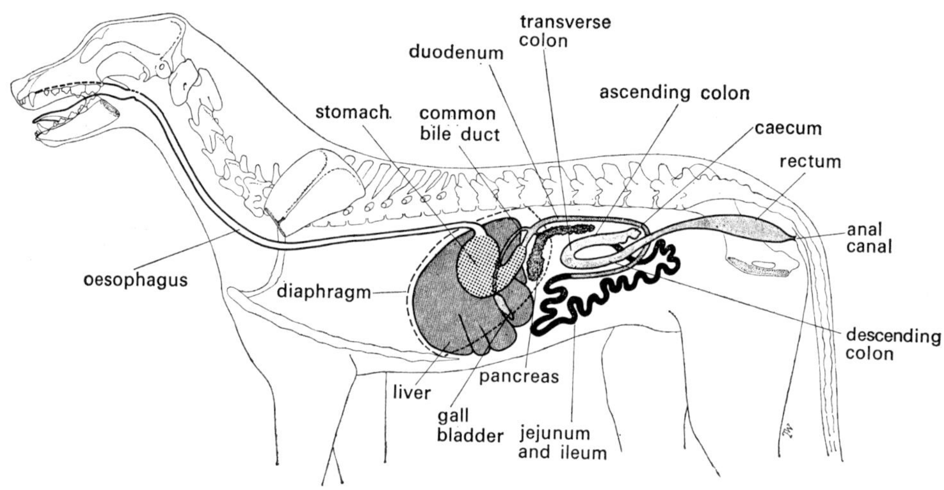

Fig.1.39. Diagram of digestive system of a dog: the intestine is longer and more coiled than shown here.

The submucous coat consists of loose connective tissue and allows movement of the mucous membrane. The muscular coat has at least two layers of smooth muscle fibres. At the cardiac and the pyloric openings, the smooth muscle layers tend to be arranged as sphincters; the pyloric sphincter is quite strong. The stomach wall is moved by its muscle layers to mix the food with the gastric juice and to pass it on to the small intestine. The movements are rhythmic segmentations which chop the food at different places by isolated constrictions and also peristalsis similar to that described for the oesophagus.

Peristaltic waves also occur in an empty stomach. These are hunger contractions and seem to be linked with a low level of glucose in the blood. (Thirst, however, appears to be more closely connected with a dehydration of the mucous membrane of the mouth and throat.) In antiperistalsis, the waves of contraction pass toward the head. This occurs in vomiting, the act of ejecting stomach contents through the oesophagus and mouth. The pylorus closes, the cardia opens and the abdominal muscles contract to press the stomach against the diaphragm and force its evacuation. Some drugs called **emetics** can cause this automatic act, which may be necessary to rapidly remove swallowed poisons.

Small Intestine

This is a long and relatively narrow tube and is the chief site of absorption. The peritoneal covering which forms the serosa is attached to the dorsal abdominal wall, the connection being called **mesentery**. Blood and lymph vessels and also nerves use the mesentery to reach and leave the intestine. For most of the intestine the mesentery is quite long and allows it to form numerous coils (Fig. 1.39). The first part of the small intestine, however, is close to the roof of the abdominal cavity; it has only a

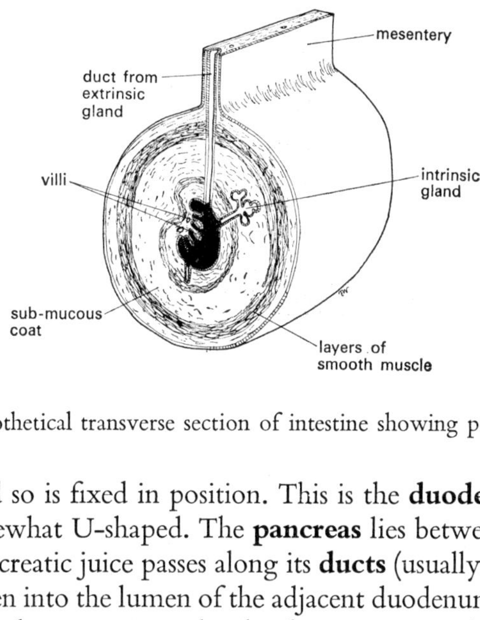

Fig. 1.40. Hypothetical transverse section of intestine showing possible structures.

short mesentery and so is fixed in position. This is the **duodenum** and the general arrangement is somewhat U-shaped. The **pancreas** lies between the limbs of the U and the secreted pancreatic juice passes along its **ducts** (usually two, but occasionally only one) which open into the lumen of the adjacent duodenum. The **common bile duct** from the liver also opens into the duodenum a very short distance from the pylorus and closely related to the pancreatic duct openings. Immediately following the duodenum, the rest of the small intestine is attached by the relatively long mesentery. These parts are the **jejunum** and **ileum.**

The mucous membrane of the small intestine is arranged in numerous fine projections called **villi** (singular, *villus*) which greatly increase the surface area available for absorption (Fig. 1.40). There is also a profusion of glands whose secretion is called *intestinal juice* (*succus entericus*). Areas of lymphoid tissue are freely distributed in the intestinal mucous membrane. The submucous coat is surrounded by two layers of smooth muscle, one encircling the tube, the other running longitudinally. The ileum, the terminal part of the small intestine, joins the large intestine. Pancreatic juice, intestinal juice and bile all combine with the chyme in the small intestine. The wall of this part of the digestive system undergoes peristalsis and rhythmic segmentation movements to ensure that food is moved from place to place, that it is brought close to the absorptive surfaces and that it undergoes a thorough mixing. Pancreatic and intestinal juices contain many enzymes used to split proteins, lipids and carbohydrates into simpler absorbable compounds. Bile supplies *bile salts* which are essential to get the fat and other lipids into a form suitable for the specific enzymes in pancreatic juice. If bile is not present, digestion of fat is markedly reduced and it can appear unchanged in the faeces. A similar result will occur if pancreatic juice is absent or deficient. Bile is also used to excrete waste products of blood pigment breakdown and these are the main cause of the colour of faeces.

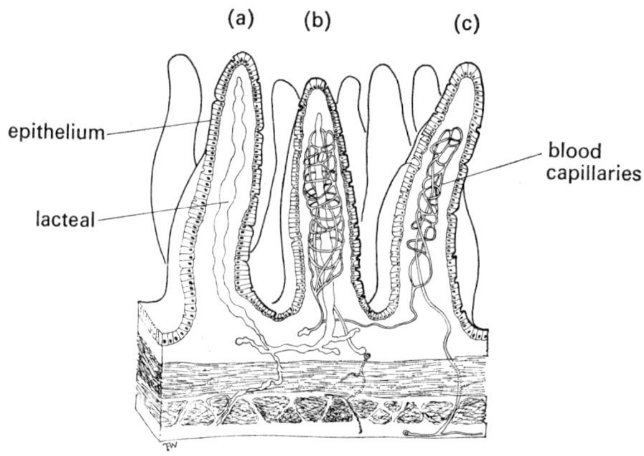

Fig. 1.41. Arrangement of intestinal villi (highly magnified): (a) shows central lacteal, (b) lacteal and blood-vascular system, (c) blood-vascular system only.

Absorption by the small intestine is facilitated by the villi. These projections have a large lymph capillary, called a **lacteal,** in their centre and this drains into lymph vessels in the wall of the intestine (Fig. 1.41). From here the lymph passes into mesenteric lymph vessels to mesenteric lymph nodes and then into a collecting chamber called the **cisterna chyli** in the roof of the abdominal cavity.

Chyle (pronounced kile) is the name often given to lymph from the wall of the intestines. Lymph leaves the cisterna chyli in the thoracic duct, a vessel that runs through the thorax to open into the large veins near the cranial thoracic aperture.

There is a plexus of blood capillaries around each lacteal and these together with other vessels of the intestine unite to form the venules and veins which join to become the **portal vein.** This enters the liver where the blood is discharged to circulate round the liver cells.

The surface of each villus is covered by the epithelial lining of the intestine. The villi are continually waving about, shortening and lengthening, either singly or in groups. Inorganic compounds and the simplified products of protein and carbohydrate digestion are absorbed through the intestinal surface and are mainly carried to the liver by the blood in the portal system. The fatty acids resulting from lipid breakdown and also very finely divided fat globules are absorbed into the lacteals of the villi. This causes the lymph in the mesenteric vessels (chyle) to appear milky-white. It passes eventually into the venous system.

Large Intestine

Most of the large intestine has a greater diameter than the small intestine. The arrangement of this region of the digestive tube is **caecum, ascending colon, transverse colon, descending colon, rectum, anal canal** (Fig. 1.39). There are no villi in the large intestine. Its main function is to absorb water from what is left of the foodstuffs and the secretions that have been added earlier in the system. There is practically no absorption of organic compounds. Mucus is secreted by the glands of the mucous membrane and bacteria flourish in this part of the gut. They split up some of the protein which is still present and the resulting products are responsible for the odour of faeces. The contents are passed on by intestinal movements caused by the muscle layers surrounding the submucosa.

The caecum is a short blind-ending sac. The ileum joins the large intestine at the junction of the caecum and ascending colon. The latter is on the right side of the abdominal cavity closely applied to its roof. The transverse colon crosses the more cranial part of the abdominal cavity and the descending colon is on the left side.

The rectum is that part of the large intestine between the cranial aperture of the pelvis and the anal canal. The region immediately continuous with the descending colon is covered by peritoneum. More caudally the limit of the peritoneal cavity is reached and so this part of the rectum is covered by fascia and connecting extrinsic muscles.

The terminal piece of the large intestine, the anal canal, is a very short length of the digestive tube that is usually closed by the action of sphincter muscles. One sphincter results from a thickening of the circular smooth muscle fibres. Around this, extrinsic striated muscles also form a sphincter, attached in part to the local skeleton. The continuation of the epithelium of the mucous membrane and that of the skin occurs at the anus, the terminal external orifice of the digestive system.

The anal sacs (para-anal sinuses) which occur at this junction are described with the cutaneous glands of the integument.

The act of passing faeces to the outside is defaecation. As the rectum fills, sensory nerve impulses pass to the spinal cord from which motor impulses are sent to relax the internal smooth muscle sphincter. However, the external sphincter is under voluntary control and is opened only when the animal decides the time and place are appropriate.

Pancreas

This organ consists of glandular tissue found in the loop of the duodenum near the roof of the abdominal cavity (Fig. 1.39). The exocrine part of it is responsible for providing pancreatic juice which passes into the duodenum via one or, more usually, two ducts. Embedded in the exocrine tissue are small islands of endocrine tissue which produce the hormone *insulin*. The secretions of this tissue are passed into the blood stream.

Liver

The liver is a large, rather flattened, gland which fits into the concavity of the abdominal side of the diaphragm (Fig. 1.39). It is divided into several lobes, which are separated peripherally.

One of the many functions of the liver cells is to produce *bile*. This is collected into small tubes, the *bile ducts*, of increasing order of size that join with one another until one main **common hepatic duct** is formed (hepatic is an adjective used in phrases referring to the liver). This joins the **cystic duct** of the **gall bladder**. The common bile duct results from this union and enters the duodenum a short distance from the pylorus. Bile is stored and concentrated in the gall bladder.

The liver has many functions other than the production of bile. Nearly all the blood which has circulated around the abdominal part of the digestive tube passes immediately to the liver in the portal vein where it comes into intimate contact with the liver cells. Much of the foodstuff that has been absorbed from the alimentary tract into the blood stream is transferred to the cells whose function is to store it and, in some cases, begin its metabolism.

Urogenital System

The urogenital system consists of the **urinary system** and the **genital system.** The urinary system is responsible for removing waste products and excess water as **urine.** The genital system includes the organs, called **gonads,** which produce the cells used in procreation. Those of the male are the **testes** and produce **sperms** whereas the gonads of the female are **ovaries** and produce **ova.** The system also includes the means whereby the male and female products can unite and in the female provides an environment in which the resultant organism can develop properly.

For part of their course, the urinary and genital systems have common use for certain structures. In the male the products of the genital system are poured into the terminal part of the urinary system and the urethra is used as a common tube to the outside. The products of the urinary system of the female use the terminal part of the genital system and here the vestibule and vulva are the shared parts of the urogenital apparatus.

The urinary system will be described first. In the case of the male this includes the complete tract that conveys the urine to the outside of the body; the description of the female urinary system will finish where it joins the reproductive tract. The male genitalia will then be described as far as its junction with the urinary system. The description of the female genitalia includes all parts of the tract.

URINARY SYSTEM

The urinary system is responsible for removing a lot of the excess water and several waste products from the body. These are brought in the blood stream to the left and right **kidneys** and in these organs they are passed into the thousands of small blind-ending **renal tubules** (sometimes called nephrons). There are in the region of half a million in each kidney of a dog. ("Renal" is an adjective used in phrases referring to the kidney.) The tubules unite and eventually one tube, the **ureter,** leaves each kidney to transport urine (the material to be excreted) to the single **bladder** (Fig. 1.42). From here the fluid is voided at intervals to the outside through the **urethra.**

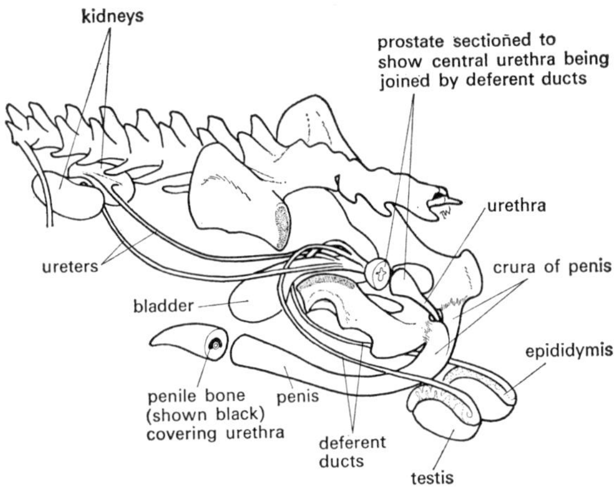

Fig. 1.42. Urogenital system of male dog.

Kidney

One kidney is found on each side of the midline ventral to the lumbar vertebrae. They lie in the abdominal cavity where they are related to the large blood vessels, the aorta and the caudal vena cava. The kidneys are between the parietal peritoneum and the roof of the abdominal cavity. The organ itself is invested in a strong **fibrous capsule** of dense connective tissue which can be stripped easily from the healthy organ.

The blind end of each renal tubule is the **glomerular capsule** and this is invaginated by a knot of capillaries known as a **glomerulus** (Fig. 1.43). Material to be excreted is filtered from the blood through the wall of the capillary and through the capsule lining. The pressure of blood in the capillaries is high and causes continual passage of filtrate. Control of local blood pressure can affect urine flow; if it falls, for example due to haemorrhage, then less urine will be passed. The volume of blood and extracellular fluid will not suffer further reduction via the kidneys until blood pressure is restored to normal level.

As the filtrate passes along the remainder of the renal tubule, water and other required substances are absorbed back through the tubule wall into the network of surrounding capillaries. There is a definite control on the amount of each that is reabsorbed from the filtrate; some substances are completely readmitted whereas very little is taken back of an unwanted compound, such as urea. As well as absorbing needed material, the walls of the tubules do empty some excretions directly into the fluid. As little as 1% of glomerular filtrate may end up as urine. The tubules empty into **collecting ducts** and these amalgamate to form eventually a few large **papillary ducts** which open into a collecting area called the **pelvis.** (This is not related to the skeletal pelvis, both names are derived from the Latin word for a basin.)

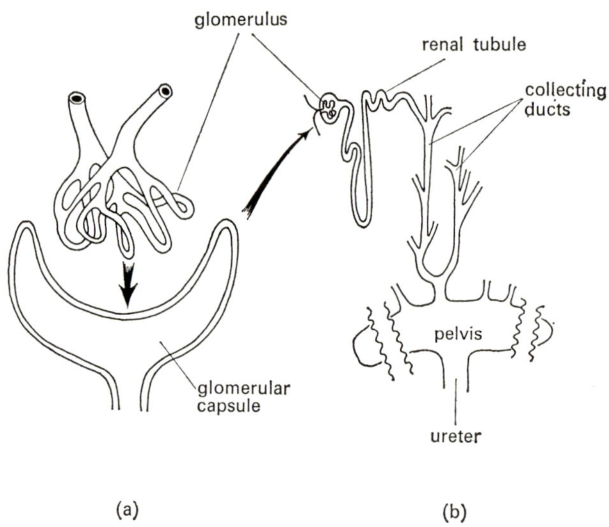

Fig. 1.43. Diagrams of arrangements of renal tubules: (a) glomerular capsule (very highly magnified with glomerulus removed; (b) remainder of tubule and connection with renal pelvis.

The pelvis, the renal blood and lymph vessels, and the nerves may be surrounded by fat and are situated in the cavity of the kidney called its **sinus.** This opens on the medial edge of the kidney at the **hilus.** The renal blood vessels and nerves pass through the hilus and here also the renal pelvis narrows rapidly to be continued to the bladder by the ureter.

Ureters

This pair of tubes conveys the urine from the kidneys to the bladder by peristalsis. They are each suspended in a peritoneal fold and consist of a lining mucous membrane surrounded by a coat of smooth muscle which in turn is covered by an adventitial coat. The ureters enter the neck of the urinary bladder at an angle that ensures that they travel for some distance in its wall (Fig. 1.42). In this way a very effective valve is formed to prevent the return of urine from the bladder into the ureters.

Bladder

The bladder is shaped something like a pear, with the more caudal narrower end being the **neck** and the other end the **apex** (or **vertex**). Between these ends is the **body.** The size, shape and position of the organ varies with the quantity of its contents, but ventrally it is usually in contact with the abdominal floor.

The mucosa is attached to the muscular coat by a very elastic submucous layer and forms many folds when the organ is empty. The muscle coat consists of fibres running in all directions, but around the neck the circular fibres form sphincters. Not all of the bladder is covered by peritoneum since the most caudal part (i.e. near the neck) is beyond the level of the peritoneal cavity. The neck of the bladder is continuous with the urethra.

When the bladder is sufficiently full, sensory nerve impulses pass to the nervous system. Motor impulses to the bladder wall cause it to contract and the innermost smooth muscle sphincter to relax. There is, however, an outer voluntary muscle sphincter that only relaxes when the animal finds it convenient.

Urethra of the Female

This is a very short tube which leaves the neck of the bladder and opens into the floor of the vestibule of the female genital tract.

Urethra of the Male

The part of the urethra lying in the pelvis has a small projection into the dorsal side of its lumen and near this there are the duct openings associated with the genital system.

The mucous membrane of the urethra is surrounded by a layer of cavernous erectile tissue. This consists of connective tissue divisions and trabeculae which condense peripherally to form a limiting layer. The spaces ("caverns") between the trabeculae are lined with endothelium and usually filled with blood. When the passages by which the blood leaves are markedly narrowed, the local pressure rises and the tissues become engorged. The turgid organs may then stiffen and in some cases become erect; for this reason the descriptive term of erectile tissue is used for those situations where such vascular engorgement is possible.

As the urethra surrounded by its erectile tissue and muscle coats leaves the pelvis it is joined by more erectile tissue, and the whole mass forms the **penis.** The urethra runs the entire length and opens at the end of this organ.

Penis

The attachment to the ischium of each side is by fibrous connective tissue and is called a **crus.** These crura (plural of *crus*) contain erectile tissue and come together uniting in the midline forming the root of the penis. Here they are joined by the urethra with its erectile coat to complete the penis.

At the free end is the **glans** of the penis and in the male cat (the tom-cat) its surface is covered by tiny curved papillae which are hard and sharp (Fig. 1.44). The penis of the tom points caudally and the urethra with its surrounding layers lies on the dorsal aspect. Ventral to this the erectile tissue of the remainder of the penis becomes partly replaced in the glans by bone (cartilage in the young cat) which stiffens the organ even when it is not engorged.

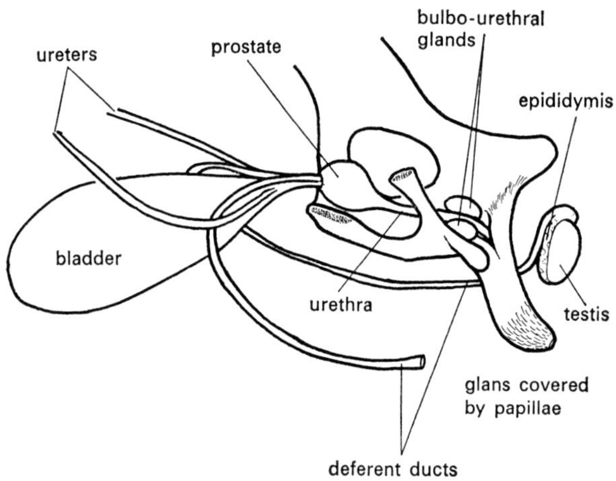

Fig. 1.44. Genital system of tom (male) cat. (The left testis has been removed.)

The penis of the dog curves cranio-ventrally at its root turning to point between the thighs. The urethra will therefore be on the ventral side. There are no papillae on the glans but there is a well-developed **penile bone** (or **os penis**) which in the dog lies dorsal and on each side of the urethra which is thus in a bony tunnel. Although the dog and cat are the only domestic mammals in which this penile bone is found, it occurs in a large number of other mammals.

The function of the cavernous erectile tissue is to stiffen the penis for insertion during copulation; it has no special use during urination.

The entire relaxed organ lies within a sheath of skin called the **prepuce.** The epithelium of the skin is continuous with that inside the prepuce. From here it is reflected on to the end of the penis and becomes continuous with the epithelium of the mucous membrane of the urethra where that tube opens to the outside.

GENITAL SYSTEM OF THE MALE

This system is responsible for producing the cells that will fertilize the ova of the female and also a suitable fluid medium for their transport and maintenance. It is another visceral system that consists of several tubes joining together to have eventually only one opening to the outside. The many blind-ending tubes are **seminiferous tubules** and into their cavities are shed the sperms which are the fertilizing cells (Fig. 1.45). These tubules are all in the paired **testes** and they collect together to form eventually the **deferent duct** (**ductus deferens**). This pair of tubes open into the urethra near the neck of the bladder and the sperms use the urethra to reach the outside of the body of the male. Accessory glands add their secretions so that sperms are part of the fluid mixture called **semen.** This is ejaculated during sexual union via the temporarily stiffened penis which has been inserted into the female genital system.

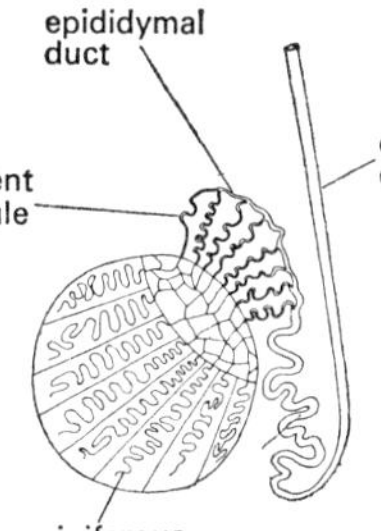

Fig. 1.45. Section of testis: there are very many more seminiferous tubules than are shown here.

The testes are surgically removed if the animal is not to be allowed to breed. It is then said to have been **neutered** or **castrated** as opposed to the unoperated animal which is called an **entire.** The erectile tissues of the penis do not develop fully if the animal has been castrated when young. There are several more of these features called **secondary sexual characteristics** which are also affected by early castration.

Testes

The walls of the seminiferous tubules consist of two types of cells: those from which the sperms are produced and those which produce fluid that is thought to be nutritive. The production of sperms is **spermatogenesis** and this involves a special method of division of nuclear material.

In the multiplication of body cells that is described as mitosis, the chromosomes are arranged as pairs of chromatids. These separate and an equal identical amount of this nuclear material goes to each of the resulting cells. The chromosomes control the morphology and functioning of the cell and every cell (except those becoming sperms and ova) in every animal *of the same species* has the same number of chromosomes. This is the species number. When fertilization occurs, i.e. the union of cells from the male and female, this would result in there being double the number of chromosomes unless at some stage in the development of the sex cells there was an alteration to the cell reproduction pattern; in fact, a reduction division.

The species number of chromosomes is always even. They can be arranged in pairs which are similar but not identical and this is what happens prior to the reduction division. One chromosome of each pair then goes to the two resulting cells; they will therefore have half the number of chromosomes. This means that the nuclear material is distributed to the two cells and in the shareout they will receive different chromosomes. A similar condition takes place in the production of ova, consequently the total chromosome count after fertilisation will still be the species number but only half of the inherited characteristics will have come from each parent. This division of nuclear material is unique to the sex cells and is said to be **meiotic** to distinguish it from the usual mitosis.

The sperm-producing cells multiply mainly by mitosis but some of those that result do not continue in this way. These enlarge considerably and are the ones that will undergo meiotic division and become **spermatids.** Multiplication for them then ceases and by a series of modifications including the formation of a tail, the spermatids become transformed into sperms. At this stage they detach from the sperm-producing wall of the seminiferous tubules and, carrying only half the species number of chromosomes, they are released into its lumen.

The tubules form a network of channels through which the sperms pass. They can then leave the testis by several **efferent ductules** which unite to form one **epididymal duct (ductus epididymis)** outside the testis.

Epididymis

The sperms are stored and mature in the ductus epididymis which slowly transports them away from the testis. This is very long but by close coiling it forms **lobules** which are attached to the long border of the testis, and it is then usually referred to as the **epididymis** (Figs. 1.42, 1.44). The epididymal duct is continued by the **deferent duct (ductus deferens)**.

Deferent Duct

Each one of this pair of tubes connects the epididymis to the urethra. At its termination the wall thickens and becomes very glandular; the secretion of the glands is poured directly into the lumen of the duct. The opening of each tube into the urethra occurs near the junction of the urethra and the bladder.

Accessory Genital Glands

These structures add their secretions to the semen, producing, in fact, most of its volume. The only accessory genital gland in the dog is the **prostate** (Fig. 1.42). The cat has, in addition, a pair of **bulbo-urethral** glands (Fig. 1.44). The prostate of the dog surrounds the urethra near the neck of the bladder; in the cat the gland is further caudal. It has several openings into the urethra and the deferent ducts pass through its substance to open near by. The prostate normally lies on the floor of the pelvis and may, when pathological, enlarge to almost fill the pelvic cavity. A gland in such a state can severely interfere with defaecation by pressure on the rectum.

In the cat the bulbo-urethral glands flank the urethra caudal to the prostrate, lying just cranial to the ischial arch.

Scrotum

The testes of the adult domestic mammals are contained in a diverticulum of the abdominal cavity called the **scrotum,** which in the cat is ventral to the anus near the ischiatic symphysis. The scrotum of the dog lies between the thighs. Smooth muscle tissue and collagenous and elastic fibres form a **septum** between the right and left halves of the scrotum and each of the pouches which are thus formed contains a testis.

Each testis is surrounded by a diverticulum of peritoneum which is called the vaginal tunic or coat (**tunica vaginalis**) as it leaves the main abdominal cavity. The deferent duct, the nerves, the blood vessels and the lymphatic vessels which are connected with the testis are also covered by the vaginal coat. These structures which pass to and from the testis, and the layer of tunica vaginalis which covers them, constitute the **spermatic cord.**

Each cord runs between the abdominal cavity and the pouch of the scrotum in a passage called the **inguinal canal.** The abdominal opening of the canal is called the **deep inguinal ring;** the other end is a slit in an abdominal muscle and is called the **superficial inguinal ring.**

The diverticulum of peritoneum remains open throughout life, and omentum or intestine may occasionally slip down it into the scrotum. This condition is called a **scrotal hernia.** A similar condition called an **inguinal hernia** occurs if the abdominal contents protrude through the inguinal canal outside, but along with, the tunica vaginalis.

GENITAL SYSTEM OF THE FEMALE

The organs of this system produce the female sex cells (ova) and provide situations in which these can be fertilized and develop during *pregnancy*. This is the period, also known as *gestation*, between the fertilization of the ova and *parturition* (the act of birth). The genital system is also arranged to receive the penis during copulation.

The time of year at which sexual union normally takes place is the *breeding season*. The bitch has two seasons in the year and during this time there is a period of sexual activity on the part of the female known as *oestrus* or *heat*. The cat has two or three seasons in the year and during each of these oestrus occurs several times. The release of ova (*ovulation*) is closely related to oestrus and the rhythmical changes undergone by the female genital system at this time constitute the *oestrous cycle*. It is unusual for signs of oestrus to appear during pregnancy.

The ova are produced by paired **ovaries** and pass into the open ends of **uterine tubes** (one of which is associated with each ovary) (Fig. 1.46). These continue into the **uterus.** If the ovum is fertilized by a sperm it becomes an **embryo** and develops in the lumen of the uterus; this undergoes marked changes during pregnancy. The uterus of a pregnant animal is said to be *gravid*. When the animal is pregnant for the first time it is *primigravid;* during later pregnancies the animal is *multigravid*. When several young are developing in the one uterus as in the dog and cat, the animal is *multiparous.*

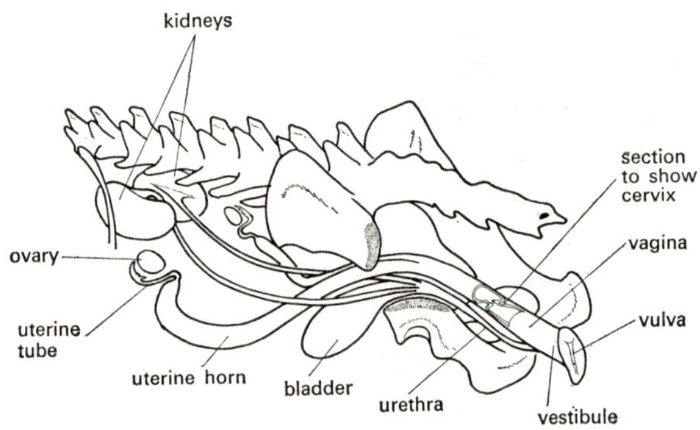

Fig. 1.46. Urogenital system of bitch.

The caudal end of the uterus is modified to form the **cervix,** through which the cavity of the female genital system continues into the **vagina.** Caudal to this the **vestibule** continues into the **vulva** consisting of a pair of lips through which the female genital system opens to the outside.

The surgical removal of ovaries to prevent breeding is **ovariectomy.** If the uterus is also removed, the operation is **ovario-hysterectomy,** more commonly called **spaying.**

Ovary (Fig. 1.47)

Each ovary consists of a framework of connective tissue which condenses peripherally. A layer of epithelial cells attached to its outer surface is continuous with the epithelium of the peritoneum. As it leaves the ovary to attach to the wall of the abdominal cavity the peritoneum is called the **mesovarium.** This helps form a pouch (**ovarian bursa**) which in the bitch completely encloses the ovary, hiding it from view even when the rest of the tract is exposed.

In the very young animal, cells in the ovary group together to form **follicles** and eventually **follicular fluid** is formed within the cluster. Some of the inner cells of the follicles give rise to the ova (eggs). Their formation resembles that of sperms in that meiosis occurs and the hereditary material is distributed evenly but not identically to the two cells resulting from the reduction division. It differs from spermatogenesis since the stored food material of the original cell is not equally shared but all goes to one which then continues to develop. The other is allowed to degenerate although it has half the original chromosomal material. The developing cell undergoes a mitotic division but again all the food material goes to one and the other yet once more degenerates. As a result a few comparatively large ova are formed whereas many small sperms are produced by the male.

The follicles move slowly towards the surface of the ovary while these events are beginning. At some physiologically opportune moment the outer surface of the follicles rupture, expelling the follicular fluid and the mature ova. This phenomenon is ovulation and in the dog and cat several ova are released at the same time. Adult ovaries will usually show follicles at all stages of development and at varying depths from the surface.

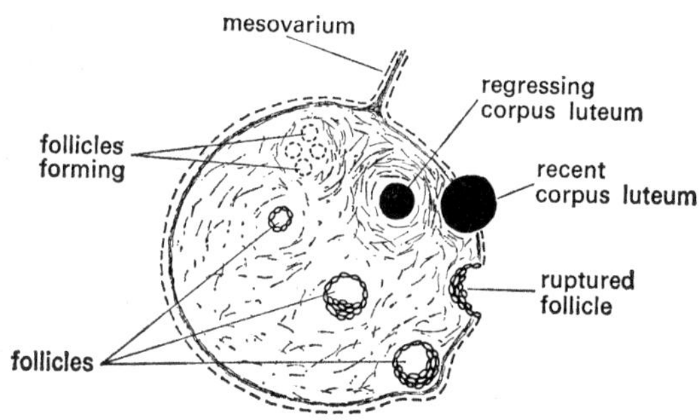

Fig. 1.47. Diagram of ovary.

Some bleeding into the ruptured follicle occurs after ovulation. The blood clot that forms is gradually resorbed and replaced by cells which grow in with their products from the wall of the ruptured follicle. This structure is called a **corpus luteum**. Each ruptured follicle is succeeded by a corpus luteum which then undergoes a slow diminution in size. However, if the ova liberated by the ruptured follicles are fertilized and so the animal becomes pregnant, the regression of the corpora lutea (plural of corpus luteum) is delayed.

Adult ovaries, then, may show not only follicles at all stages of development and at varying depths from the surface, but also corpora lutea at different levels of maturity and degeneration.

Uterine Tube (Fig. 1.46)

The ova are expelled from the ovary into the peritoneal cavity. However, the open end of a uterine tube (also called a Fallopian tube) is very close to the ovary and the ova are passed along this and into the uterus. The ovarian end of the tube flares out and may be split into irregular processes called **fimbriae.** The uterine end of the tube opens into the uterus.

It is in the uterine tubes that the sperms usually fertilize the ova. A large number of sperms surround the small number of ova and eventually a single sperm penetrates into each egg. This seems to affect the surface of the ovum so that no more sperms can then enter. The nuclear material contained in the sperm begins to separate out and so does that of the female. The sperm has also provided a centrosome apparatus and this develops into a spindle exactly as in ordinary mitotic divisions. The chromosomes from the male and the female arrange themselves on the spindle and mitotic division starts the ever-increasing production of cells that will constitute the new animal.

Uterus (Fig. 1.46)

The entire uterus is somewhat Y-shaped with a pair of **uterine horns** joining to form a single **uterine body.** Each horn is about five times the length of the body. The uterus undergoes tremendous changes in shape and position during pregnancy and afterwards it never completely returns to its non-gravid morphology. It lies usually in the abdominal cavity but in the young animal some of it may be in the pelvis.

In structure it resembles other parts of a visceral system. The mucous membrane forming the inner layer is called the **endometrium** and the muscle layer the **myometrium.**

Probably the most important function of the uterus is to retain the embryos within the body of the mother and these are distributed in the two horns. As the fertilized ova develop they each produce a group of structures called **foetal membranes**; during the later parts of embryonic life the developing organism may be known as a **foetus.** In addition to providing a container for fluid in which the embryo develops, the foetal membranes form an intimate attachment to the endometrium whilst remaining in complete continuity with the embryo. The foetal membranes have an extensive blood supply and in this way the local blood streams of the mother and of the embryos are brought very close together (**but do not intermingle**) and an exchange of nutrient and waste material can take place between the mother and the offspring. This arrangement of embryonic and maternal tissue constitutes a **placenta,** having a **foetal** and a **uterine** part.

In the dog and cat each placenta forms a broad ring with the inside encircling the foetal membranes. The blood vessels and other attachments to the foetus come together to form the **umbilical cord** which enters its abdominal region; apart from this connection the developing animal floats freely in the foetal fluids. At parturition the foetal membranes are usually expelled shortly after the young; hence the origin of one of their names, *the after-birth.*

The cavity of the body of the uterus connects with that of the vagina through the

cervical canal. The thickened walls reduce the passage and act as a sphincter which relaxes only during oestrus to allow the passage of sperms and during parturition to allow the expulsion of the young. During pregnancy the cervical canal is closed by muscular contraction and by a plug of mucus. The peritoneal suspension of the uterus and ovary is part of the **broad ligament.**

Vagina

The vagina extends from the cervix to the **external urethral orifice,** the opening of the urethra into the floor of the female genital system. The vagina is a highly dilatable part of the tract and lies entirely in the pelvis. Only the cranial part has a peritoneal covering forming its serosa. The caudal part is surrounded by connective tissue called **pelvic fascia.**

Vestibule

The vestibule extends from the vagina to the external opening of the female urogenital system. Since the external urethral orifice is its cranial limit the vestibule is a part that is common to the genital and the urinary systems. Muscle fibres in the wall of this part of the tract form a very strong sphincter mechanism.

Vulva

This vertical slit marks the external opening of the urogenital system and consists of a pair of **lips** which join dorsally and ventrally. A small knob-like structure called the **clitoris** formed partly of cavernous erectile tissue is found just inside the ventral angle of this vulvar cleft.

MATING

The female will only accept the male during oestrus. This occurs first sometime after about 6 months of age. Just prior to every oestrus, the vulva of the bitch becomes swollen and there is a haemorrhagic vulval discharge. Although the male may be attracted he is not allowed to serve (mate). After about a week the discharge is replaced by a clear amber-coloured secretion and the female positively invites **coitus,** the act of sexual union. This stage also lasts for about a week; thereafter the vulva returns to normal size and mating is no longer allowed.

If conditions are favourable, the dog mounts and pushes the penis between the lips of the vulva. Thrusting movements follow and the penis becomes engorged with blood. Semen is being ejaculated into the female at this time. The sphincter muscles around the female vestibule hold the male in position even after ejaculation is complete; this constitutes the **tie** that often (but not always) occurs with dogs. Engorgement of the genitalia will gradually reduce and the animals will then separate.

The cat also becomes sexually mature after about 6 months but the oestrous cycle is different from that of the bitch. During each of the two or three breeding seasons of each year, the cat comes into oestrus about every 2 weeks and stays in this condition for about 3 to 6 days. Inviting postures such as raising the hindquarters and flattening the back accompanied by "calling" usually occur for a day or two before she will accept the tom. Mating can then occur several times a day for the period of oestrus. The mating posture and realignment of the penis (which at other times points caudally) enables the vulva to be entered. Ejaculation is immediate and the animals soon separate.

Sperms move very rapidly and may be found in the uterine tube within half a minute of being deposited near the cervix.

PREGNANCY AND PARTURITION

For the dog and cat, pregnancy is about 9 weeks. After about a month the embryos can be palpated through the abdominal wall like a string of spherical swellings. In the bitch each enlargement is about an inch in diameter and in the cat approximately three-quarters of an inch at that time.

About 2 weeks before parturition the mammary glands begin to get markedly enlarged and this continues to the end of pregnancy. Just before birth they produce a watery secretion and this is then followed by milk.

At parturition the tissues around the pelvis relax and the external genitalia become swollen. Muscular contractions of the uterus ("labour") begin and increase in strength and frequency. Some of the foetal membranes containing foetal fluid are presented at the vulva, forming the so-called water-bag. This bursts and is soon followed by the expulsion of the first of the young, which is usually nuzzled by the mother who licks off any enclosing membranes. The remainder of the afterbirth of that new-born usually follows within minutes and the animal itself soon finds the way to a teat. A repeat performance occurs for each of the young but the intervals at which they appear are extremely irregular.

More details on breeding are given in a later section.

Vascular System

This is an arrangement of tubes for the circulation of fluid. Two parts can be recognized and considered separately, although they are very closely related and are connected. The *blood-vascular system* conveys blood throughout the body; it is sometimes called the cardio-vascular system. ("Cardiac" is an adjective used in phrases referring to the heart.) The *lymph-vascular system* carries lymph and eventually opens into the blood-vascular system. These systems are also described as the circulatory systems; there are, however, other regions which can be said to constitute a circulatory system.

BLOOD-VASCULAR SYSTEM

In the section on connective tissue, blood was described as circulating in a continuous system of tubes called blood vessels. The organ which plays a major role in causing circulation is a mass of muscle associated with a restricted part of this system of tubes; the structure is the **heart.** As blood is carried away from the heart, the vessels split into branches with smaller diameters and thinner walls than the parent vessel. With every branching the total diameter of the resulting vessels increases. At the level at which there is an interchange of fluid between the inside and the outside of the vessels, they are very small in diameter and the walls consist almost entirely of a single layer of epithelial cells constituting the endothelium. At this level they are called **capillaries.** The first parts of the vessels carrying blood from the heart to the capillaries have quite thick walls of smooth muscle and elastic fibres and are called **arteries.** Between these and the capillaries they are known as **arterioles** and have thinner walls and smaller diameters than arteries.

The large arteries form a pattern that is fairly constant in animals of the same species and there are often striking similarities between animals of different species. The arterioles can contract rhythmically and control the flow of blood into the capillaries. In this way the supply to major sections of the body is regulated so that each tissue gets the amount it needs to function properly. Constriction and dilatation of the blood vessels is controlled by the rate of motor nerve impulses to the smooth (involuntary) muscle of their walls. Arteries may unite with one another to form **anastomoses** and the smaller the vessels the more frequently they occur. The anastomosis may be by means of a network called an **arterial plexus.** Because of this arrangement the blockage of one vessel does not necessarily cut off the blood supply to a region; using the anastomotic pathways, a *collateral circulation* is set up.

Capillaries form a complex network in nearly all the organs of the body; on the whole the more active the organ the smaller the spaces between the capillaries forming the strings of the net and the larger its supply of blood. The term *capillary bed* is also used for the network. It is at this level that nutrients and waste products leave or enter the blood. The capillary wall acts as a semi-permeable membrane, being permeable to some, but not all, of the constituents of blood. The part of blood that can diffuse into and out of the lumen is tissue fluid and this is the transfer medium for the nutrients and waste products of the body cells.

Blood passing on from the capillaries returns to the heart through vessels called **venules,** which gradually increase in diameter. Their walls, however, are very thin, the endothelium being supported only by a small amount of collagenous connective tissue. The venules unite to form **veins** and these have a wider lumen and thinner walls than the corresponding arteries. Some veins, especially those in the limbs, have a system of **valves** which open towards the heart and prevent a backflow of blood. Each valve usually consists of a pair of flaps (*cusps*) formed by a fold of the endothelium strengthened by a small amount of connective tissue. When a limb is moved or even when a muscle contracts, the blood in the local veins is compressed. Because of the valves, it is only able to flow towards the heart. Veins, like arteries, anastomose very freely with one another; they may thus form **venous plexuses.**

Some veins are called **sinuses**: for instance, the large vessel which receives smaller veins from the tissues of the heart itself is called a sinus. So also are the veins in the cranial cavity and those in the vertebral canal. It is best, where possible, always to use the term **venous sinuses** for these structures, to distinguish them from other recesses of the body which may be called sinuses (e.g. para-nasal sinuses). The venous side of the blood-vascular system acts as a reservoir for blood, holding it in the plexuses and sinuses as well as in the large veins. If it is required rapidly, the vein walls are constricted and transfer the blood to where it is needed.

Some veins break up into a plexus of capillaries instead of continuing directly into main venous trunks. This is a *portal system* and ensures that material absorbed from one region by the first capillary network can be transferred to another region by the second (portal system) capillary network without having to circulate very far or without being widely distributed. The blood leaves the portal system in venous trunks.

Cavernous erectile tissue consists of connective tissue partitions separating intercommunicating spaces which can be filled with blood. The spaces are lined with endothelium and in some cases will act as capillaries, occurring between arteries and veins; in other cases the cavernous erectile tissue occurs as part of the course of a vein. Engorgement of the spaces with blood causes a stiffening and hardening of the tissue. (Cavernous erectile tissue has been described in the section on the urinary system.)

In some regions of the body the arterioles and venules are in direct communication by **arterio-venous anastomoses.** Blood can thus by-pass the capillary network.

Heart

This can be considered in effect as a localized increase in the muscle layer surrounding the endothelial lining of the blood-vascular system. It is situated in the mediastinum of the thoracic cavity and there forms an invagination into a sac of tissue called the **pericardium** which is attached to the sternum and to the mediastinal pleura (Fig. 1.48). The sac has a continuous layer of epithelial cells on its inner surface; part is closely attached to the heart muscle and this region of the epithelial cells is considered as the outer layer of the heart wall and is called the **epicardium.** The inner surface of the sac produces serous *pericardial fluid* and is also termed the **serous** pericardium. This is surrounded by the **fibrous layer** of the pericardium which is continuous with adjacent tissues and with the external coat of the vessels entering and leaving the heart. In life the inner surfaces of the pericardium are separated only by a thin film of pericardial fluid; nevertheless, the potential space is called the **pericardial cavity**.

The wall of the heart consists of three layers. The outermost is the **epicardium** which has just been described. The innermost is the **endocardium**, consisting of a layer of epithelial cells; this is continuous without a break with the epithelial lining (the endothelium) of blood vessels attached to the heart, the whole presenting a very smooth surface lining the blood-vascular system. The endocardium is connected by a thin layer of loose connective tissue to the muscular middle layer of the heart wall. This is the **myocardium** and consists entirely of cardiac muscle cells; these were mentioned with muscle tissue.

The heart has right and left halves (which, however, are not strictly in the right and left halves of the body); in the adult there is no communication between the cavities in each half, which are kept separate by a muscular division. Each half has two chambers, an **atrium** and a **ventricle** (Fig. 1.49).

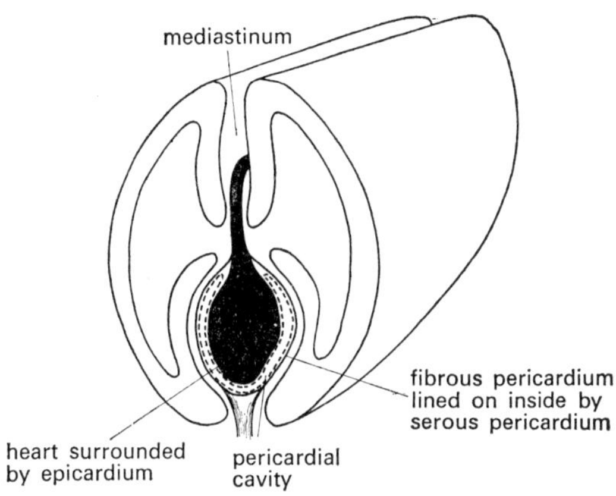

Fig. 1.48. Heart in pericardium within mediastinum. (Heart and vessel represented in black.)

The blood enters an atrium and is then forced through a corresponding **atrio-ventricular valve** into a ventricle. The atrioventricular valve of each side of the heart consists of a number of flaps or cusps lined on each side by continuous endocardium enveloping a thin layer of connective tissue. The free edge of each cusp is attached to the inside of the muscular wall of the ventricles by fibrous threads (**chordae tendinae**) covered by endocardium. In this way the blood is allowed into the ventricles but the reverse flow is prevented by the cusps meeting together to form a barrier; the chordae tendinae prevent the cusps being turned inside out even under the great pressure to which they are subjected.

Blood leaves the ventricles through great vessels: from the left part of the heart through the **aorta**; from the right through the **pulmonary artery**. The reverse flow of blood from each of these vessels is prevented by a valve at the junction with the ventricle. There are three cusps in each of these valves; their connective tissue is covered on each side by epithelial cells which will be called endocardium on the heart side and endothelium on the vessel side. There are no fibrous threads attaching to the edges of the cusps of these aortic and pulmonary valves.

When the blood leaves the right ventricle in the pulmonary artery it is carried to the lungs (Fig. 1.50). Here it is oxygenated and returns via a few **pulmonary veins** to the left atrium. From this chamber it passes through the left atrioventricular valve (sometimes called the mitral valve) into the left ventricle. The oxygenated blood is then forced through the aortic valve into the aorta to spread throughout the entire body with the exception of a very few restricted areas. The oxygen will be given up to the tissues and the blood will take up the waste carbon dioxide and return to the heart via the **venae cavae.** These are large veins which drain the deoxygenated blood into the right atrium. From here it passes through the right atrioventricular valve (sometimes called the tricuspid valve) to the right ventricle and so again through the pulmonary valve.

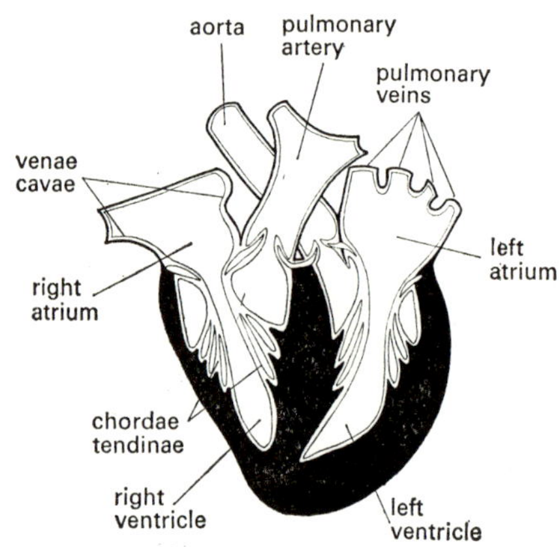

Fig. 1.49. Section of heart.

Systemic Circulation (Figs. 1.51, 1.52)

The flow of blood from the heart via the pulmonary artery to the lungs and its return through the pulmonary veins to the left atrium is the pulmonary circulation. The path from the aorta and back through the venae cavae is the systemic circulation.

As soon as the aorta leaves the heart it gives off two **coronary** arteries whose sole function is to supply the heart with oxygenated blood. Much of the venous return is through cardiac veins which join to form the **coronary sinus.** This opens into the right atrium. Some small veins open directly into the heart chambers.

The next arteries that arise from the aorta (and this is still near to the heart) are vessels which will supply the neck, the cranial end of the thorax, the head and the forelimbs. These originate very close to one another usually as two main branches which then give regional vessels. The supply to the head uses the paired **common carotid** arteries (one on each side of the neck) which, on reaching the jaw, split into several branches to the superficial and deep structures (including the brain). The main returning blood leaves the head as several veins which unite just caudal to the mandibles to form the left and right **external jugular** veins. These are large vessels closely related to the common carotid arteries on the ventral side of the neck. The veins are the more superficial and lie directly under the skin. If pressure is applied at the base of the neck to dam back the venous blood and prevent it continuing to the heart, these veins will become engorged, enlarged and stiffened. They are then convenient for **venipuncture** (entering with a hypodermic syringe needle), either to obtain a blood sample or to give an intravenous injection.

The vessels inside the thorax which will supply the forelimbs are the pair of **subclavian** arteries. One runs to each limb leaving around the first rib through the cranial thoracic aperture. There the name of the vessel is changed to **axillary** artery and this continues to the forelimb, dividing up into many more named arteries. The venous return from the forelimb can be divided into deep and superficial vessels.

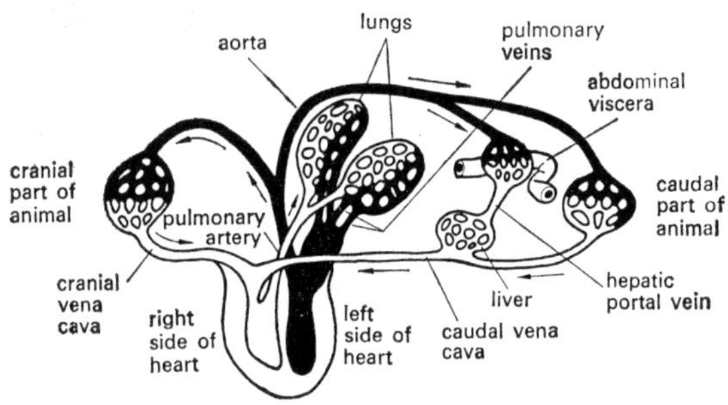

Fig. 1.50. Generalized pattern of blood circulation.

The deep ones run very close to the arteries that supply the limb and usually have similar names; the superficial ones are subcutaneous. One of these is the reasonably large **cephalic** vein which runs proximally on the cranial aspect of the radius and presents another site for venipuncture. Pressure can be applied on the cranial side of the elbow joint to cause venous enlargement.

Arteries to the neck and cranial part of the thorax radiate out to supply these regions and the returning veins are found very close to them. These veins join those from the forelimbs and the head; the resulting large vessel is the single **cranial vena cava** which empties directly into the right atrium.

The aorta leaving the heart curves to reach the ventral surface of the vertebral column at about the fourth thoracic vertebra and continues in this relation as far as the lumbo-sacral junction. At approximately each vertebra a pair of vessels is given off dorsally to supply the vertebral column and adjacent muscles, the spinal cord and the local region of the body wall. Within the thorax relatively small arteries run to the lungs to supply these structures with oxygenated blood. (Although this is where oxygenation takes place, the supporting connective tissues of the lung require oxygenated arterial blood for their nutrition. Blood in the pulmonary arteries comes to the lungs to receive, not to release, oxygen.)

Within the abdominal cavity, the aorta continues to give dorsal segmental vessels and it also supplies the abdominal part of the digestive tract through three ventral midline unpaired vessels, the **coeliac, cranial mesenteric** and **caudal mesenteric** arteries. The venous return from this system will contain a large amount of the absorbed results of digestion and the veins unite to form the large **portal** vein which enters the liver. Here it breaks up into a second set of capillaries which penetrate the hepatic tissue. The abdominal part of the aorta also gives paired **renal** arteries to the kidneys and **spermatic** or **ovarian** arteries to the gonads.

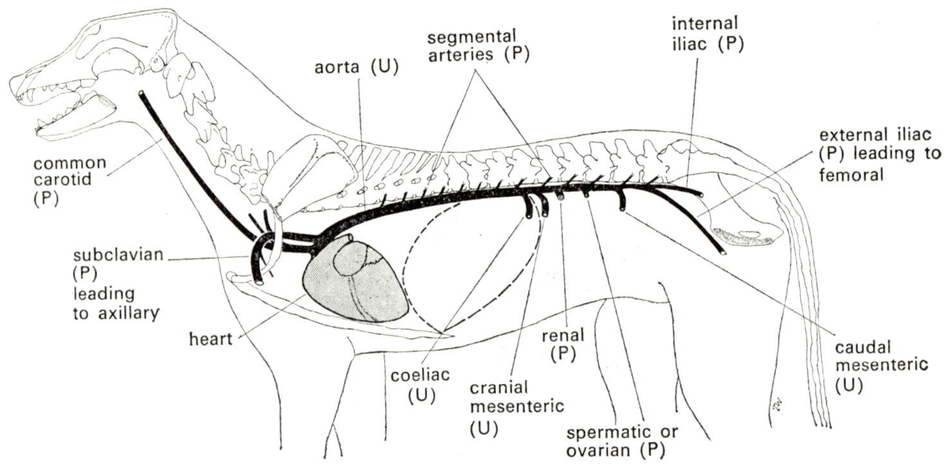

Fig. 1.51. Arterial pattern of a dog. (P = paired vessel, U = unpaired vessel.)

The termination of the aorta is by splitting into left and right **internal iliac** arteries supplying the pelvic contents and left and right **external iliac** arteries which supply the wall of the pelvis and also give a **femoral** artery as the main supply to each hindlimb. (This is the one recommended as a site for feeling the pulse.) As in the forelimb the hindlimb drainage is superficial and deep and there is also a convenient vessel, the **saphenous** vein, on the lateral side of the distal end of the tibia that can be used for intravenous injections.

The hindlimb and pelvic veins unite to form the large **caudal vena cava** near the lumbo-sacral junction. It is closely associated with the aorta in the abdominal cavity. The venous return from the kidneys, gonads and all the body segments that have been supplied by the corresponding arteries opens directly into the caudal vena cava. That from the abdominal part of the digestive system forms the portal vein and only after it has passed through the hepatic capillary bed does this venous blood enter the vena cava. Whereas the aorta is adjacent to the vertebral column throughout the caudal two-thirds of the thorax, the caudal vena cava on reaching the liver turns ventrally and passes through the diaphragm near its centre point. As it travels through the edge of the liver it receives numerous **hepatic** veins draining that organ. In its thoracic course the caudal vena cava receives no more tributaries but empties into the right atrium. The venous drainage of the dorsal part of the thoracic wall and the corresponding part of the vertebral column is by a series of segmental vessels into an unpaired **azygos** vein which does not have a corresponding artery. This runs on the right side, dorsally the length of the thorax and discharges its blood into the cranial vena cava.

Heart Beat

Most of the force necessary to drive the blood through the complex circuit comes

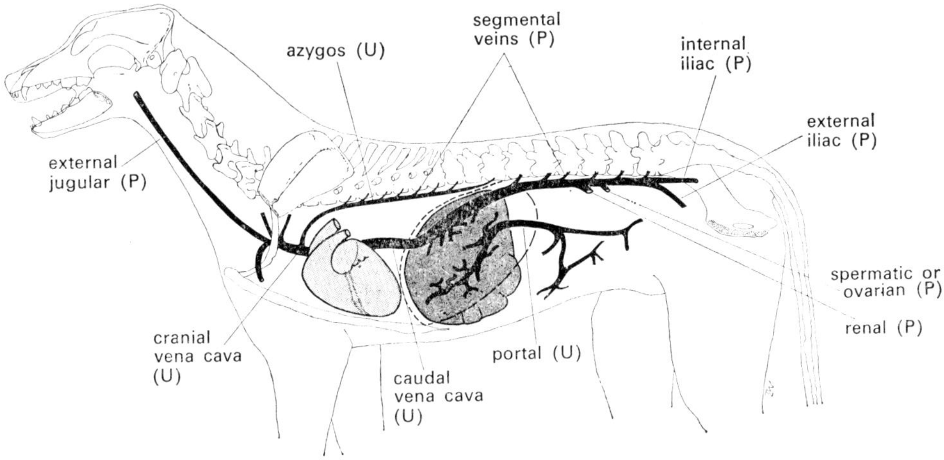

Fig. 1.52. Venous pattern of a dog. (P = paired vessel, U = unpaired vessel.)

from the cardiac muscle itself which has the intrinsic property of rhythmic contraction.

The muscle in the different parts of the heart contracts in a definite sequence. Initiation and control is the responsibility of a group of modified muscle cells forming the **conduction system.** The beat appears to be started by a mass of specialized fibres, the **sinuatrial node**, in the wall of the right atrium. The impulse then passes to the **atrioventricular node**, which is a collection of the special muscle cells in the wall between the atria. From here they form an **atrioventricular bundle** which soon splits to give one limb running in each ventricle in opposite sides of their common (interventricular) wall. The conducting system ends by merging into the regular cardiac muscle tissue.

The spread of the impulse through the heart sets up an electrical current in the surrounding fluids. This can be detected on the surface of the body by a special instrument called an electro-cardiogram (ECG) recorder and will show whether or not the heart is functioning normally.

The central nervous system has an overriding control on these automatic cardiac contractions. In this way heart activity may be markedly increased in stressful situations such as exercise, excessive heat and disease.

The right and the left atria contract together to force blood into the respective relaxed ventricles. The phase of contraction is *systole* and *atrial systole* has just been described. When the blood is forced out of the ventricles this is *ventricular systole*. The relaxed filling periods which follow systole are called *diastole*. The sequence of events between any particular phase and its next occurrence is a *cardiac cycle*: this constitutes a complete *heart beat*.

The number of heart beats per minute is the *heart rate* and is faster for smaller animals than for larger ones. A resting small dog may have a heart rate of 120 beats per minute whereas in a large one it may be 80 or less. The cat varies between about 110 to 130. Young animals have a faster rate than old ones, and exercise, excitement, high environmental temperatures can all have an accelerating effect.

Two definite sounds are produced during each heart beat. The first is related to ventricular systole and is produced by the contraction of the muscle of the ventricle and the vibration of the atrioventricular valve flaps and the chordae tendinae. The second sound is related to the vibrations of the aortic and pulmonary valves after their closure and this will coincide with the start of ventricular diastole.

Blood pressure

This usually means pressure in the arteries and is the force that makes blood flow through the vessels. It is governed by the beat of the heart, the volume of the blood, the resistance and elasticity of the blood vessels. It is measured like barometric pressure in millimetres of mercury.

The pressure is highest at systole and this is the systolic pressure; diastolic pressure is the lowest. The mean pressure is the average of the systolic and diastolic pressures over a given period of time and for the dog is about 150, for the cat about 160 mm of mercury. Blood pressure in capillaries and veins is very low.

Pulse rate

Each beat of the heart is reflected in the arterial blood pressure and this causes a wave of expansion and elongation of the arterial walls, which starts at the aorta and spreads over the entire arterial system. This is the **pulse** or **pulse wave** and it may be felt in many of the superficial arteries. In the dog and cat, the most convenient site is on the medial side of the thigh, where the large femoral artery is virtually subcutaneous. The pulse rate will be the same as the heart rate but the experienced clinician can deduce a lot of other information on the heart and circulation by palpating the arterial pulse.

Heart failure

The body tissues often rapidly increase their oxygen requirements; for instance, muscles during exercise may need up to fifteen times as much as they use when resting. Some of this can be met by a better use of the oxygen carried in the blood, but an increase in cardiac output will probably also be needed. Cardiac output is the volume of blood pumped out by a ventricle per minute and depends on the heart rate and on the output of a ventricle at each beat. The heart may well have sufficient reserve to accomplish this. If it is unable to cope blood will accumulate in the pulmonary system and the right atrium and the condition is that of heart failure.

Circulatory shock

In this very serious condition, there is a marked reduction in blood volume passing through the heart. This may be due to blood loss through haemorrhage, plasma loss from wounds and burns, increased water excretion from the urinary and digestive systems, and decreased water intake. Sometimes blood remains pooled in the venous system and does not return to the heart. Cardiac output is insufficient to supply the tissues and this results in inadequate nutrition and an accumulation of waste products. The heart itself becomes starved and unable to work and, furthermore, the deprived brain is not able to respond correctly to danger signals from sensory nerves monitoring the condition of the internal environment.

LYMPH-VASCULAR SYSTEM

The tissue fluid bathing the cells can enter the blood stream by two routes. The direct way is through the thin walls of the capillary blood vessels. A very important alternative that is extensively used is the capillary lymph vessel network which also permeates the tissues. Once the tissue fluid has passed into this alternative set it is called **lymph** and these capillaries join up to form larger **lymph vessels.** They eventually discharge their fluid into the system of blood vessels. However, before the lymph drains into the blood it passes through *lymphoid (lymphatic) tissue* somewhere along its course. This may be massed together in a connective tissue capsule to form a lymph node or it may be scattered diffusely throughout various organs such as the intestines. The nodes act as filters to hold back bacteria, dust and other foreign matter from entering the blood. Lymph tissue also produces lymphocytes (a very important group of white blood corpuscles which also circulate in the lymph) as well as substances called **antibodies** used to neutralize the effect of bacterial infections. The lymph-vascular system (also called the lymphatic system) includes the lymph vessels and the lymphoid tissue.

Lymph Vessels

The lymph capillaries, like blood capillaries, are endothelial vessels formed of epithelial cells. The blind-ending terminal tubes join together to form networks which combine to form lymphatic vessels of increasing size. These resemble veins in their structure and also possess numerous delicate valves with one or two cusps directing the lymph away from the tissues and towards the vein into which it is finally discharged. The flow of lymph is similar to the venous return from the extremities. Muscle action moves the fluid which can only go in one direction because of the valves. Eventually two major vessels can be recognized: the thoracic duct and the right lymphatic duct.

The **thoracic duct** is the main collecting channel and can be traced through the thorax from an expanded end called the **cisterna chyli** which lies partly in the abdominal region. The cisterna chyli receives lymph from the hindlimb and the lumbar region in addition to that from the abdominal organs. Chyle from the wall of the intestines performs yet another important function of lymph, being responsible for transporting a major fraction of the absorbed fats. The products of lipid digestion enter the lacteals in the intestinal villi and pass through mesenteric lymph vessels and nodes to reach the cisterna chyli. After receiving many vessels from other areas, the thoracic duct opens into one of the great veins which join the right atrium.

The **right lymphatic duct** drains the lymph from the right forelimb and the adjacent part of the body. It opens into the venous system near the thoracic duct or even into the thoracic duct. A pair of **tracheal ducts** carry lymph from the head region and these open into the above-mentioned vessels or near them into the venous system.

Lymph Nodes

These encapsulated masses of lymphoid tissue vary tremendously in size and shape. Several vessels carry lymph to each node entering at various points through the capsule. Connective tissue divides the inside of the node into a series of compartments which are filled with lymphoid tissue. After filtering slowly through the lymphoid tissue, the lymph leaves in a small number of vessels which originate from one area, the **hilus**, of the node.

Each region of the body and each viscus has lymph vessels leaving which pass through at least one node before entering the venous system. Since they are important defences against the spread of disease, the condition of the nodes can help in deciding its nature and extent. Whilst many may only be seen at operation or post-mortem examination, some can be felt through the skin.

The group of **mandibular** lymph nodes lying just caudal to the junction of the ramus and body of each side of the lower jaw can be palpated and these receive lymph from much of the head. This can be called the drainage region of the mandibular nodes. The lymph from these and from the remainder of the head all passes to the very large **retropharyngeal** lymph nodes which lie close to the pharynx. They are too deep for palpation and it is from these that the tracheal ducts arise which carry the lymph along the neck. Another node that can be felt through the skin is the **superficial cervical** lymph node (also called the prescapular) and this lies at the base of the neck on each side just cranial to the scapula. Lymph from the lateral surface of the neck and from the forelimb drains through this node.

A superficial node involved in hindlimb drainage is the **popliteal** and this lies subcutaneously caudal to the stifle joint. All the lymph from the hindlimb and also from the caudal mammary glands, or penis, and adjacent skin passes through **superficial inguinal** nodes. These lie dorsal to the mammary glands or penis, between the thigh and the abdominal wall.

Within the thorax, **bronchial** lymph nodes associated with the major bronchi drain the lymph from the lungs and this, together with that from the remainder of the thoracic viscera and from the thorax, passes through **mediastinal** nodes to reach the thoracic duct. Lymph from abdominal viscera drains through their specific nodes, **mesenteric**, **hepatic**, **colic**, etc., before reaching the cisterna chyli from where it passes along the thoracic duct.

Lymph Follicles

Masses of lymphoid tissue, usually associated with mucous membrane may occur as small discrete areas but they are also found grouped together as large patches called follicles.

Tonsils

These have been mentioned in the description of the pharynx in the section on the digestive system. They help form a complete ring of lymphoid tissue around the opening of the mouth into the pharynx.

Spleen

This organ is closely adjacent to the stomach in the abdominal cavity. It is, however, a haemopoietic organ and contains regions of lymphoid tissue. Its functions are still imperfectly understood. In addition to the blood-cell formation and destruction carried out by all haemopoietic tissue the spleen is a very efficient storage area for blood, a function that produces considerable variations in its size.

Nervous System

In the notes on nervous tissue, the neuron (nerve fibre) is described as a cell body with processes. The processes carrying impulses to the cell body are called dendrites (dendrons) whereas the one process that carries impulses away from the cell body is called an axon. When the impulse passes from one neuron to another it does so at a synapse. The impulse can only pass one way across the synapse. The axon termination may be composed of a very large number of filaments and these will not necessarily all synapse with one neuron; in fact, the termination of one neuron, by virtue of its large number of terminal filaments, will usually synapse with a large number of other neurons. Conversely, any neuron may receive impulses (via synapses) from many other neurons. This arrangement of terminations allows extensive interraction and integration of impulses.

The function of the nervous system is to receive stimuli from the environment (inside and outside the body), to analyse and integrate these stimuli and then cause such response by the tissues of the body as is necessary. The stimuli are received by neuron processes which may be free endings or may be attached to more complicated structures. The receptors are known as **sensory nerve endings** and the processes which transmit the impulses are **sensory fibres.** The first part of the fibre will be a dendrite and this will end at the cell body. The impulse will then be carried by the second part of the neuron, the axon. If a response is evoked, an impulse has to be transmitted to muscle tissue or to a gland. The neuron process leaving the central nervous system and carrying this impulse is a **motor fibre.** The simplest functional unit of the nervous system consists of a sensory unit synapsing with a motor unit. At least one other neuron is usually involved and conveys the impulse from the sensory to the motor unit; such a neuron is an **intercalated** or **connector** neuron.

A further classification of fibres is made which relates to the structures in which the sensory and motor nerve endings are found. Internal organs, smooth muscle, glands and mucous membrane are considered to be innervated by **visceral** motor and sensory fibres. All other structures are innervated by **somatic** motor and sensory fibres.

Somatic sensory fibres have receptors in, or close to, the skin which are activated by stimuli such as pain, pressure, heat and touch from the outside environment. There are also receptors in muscles, tendons and joints which are sensitive to alterations in their state, tension and position. **Special somatic** sensory fibres have highly specialized endings and carry impulses from organs responsible for sight, hearing and balance.

Somatic motor fibres: the impulses pass along these neurons from the central nervous tissue to skeletal muscle cells.

Visceral sensory fibres: stimuli are received from blood vessels, mucous membranes and viscera. Those carrying stimuli relating to smell and taste are often referred to as **special visceral** sensory fibres.

Visceral motor fibres: these are distributed to involuntary muscle cells and to glands.

The visceral sensory fibres, the visceral motor fibres and their connections within the central nervous system are often said to form the **autonomic nervous system.** The term means self-governing, and refers to the fact that bodily processes (for example, blood circulation and digestion) involving the visceral sensory and motor neurons, etc., are not under the control of the will.

The somatic and visceral fibres together with some connective tissue, make up the nervous system. This is a functional classification. It is often convenient to use a topographical division and so the part of the system which is situated in the midline of the body closely related to the vertebral column and the skull is called the **central nervous system** and this includes only the brain and spinal cord. All the other nervous tissue constitutes the **peripheral nervous system.** It is essential to understand that both somatic and visceral neurons appear in the central nervous system and that both somatic and visceral neurons are present in the peripheral nervous system.

Further, that a somatic or a visceral nerve fibre can be part of the peripheral nervous system, continue into the spinal cord or brain and so become part of the central nervous system; similarly somatic and visceral fibres can leave the central nervous system and then continue in the peripheral nervous system.

CENTRAL NERVOUS SYSTEM

This topographical unit of the nervous system consists of the **brain** located in the cranial cavity and the **spinal cord** in the vertebral canal. In addition to the protection afforded by these skeletal structures, the central nervous system is enveloped in three tubes of protective membranes called **meninges**, between two of which there is a layer of liquid, the **cerebro-spinal fluid** (CSF).

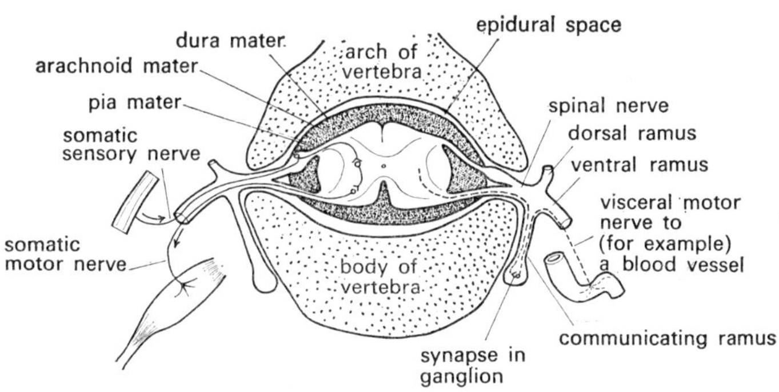

Fig. 1.53. Section of spinal cord within vertebral canal.

The outermost of the protective membranes is the **dura mater**: this is tough and fibrous and within the head it is interwoven with the periosteum on the inner surface of the bones of the cranium. In the vertebral canal the dura is quite free from the local periosteum and is surrounded by fat and blood vessels occupying the **epidural space** (Fig. 1.53). The innermost of the protective membranes is the **pia mater**; this is closely applied to the central nervous system. It is a delicate but very vascular membrane and follows all the gross irregularities of the brain and spinal cord. The meninx (singular of meninges) between the dura mater and the pia mater is called the **arachnoid** and consists of a network of delicate collagenous fibres. The **subarachnoid** space between the fibres is occupied by the cerebro-spinal fluid.

Spinal Cord (Fig. 1.53)

This extends from the foramen magnum of the cranium as far as the caudal lumbar/cranial sacral region. The caudal end of the tube of dura mater is about mid-sacral region, but the spinal cord does not extend quite so far.

At an early stage of development, the body of the embryo is partly segmented and each segment has its own muscles, blood supply and sensory and motor nerve fibres. A **spinal nerve** is formed by the sensory and motor fibres between the spinal cord and each one of these segments. The nerve uses the intervertebral foramen between adjacent vertebral arches to enter and leave the vertebral canal. There are a pair (a left and a right) of nerves related to each vertebra. In the case of the cervical region there are eight pairs although there are only seven vertebrae; this is because the first pair emerge through the arch of the first cervical vertebra (the atlas). All the other spinal nerves emerge caudal to a vertebra. There are only a few coccygeal spinal nerves, restricted to the more cranial coccygeal intervertebral foramina. Each spinal nerve is attached to the spinal cord by a **dorsal** and a **ventral root**; the attachment

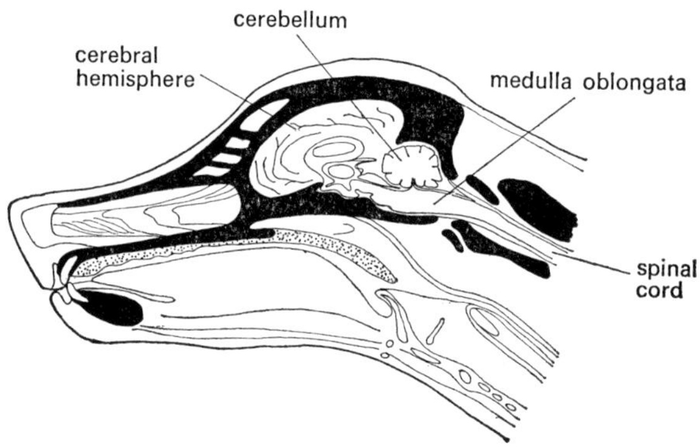

Fig. 1.54. Median section of dog's head. Solid black represents bone.

consists of a series of filaments (Fig. 1.55). The dorsal root has a localized swelling, the **dorsal root ganglion**, which lies close to, or in, the intervertebral foramen.

A transverse section of the cord shows the ventral part separated into halves by a **ventral median fissure** containing pia mater and blood vessels. The dorsal part is also separable into halves by the **dorsal median septum**; this connective tissue partition can usually only be seen under magnification. A very narrow bore **central canal** runs the length of the cord, in the area between the ventral median fissure and the dorsal median septum. In life, this contains cerebro-spinal fluid.

The nerve fibres that help to form the spinal cord tend to run in recognizable regions. Since many of the fibres are covered by a fatty material called *myelin*, the regions are fairly clearly defined and form the peripheral **white matter** of the cord. The more central region consists mainly of cell bodies, but there are also many nerve processes. This is the **grey matter** and although usually considered to be H-shaped it will vary with the region of the cord.

The spinal cord is formed entirely of neurons, comprising cell bodies together with their dendrites and axons and also a relatively small amount of supporting tissue.

Brain

The spinal cord is continued rostrally by the brain without any abrupt change. Like the cord it is formed of neurons, but the grey matter of the brain tends to be separated into discrete areas by tracts of (white) fibres connecting different regions. The brain has to deal with more complex activities than the spinal cord and so certain regions are greatly enlarged by bulges of nervous tissue superimposed on the otherwise simple tube. A transverse section of the *spinal cord* shows the white matter enclosing the more central grey matter. In certain parts of the *brain* grey matter is found on the outer surface of the white matter. The central canal of the spinal cord continues rostrally in the brain tissue, where it expands and has diverticuli to produce a relatively large **ventricular system** still filled with cerebro-spinal fluid. It is actually into the ventricular system that this fluid is produced.

The brain can be divided into a **hind-brain** continuous with the spinal cord, a **mid-brain** and a **fore-brain.**

Hind-brain. The part of the hind-brain continuous with the spinal cord is the **medulla oblongata** (Fig. 1.54). It merges with the spinal cord and has similar markings. The dorsal surface is at first similar to that of the cord; it does, however, rapidly widen and then narrow again. The amount of tissue over the rostral continuation of the central canal suddenly decreases and the space itself is expanded in the widest part of the hind-brain. This enlarged part of the channel in the medulla oblongata is the **fourth ventricle.** It has a thin roof and is bounded on each side by large tracts of fibres entering and leaving the **cerebellum** (Fig. 1.54). This is a globular mass of nervous tissue with a surface of ridges separated by furrows; it is concerned with the maintenance of balance and equilibrium by co-ordinating muscular activity. The cerebellum lies on the dorsal aspect of the hind-brain over the fourth ventricle and it is attached to the remainder of the hind-brain by three pairs of **peduncles.** These are fibre tracts.

Mid-brain. The dorsal surface of this short length of the brain is covered by the overhanging fore-brain. The ventricular system is continued rostrally through the mid-brain by the **cerebral aqueduct.**

Fore-brain. The fore-brain consists of a mid-line portion flanked by two lateral expansions, the right and left **cerebral hemispheres** (Fig. 1.54). The midline portion and each hemisphere encompass parts of the ventricular system; the **third ventricle** is a laterally flattened fluid-filled space in the midline and diverticuli of this (called **lateral ventricles**) occupy part of each cerebral hemisphere.

The ventral surface of the midline portion consists mainly of the **optic chiasma** which is a cross-shaped arrangement of nerve fibres associated with the eye, and the **pituitary gland** (an endocrine tissue attached by a short stalk).

The cerebral hemispheres are large masses joined to each other by a band of nerve fibres. The surface resembles that of the cerebellum in being arranged in ridges and grooves. The nerve cell bodies form the peripheral layer of the cerebral hemispheres and so in sections the grey matter appears outside the white matter. However, embedded in the central area of white matter are collections of nerve cell bodies. The most rostral parts of the cerebral hemispheres, and hence of the brain, are the **olfactory bulbs.** These paired structures are closely applied to the plate of bone separating the brain from the nasal chambers and convey the stimuli concerned with the sense of smell.

The attachment to the spinal cord of motor and sensory fibres forming spinal nerves has already been described. Motor and sensory fibres are also attached to specific regions of the brain to form **cranial nerves**. Spinal and cranial nerves constitute the peripheral nervous system.

PERIPHERAL NERVOUS SYSTEM

There are four basic functional types of fibres that can make up a cranial or a spinal nerve: somatic sensory, somatic motor, visceral sensory and visceral motor. Not all nerves contain all functional types; some nerves contain additional special functional types.

Somatic motor fibres leave the spinal cord through the ventral root of every spinal nerve and somatic sensory fibres enter through every dorsal root. In fact, the swelling on the dorsal root (the dorsal root ganglion) is caused by the collection of cell bodies of the sensory fibres forming that root. It is likely that the dorsal roots of many of the spinal nerves also contain visceral sensory fibres. The distribution of the visceral motor fibres differs slightly from the other functional types. The ventral roots of the thoracic and lumbar spinal nerves contain visceral motor fibres. These are also called **sympathetic fibres,** but it is important to remember that they are visceral motor. The ventral roots of some of the sacral spinal nerves and the corresponding parts of some of the cranial nerves also contain visceral motor fibres; these cranio-sacral fibres are **parasympathetic**. To summarize: sympathetic nerves are visceral motor fibres that leave the central nervous system in the ventral roots of the thoracic and lumbar spinal nerves; parasympathetic nerves are visceral motor fibres that leave the central nervous system in cranial nerves and in the ventral roots of some sacral nerves. There are many functional differences between sympathetic and parasympathetic fibres. Some structures receive visceral motor innervation from both sympathetic and parasympathetic divisions.

As a general rule it can be taken that the parasympathetic fibres are concerned with maintaining smooth muscle tone and glandular secretions sufficient for the ordinary normal state of the animal. Sympathetic stimulation is often associated with states of excitement, as suggested by the phrase, "fight, flight and frolic". Physiological phenomena commonly experienced at these times, e.g. increased heart rate, more rapid respiration, are usually due to the increased activity of the sympathetic system.

Spinal Nerves (Fig. 1.55)

The dorsal and ventral roots fuse to form a **mixed** spinal nerve which then divides into a dorsal and a ventral **ramus**. The dorsal rami are usually smaller than the corresponding ventral rami and retain more or less their segmental pattern of innervation.

The ventral rami carry fibres that innervate the limbs and the ventral and lateral parts of the neck and trunk. In the cervico-thoracic and the lumbo-sacral regions the ventral rami of adjacent nerves form a network or plexus where the nerve fibres related to different segments of the cord intermingle. The fibres innervating the limbs enter or leave the plexus peripherally as named, but not segmentally distinct, nerves.

All spinal nerves have a **visceral ramus**, or **communicating ramus** (ramus communicans), as a branch of the ventral ramus. This originates close to the continuation of the ventral ramus with the mixed spinal nerve and consists of visceral

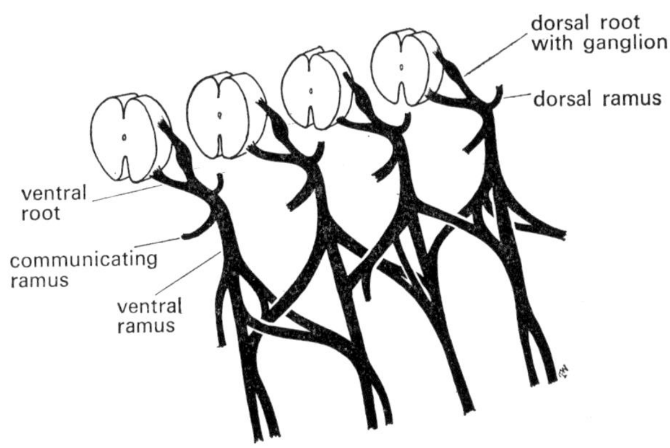

Fig. 1.55. Formation of plexus by ventral rami of adjacent nerves.

motor and visceral sensory fibres. Visceral motor fibres always have a synapse interposed between the central nervous system and the structure they supply. The synapses occur close to or with the cell bodies; collections of these synapses are therefore associated with collections of cell bodies. Where large groups of cell bodies are found in the peripheral nervous system they cause a swelling called a **ganglion** and these synapses of visceral motor fibres occur in ganglia (plural of ganglion) on the course of the communicating rami. In the thoraco-lumbar region, sympathetic nerve fibres connect up these ganglia and form a *sympathetic chain* which lies on either side of the vertebral bodies.

Cranial Nerves

The nerves are numbered as they arise from the brain from the most rostral I to the most caudal XII. Although this is a matter of convenience it does not explain the fibre types involved, nor how the nerves are distributed. The nerves do not attach to the brain with regular dorsal and ventral roots, nor do many have both motor and sensory fibres. Special sensory and special motor fibres are found in the cranial nerves.

All the nerves innervate only structures in the head region with the exception of the vagus (X) nerve; this also supplies thoracic and abdominal organs.

Three nerves are concerned entirely with special senses: the olfactory (I) for smell, the optic (II) for sight and the vestibulo-cochlear (VIII) for hearing and equilibrium. Three nerves convey motor fibres to muscles of the eyeball: oculomotor (III), trochlear (IV) and abducens (VI). Another nerve with only motor fibres is the hypoglossal (XII), which supplies the muscles of the tongue. The remaining nerves are mixed, being formed of motor and sensory fibres. The trigeminal (V) carries the general sensory fibres of the head and also motor fibres to some of the muscles of mastication. The facial (VII) carries mainly motor fibres to the non-masticatory muscles of the head. The glosso-pharyngeal (IX), vagus (X) and accessory (XI) carry motor and sensory fibres for the mouth, the pharynx, larynx, heart, lungs and abdominal organs.

Reflex Arcs

A reflex action is a fixed involuntary response which is always similar for a given stimulus. The reflex arc is the nerve pathway along which the stimuli travel; from the source of the sensory stimulus to the central nervous system, the route within the central nervous system, the motor nerve to the responding structure. Any arrangement whereby only one sensory nerve and one motor nerve (and therefore only one synapse) is involved must be a reflex arc. Where an intercalated nerve is present and this has other intercommunications, it is possible that the response would not always be the same; this would not be a reflex.

The definition stresses that the act is involuntary, but the animal may nevertheless be conscious of what is happening. If the pad is pricked, the animal will reflexly draw it away from the point, but it will become aware of the pain. The first part of this is called the **flexor reflex** and is an example of a normal **spinal reflex**; that is, one where the complete circuit is within the spinal cord. It can take place even if the cord is cut through, provided the damage does not occur at the segments used by the reflex. For the hindlimb flexor reflex, this would be approximately four to seven lumbar and the three sacral segments and if the cord is damaged more cranial than this a hindlimb flexor reflex will still probably be present.

There are several other basic limb reflexes which are restricted to the spine but more complex reflexes pass through centres in the brain. Respiratory, digestive and cardiovascular reflexes are in this category, using the autonomic (visceral) nerve pathways and not reaching the level of consciousness. Nevertheless, any given stimulus still causes the same fixed response.

SPECIAL SENSES

Vision, hearing, balance, smell and taste are special sensations and particular regions of the body are specifically modified to receive stimuli related to them. The stimuli are transmitted to the central nervous system by cranial nerves; to be quite accurate, in the case of vision and smell the sensory organs are extensions of the brain itself.

Vision (Fig. 1.56)

The **eye** is specially adapted for the reception of visual impulses. This globular mass lies in the orbit and can be moved freely in many directions. This is accomplished by a group of ocular (eye) muscles of voluntary fibres. Each muscle has one attachment to the periphery of the eyeball. The other ends of the muscles are grouped together in the depth of the orbit to attach to the skull. It is most unlikely that any one

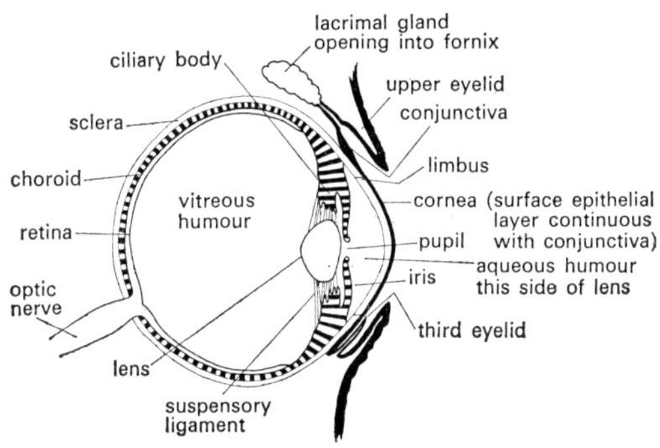

Fig. 1.56. Section of eye.

of the group operates on its own but by complex co-ordination the delicate movements of the entire eyeball within the orbit are achieved. The eye consists of three main layers which enclose two compartments, one containing a liquid called **aqueous humour**, the other a gelatinous mass known as **vitreous humour.**

The outermost layer is the tough, fibrous protective **sclera** which over the front of the eye becomes transparent and forms the **cornea.** The junction between the sclera and the cornea is the **limbus.** Immediately inside the sclera, the **uvea** forms a very vascular pigmented layer. It does not extend as far as the cornea but just behind the limbus it projects towards the centre of the eyeball as the **ciliary body.** This leaves a circular orifice which is occupied by the transparent biconvex **lens**: the circumference of the lens is attached to the ciliary body by the fibres of the **suspensory ligament.** The ciliary body, the suspensory ligament and the lens divide the interior of the eyeball into two regions. The aqueous humour fills the space between the cornea and this division; the vitreous humour fills the other region. The part of the uvea between the vitreous humour and the sclera is the **choroid.** In this there is a special arrangement of iridescent cells called the **tapetum.** This is a light-reflecting area which in the dog varies in colour from green through yellow to pink. In the cat it is an even brighter more colourful metallic yellowish blue or green. This is the surface that causes eyes to "shine in the dark", or to be more accurate, reflect the small amount of light that is present. Another part of the uvea projects as a septum between the ciliary body and the cornea: this is the **iris** and it has a central orifice called the **pupil.**

The sensory endings which receive visual stimuli form the **retina**; this is the innermost of the three main layers of the eye and is found between the vitreous humour and the choroid. Light passes through the cornea and is directed by the lens on to the sensory nerve endings of the retina. Focusing is achieved by the action of the ciliary body working through the suspensory ligament to change the curvature of the lens. The amount of light entering through the lens is controlled by the smooth muscle content of the iris which is able to vary the size of the pupil. The stimuli pass from the sensory endings of the retina along fibres which emerge from the eyeball as the optic (IInd) cranial nerve.

Most of the eyeball is within the orbit of the skull. The rest of it is protected by **eyelids** which can completely cover this part. The upper and lower eyelids of hairy skin converge at the medial and lateral **canthi** (singular canthus) or angles. Deep to these a third eyelid occupies the medial canthus. The epithelium of the skin on the outer surface of the lids is continuous with that of the **conjunctiva** of the under surface. This is reflected on to the eyeball and the epithelium continues over the cornea (where it is transparent) as its surface layer and over the third eyelid; this is in keeping with the concept that epithelium covers the entire surface of the body. The angle formed by the reflection of the conjunctiva is the **fornix.** The third eyelid consists of a plate of cartilage projecting from the medial canthus with its free lateral edge covered on its inner and outer surface by conjunctiva.

The corneal surface must be kept constantly moist and this is achieved by **lacrimal fluid** produced by the **lacrimal gland.** It is situated on the dorso-lateral surface of the eyeball and the secretion passes through several small ducts into the fornix of the upper eyelid. The fluid spreads over the entire area (helped by the eyelids sweeping over the eyeball) and then collects in the medial canthus where it drains into a small tube, the **nasolacrimal duct.** The opening for the duct is in a small depression in the lacrimal bone; note that the bone gets its name because this is where lacrimal fluid is collected and not because of any direct relationship with the lacrimal gland. The nasolacrimal duct passes through the bones of the face to open into the nasal chamber. This is where lacrimal fluid normally drains to; if there is excessive production or deficient drainage it will spill over the eyelid and may then be called **tear** fluid or tears. The fluid can have an irritating scalding effect on the skin it then runs over.

Hearing and Balance (Fig. 1.57)

These stimuli are received by endings in the **ear**, which is clearly divisible into three parts: *external, middle* and *inner.*

The external ear starts at the **pinna**, a funnel-shaped collection of cartilages covered by skin, which can be turned in various directions so that its concavity can collect air vibrations. The funnel leads to the **external acoustic meatus**, a short tube which is firmly fixed to the temporal bone. The deepest part of the meatus is closed by the **tympanic membrane.**

The middle ear is in the temporal bone and houses three small bones or ossicles which form a chain stretching from the tympanic membrane to the **vestibular window** opposite. The auditory tube also opens into the middle ear cavity. The other end of this tube opens in the pharynx; in this way the pressure on both sides of the tympanic membrane will be atmospheric and therefore the same.

The inner ear is also in the temporal bone and consists of a sealed bag of fluid called the **membranous labyrinth** which fits into excavations called the **bony labyrinth.** This consists of three main parts. The central part is the **vestibule** and on one side of

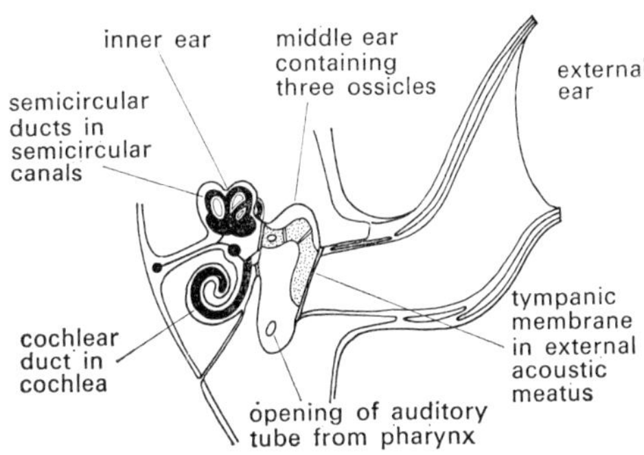

Fig. 1.57. Section of ear.

this are several openings of **semicircular canals.** Another tube that opens into the vestibule is the **cochlea**: this is coiled on itself in the form of a spiral. The bony labyrinth is filled with the fluid **perilymph** and the membranous labyrinth floats in this. However, it is not freely movable. Three tubular hoops form part of one side of the membranous labyrinth; these are **semicircular ducts** and they fit accurately into the semicircular canals of the bony labyrinth. There is also a **cochlear duct** which forms another part of the membranous labyrinth and this fits inside the cochlea of the bony labyrinth. The membranous labyrinth is filled with the fluid **endolymph**; this does not mingle with the surrounding perilymph.

The cochlear duct is concerned with hearing and the stimuli are transmitted to the brain by sensory fibres in the vestibulo-cochlear (VIIIth) cranial nerve. The remainder of the membranous labyrinth is affected by movement; sensory fibres carrying stimuli relating to equilibrium, posture, etc., also form part of the vestibulocochlear (VIIIth) cranial nerve.

Smell

The **olfactory system** is concerned with smell. The sensory nerve endings are scattered in part of the mucous membrane covering the turbinates in the nasal cavity.

The fibres do not form a compact nerve but run through the several holes in the ethmoid bone direct to the brain. They are considered to form the olfactory (Ist) cranial nerve.

Taste

The sensory nerve endings are associated with special organs called **taste buds.** These are mainly scattered over the tongue but they also occur in the mucous membrane of the palate, pharynx and larynx. The fibres carrying stimuli associated with **gustatory** sensation (i.e. taste) form parts of the facial (VIIth), glossopharyngeal (IXth) and the vagus (Xth) cranial nerves.

Endocrine System

One of the functions of the nervous system is to stimulate a specific cell or group of cells to perform a particular limited action. Endocrine glands produce **hormones,** secretions which are spread by the blood system to have more prolonged regulatory effects on their target tissues, organs or systems. The actions are extremely complex and very few are well understood. Some of the endocrine functions of the thyroid, parathyroids, adrenals, pancreas, gonads and pituitary will be outlined.

Thyroid

The thyroid gland flanks the first few tracheal rings. Its hormone requires iodine as an essential component and it has a general effect on many of the body systems especially on oxidative processes. It is necessary for normal growth and young animals deficient in this hormone (the condition of *hypothyroidism*) suffer a form of dwarfism. In the adult a lowered metabolic rate is one of the main results and the animal becomes fat and sluggish. When excess hormone is produced (*hyperthyroidism*) there is a marked increase in metabolic rate.

Parathyroids

There are usually two main parathyroid glands on each side. They are very small and are in very close anatomical relationship with the thyroid gland. The secretion is extremely important in maintaining a correct balance of calcium in the body. Excessive production results in an abnormal excretion of calcium with at least a resultant weakening of the skeleton.

Adrenals

These paired glands are anatomically closely related to the kidneys. They have an inner *medullary* region and an outer *cortex* each of which produces its own hormones; there is no connection between these secretions.

The hormones of the adrenal medulla have the same effects as stimulation of the sympathetic nervous system, those of "fight, flight and frolic". Sympathetic nerve stimulation of the adrenal medulla causes it to release the hormone and so the nerve effect will be supplemented by that of the secretion.

The numerous hormones produced by the adrenal cortex can be divided into three groups. One regulates inorganic balance (especially sodium, chlorine and potassium) in the extracellular fluids by controlling kidney tubular activity. The second group enhances the animal's resistance to disease conditions and to stress resulting from excessive exercise, extreme temperatures, etc. The third group helps control the development of male sexual characteristics.

Pancreas

This gland plays an important role in its exocrine production of pancreatic juice for intestinal digestion. Small patches of endocrine tissue form the **islets of Langerhans** which are responsible for secreting **insulin.** This hormone lowers the concentration of glucose in the blood and extracellular fluids by assisting its transfer to the interior of cells. In its absence, glucose cannot be used and so it is excreted: lipid and protein are therefore called upon to provide energy, resulting in a wasting-away of tissues.

Male Gonad

The walls of the seminiferous tubules in the testes consist of two types of cells: those producing sperms and those supplying nutritive materials. The latter also secrete the hormone **testosterone**, and this is responsible for the development of male sexual characteristics. There are several other hormones associated with these features and as a group they are called **androgens.** Castration prevents the circulation of testosterone from the gonads and if performed while the animal is still sexually immature it will stay that way. None of the remaining genitalia will develop fully nor will the accessory sex glands. The animal will not show any mating activities. If castration is performed after sexual maturity, the major result of the lack of testosterone will show in an increase in depot fat due to a lowered metabolic rate.

Female Gonad

The developing ovarian follicles produce an **oestrogenic** hormone, that is, one that is concerned with the signs of sexual desire. Oestrogens (as they are commonly termed) are also produced by other endocrine glands. They are responsible for preparing the genitalia for coitus and for the appearance of sex characteristics of the female, such as the development of the mammary gland.

A corpus luteum is formed after a follicle has ruptured and this secretes another hormone, **progesterone**, which is concerned with the maintenance of pregnancy. Under its control, the uterus prepares to support the fertilized ova and local muscular activity is reduced so as not to dislodge them. It continues the stimulation to the mammary gland that was begun by oestrogens.

Pituitary

This small gland is attached in the midline to the ventral surface of the mid-brain. It is sometimes called the **hypophysis** and there are two major hormone producing areas, the **anterior pituitary** (or **adenohypophysis**) and the **posterior pituitary** (or **neurohypophysis**). Between them these two produce a large number of hormones, many of which control the secretion of other endocrine organs.

Anterior pituitary. Two of the hormones produced have a direct controlling influence on other ductless glands. *Thyrotropic* hormone regulates the thyroid and *corticotropic* hormone (adrenocorticotrophin, ACTH) affects the secretions of the adrenal cortex. A *growth* hormone promotes the development and enlargement of all body tissues; an insufficiency results in dwarfism, an excess produces giant animals. The anterior pituitary also produces a group of *gonadotropic* (affecting the gonads) hormones: *follicle-stimulating* (FSH), *luteinizing* (LH) and *luteotropic* (LTH). The follicle stimulating hormone initiates the growth of ovarian follicles and helps the ovaries to secrete oestrogens. In the male, FSH stimulates the growth of the germinal epithelium of the testes. Luteinizing hormone causes the ovarian follicle to rupture and influences the secretion of progesterone by the corpus luteum. Its effect on the male is to cause the testes to secrete testosterone. Luteotropic hormone is associated with the initiation and maintenance of milk secretion.

Posterior pituitary. Strictly, the hormones are only stored in the neurohypophysis. They are secreted deeper within the brain tissue and are conducted to this site from whence they are released. The two important substances are the *antidiuretic* hormone and *oxytocin*. The former acts on the kidney to prevent excessive water loss and oxytocin causes the uterus to contract and also affects mammary gland tissue to release milk.

CHAPTER 2

Principles of Animal Management, Hygiene and Feeding

(a) RESTRAINT AND HANDLING

G. SUMNER-SMITH, BVSc, MSc, FRCVS

Introduction

To love animals, does not mean, unfortunately, that your love will be reciprocated, hence the necessity for restraint. But if love of animals can, as it should, comprehend a knowledge of animal psychology and behaviour patterns the first stages in the act of restraint will have been learned. Recognition of instinctive behaviour patterns in the dog and cat when faced with stress is essential to a rational approach to handling of animal patients in hospital.

Biting or scratching through fear is the main hazard in nursing the domestic dog or cat, and to understand and alleviate that fear is one of the main duties of the RANA. Although the main emphasis of this section is on the actual manual techniques of restraint it should never be forgotten that the more knowledge the RANA acquires of instinctive behaviour and breed characteristics the less will be the necessity to resort to the cruder methods of restraint.

Approach

The approach to a patient is of primary importance, as it should be remembered that the strange sites, noises and more particularly odours of a veterinary hospital may make even a normally placid patient nervous.

The RANA who is able to make friends with her charge will find it easier to restrain the animal for treatment or examination.

The Restraint of Dogs

Approach the dog with a kind and quiet word and present the back of one closed hand for inspection; the lead and collar is taken in the other hand. Before taking charge of an animal it is essential to check that the collar is fastened on a hole that is sufficiently tight, and is not likely to slip over the dog's head should it struggle on parting from the owner. The owner should be instructed to leave the dog with the RANA, rather than the RANA take the dog from the room before the owner leaves. The dog will usually submit to being led away once the owner is out of sight. On occasions it may be considered desirable to leave the lead attached to the animal's collar when it is placed in a kennel. Should the animal later be reluctant to leave the kennel it will be far easier to reach the lead with hand or broom handle than to attempt affixing the lead whilst the animal is still in the kennel. This is particularly advisable when the patient is unco-operative, but the danger of an animal becoming entangled should always be borne in mind and the RANA will decide in the circumstances which course is to be taken.

HANDLING

When it becomes necessary to lift the dog onto the examination table the collar is grasped in the left hand, the RANA standing by the animal's left foreleg, and facing in the same direction. The right arm is passed over the back and the hand under the sternum. The hand takes the weight of the dog as it is lifted, the left hand controlling the head. The left arm should be tensed in order to respond to any sudden attempt on the part of the dog to struggle or turn on its handler. Assistance will be necessary when lifting large dogs and this may be performed by a second person standing directly behind the animal, grasping both stifles to aid the lift. Patients should never be lifted by a hand or arm under the abdomen. The small, wriggling and unco-operative dog may be picked up by first covering with a blanket that has been folded a number of times, or by the handler wearing thick pruning gloves.

MUZZLING

When handling a strange dog a muzzle should be applied if there is the slightest doubt as to the docility of the animal. A muzzle may be made of leather or wire; but in veterinary practices it is usual to apply the tape muzzle (see Figs. 2.1 and 2.2). This muzzle may be discarded after use as a point of hygiene and it is not necessary to stock the large range of sizes that are required when using the fixed type. The tape may usually be applied without a lot of fuss if the approach is gentle and reassuring. Occasionally, it is necessary to have an assistant hold the forelegs if the animal attempts to remove the tape with its claws. The tape should be secured in position by a bow to aid a quick release. Whilst a tape may be applied to most breeds, it will be readily appreciated that one cannot apply same to such breeds as the Pug and Pekinese, and for these animals the use of a hand towel is recommended. The towel is rolled lengthways, passed under the neck, and the two ends held firmly close to, and behind the patient's head.

HOLDING FOR EXAMINATION AND MEDICATION

Seven methods will be described.

1. The RANA stands in front of the patient who is already standing on the examination table. The collar is grasped on each side of the head, just below the ears, with the heel of the palms pressed firmly against the dog's cheek bone on each side of the patient's head (Fig. 2.3).

2. The left arm is passed under the patient's neck and the palm of the hand pressed firmly on its right shoulder blade—the patient being hugged against the RANA.

The right hand either forces the rear quarters to the sitting position, and holds them there; or supports the body in the standing position behind and under the quarters. The method will be determined by the position required, and it is of course possible to stand on the other side of the animal and reverse the procedure, should such be required.

3. In order to restrain an animal on its side, the patient should be grasped by the far side opposing front and hindlegs, lifted from the table, lowered slightly and then rolled on its side as the table is approached again. The operator's chest aiding in pressing the animal on to the table. Ideally, this movement should be performed by one person, enabling a second person to pass one arm over the neck and grasp the underneath foreleg and the other over the lumbar region and grasp the corresponding under hindleg.

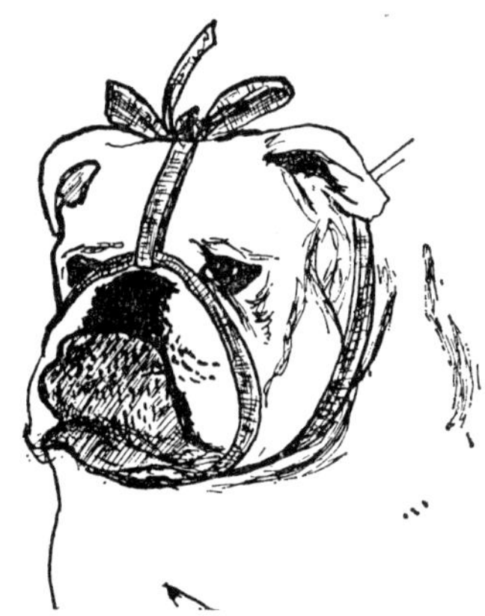

Fig. 2.2. Tape muzzle applied to "bull"-nosed dog.

4. Restraining an animal on its back is accomplished by rolling from method 3, and holding each pair of fore and hind legs in the hands. Naturally it is necessary to have the assistance of another when a large dog is being handled.

5. Small and medium-sized dogs may be sat on the knee of a RANA sitting on a chair with all four legs presented to the examiner. The animal's back is placed against the restrainer's chest, and the forelegs are grasped behind the elbow holding the legs in the extended position.

6. The administration of intravenous injections necessitates that the animal be held as still as is possible. Method 2 is recommended as being the best position with the patient in the sitting position. The dog's elbow is grasped in the palm of the right hand and the thumb passed over the radius to compress the vein (Fig. 2.4). Once the surgeon has entered the vein the pressure on the vein is released, but the leg is still steadied by the hand. Alternatively, a length of size 1 drainage tubing is wound around the foreleg above the elbow and the two ends are held in the right hand (Fig. 2.5). This raises the vein admirably, and in the small dog does not cover too much of it, whilst allowing the hand to maintain its restraining pressure on the flank and rear quarter. Once the vein has been entered, one end only is released. The

tourniquet method is recommended as being preferable to raising the vein with the thumb.

The holding of small dogs by the "scruff" of the neck has little to recommend it and in the presence of an owner is a poor advertisement, apart from the danger of luxating the eyeballs of some breeds.

7. Should it be necessary to administer an intramuscular injection to a relatively large and unruly dog, it may be carried out by the following method. A noose is passed over the dog's head and the free end is then passed through the bars of a cage or similar fixture. A hind leg may then be grasped to administer the injection while the animal is being pressed against the side of the cage (Fig. 2.6).

The Difficult Dog

Little has been said regarding the handling of obstreperous and vicious patients, and it will be appreciated that even to administer a sedative, the animal must generally be handled and the majority will not take anything hidden in food whilst they are in a strange environment.

Two points are most important: firstly, the patient must not be allowed to escape, and secondly, that those attending are not injured. Once a muzzle has been applied firmly most of the battle has been won. However, the application of that muzzle may be most hazardous. Should trouble be anticipated it is as well to have the owner affix two strong leads before the animal is admitted. This permits some restraint of the head by two operators pulling in opposing directions whilst a third attempts to apply the muzzle from the rear. Should an approach from behind not be successful the patient may be backed into a wall, and then approached from the front, whilst being restrained by two leads pulling in opposite directions. Two muzzles should be applied. The first should be of soft rope or cord, according to the size of the dog, as a tape tends to fold too easily when being dangled in front of the dog. This method is necessary as one may only hold the rope by its ends, because the operator's hands will be too close to the animal's jaw if the loop is held. Once the first muzzle has been applied a second tape muzzle may be applied in the routine manner.

The more vicious animals will necessitate resort to the dog catcher (Fig. 2.7). The dog catcher restrains the animal's head and enables it to be kept out of reach of the operator's person whilst an assistant applies the muzzle. It may also be used in conjunction with a lead or noose pulled in the opposite direction. Pressure on the noose should be eased slightly once the muzzle has been applied, so as not to cause distress and avoid the danger of choking the patient.

The Restraint of Cats

In general, cats require a slightly different approach to the dog. A firm, confident attitude is necessary as the cat will often adopt, on the approach of a stranger, an instinctive defensive posture, which looks alarming. This usually collapses once a hand is put confidently on the cat. However, the RANA should normally reassure the animal, before picking it up, by gently stroking the head and talking quietly.

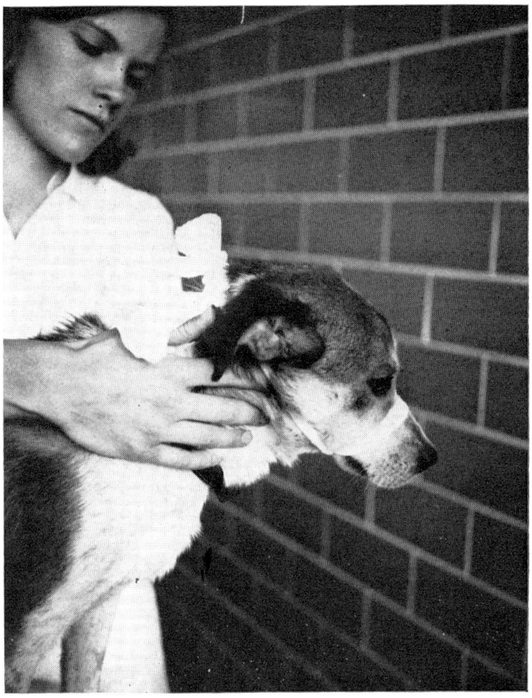

Fig. 2.1. Tape muzzle applied to "normal"-nosed dog.

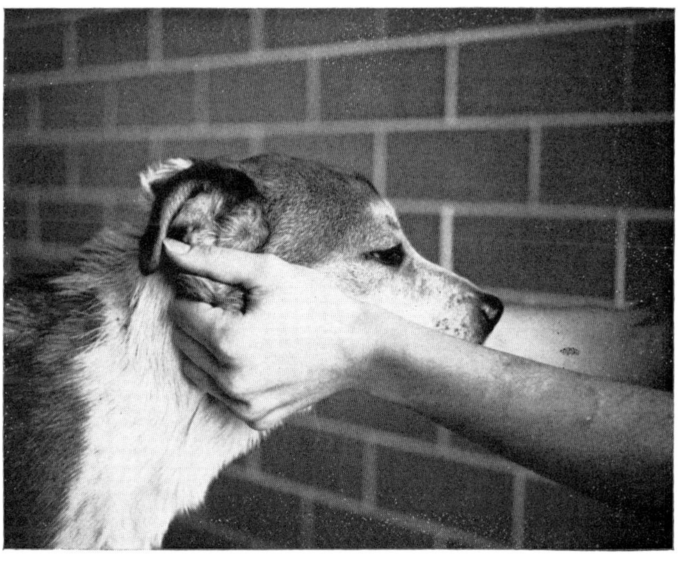

Fig. 2.3. Holding for examination—method (1).

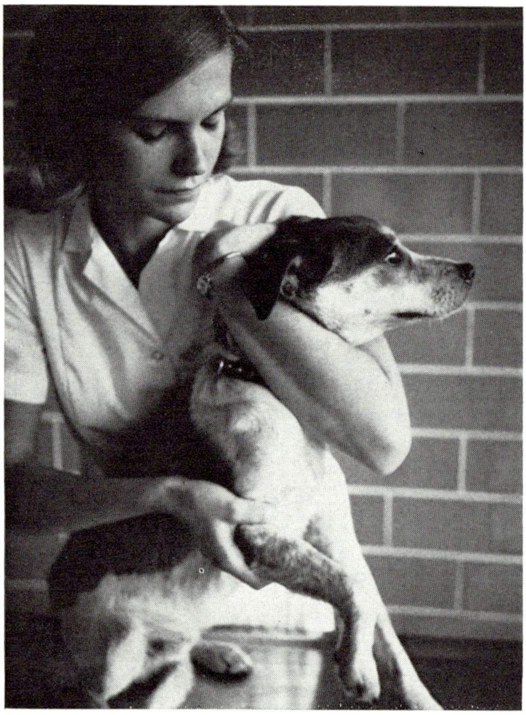

Fig. 2.4. Restraint for intravenous injection in forelimb.

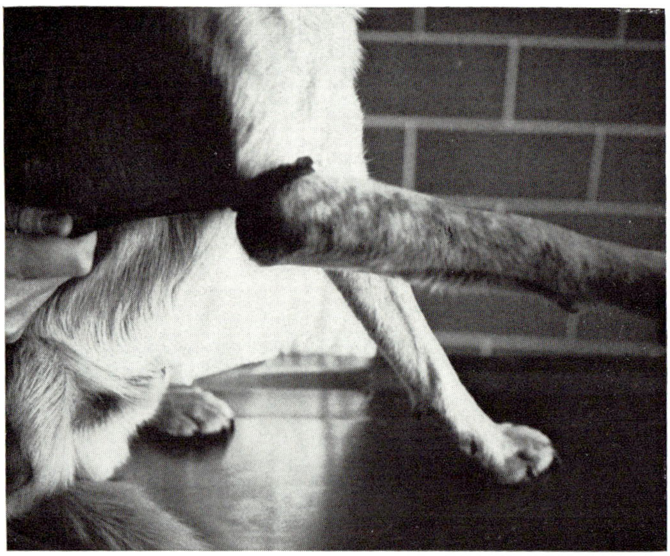

Fig. 2.5. Alternative restraint method for intravenous injection (to raise vein).

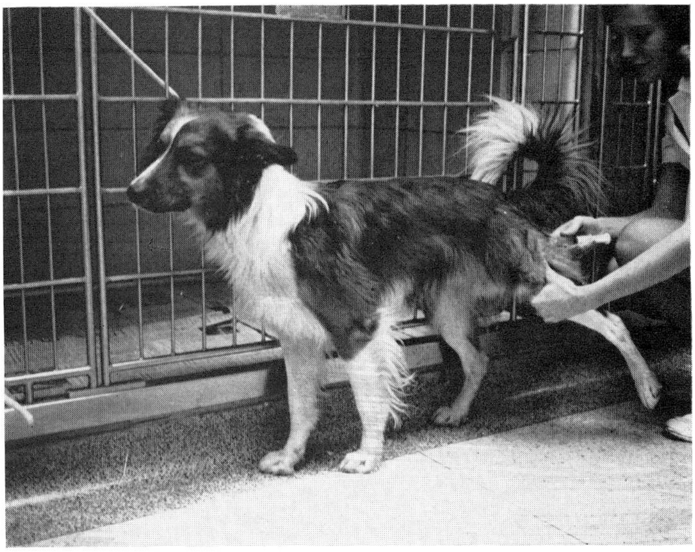

Fig. 2.6. Restraint method for intramuscular injection.

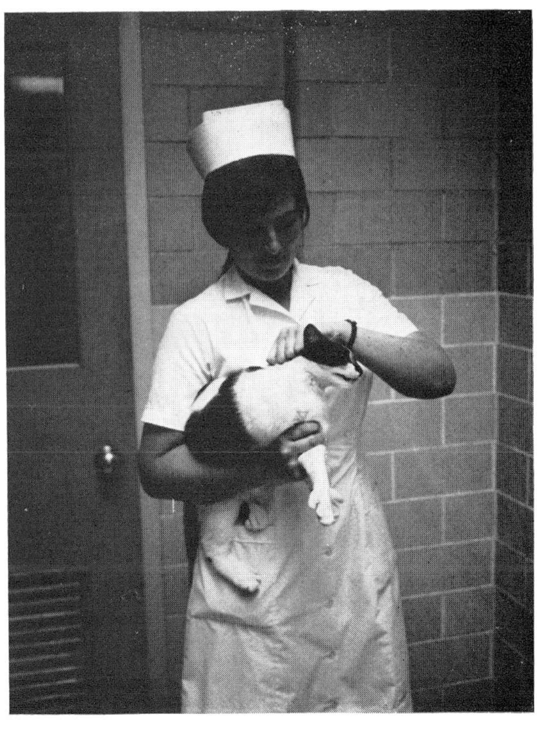

Fig. 2.8. Handling a cat prior to examination.

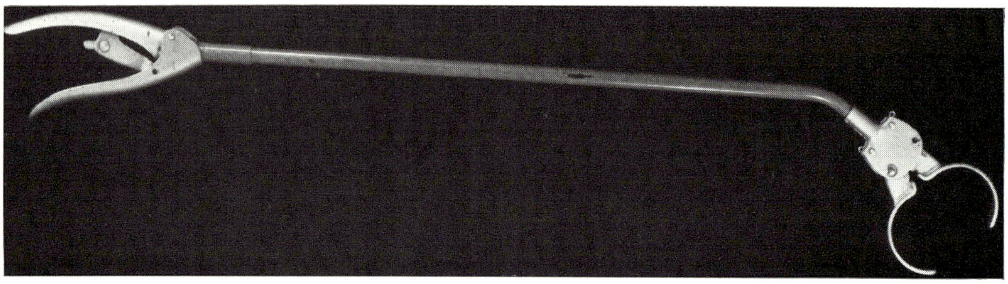

Fig. 2.9. A cat catcher. (By courtesy of Vestric Ltd.)

HANDLING

Once the RANA has decided that her patient is reasonably passive, the animal may be lifted by passing the arm over the chest and the hand under the sternum, with the other hand used to lightly grip the scruff of the neck. Alternatively, if the cat is being taken from a cage, it may be lifted by grasping both elbows from the front, and when free of the cage it is then tucked under one arm, with the hand holding the forelegs (Fig. 2.8). However, before a cat is removed from a basket or cage it is essential to ensure that all doors and windows are closed or are escape-proof. There is no more embarrassing situation than reporting to an owner that his pet has been lost, and there is no excuse for this. For the same reason a cat should only be moved from one room to another within a proper basket and not carried loose. Similarly,

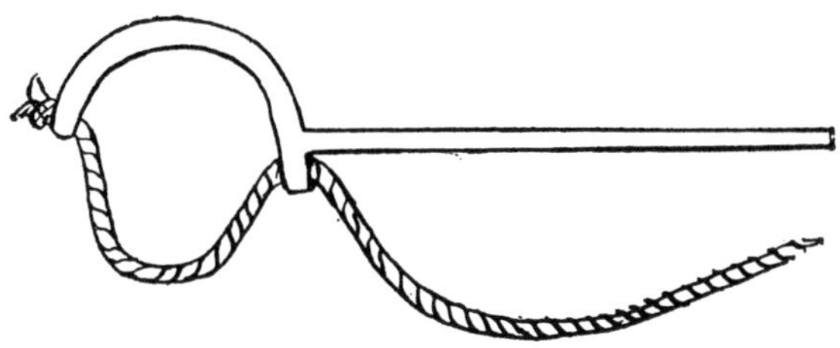

Fig. 2.7. The dog catcher.

the animal should be placed in a basket by the owner at reception, and not handed over to the RANA's arms. When a cat is to be removed from a basket the lid should be raised gently and if the animal does not appear to be vicious, the hand is slipped inside to hold the cat, before the lid is folded right back.

HOLDING FOR EXAMINATION AND MEDICATION

Five methods will be described.

1. The cat is placed on the examination table and one hand is slipped underneath the chin, and if necessary the other hand supports the rear.

2. Administration of intravenous injections may be effected in a similar manner to that used for the dog, the left hand holding the head and the right hand holding the far side foreleg or tourniquet, while the cat is held against the RANA's side by the forearm. Although it is common practice for cats to be held by the "scruff", many appear to resent this restraint far more than simply having the head held by a hand under the jaw. The RANA will decide on the most suitable method for the case in hand, as the more obstreperous will require seizing by the "scruff".

3. Should a cat resent examination of parts of the head and attempt to claw the operator's hand, a small towel may be held round the neck in the form of a bib. The cat's claws become caught in the towel when it tries to reach the operator. The method is not intended for a truly vicious animal, but is useful when the cat is a normal patient, but unused to having its mouth and ears examined.

4. Cats and kittens are commonly wrapped in a large thick towel when it is desired

to administer a local anaesthetic or dress a particular area, the area in question being left exposed. Great care should be taken that adequate ventilation exists via the head end of the roll. When a male cat is to be castrated, under local and not general anaesthesia, this method may be employed. The cat is held on its back within the roll, and the hind legs and tail are exposed. The legs are held by the hocks, the tail being tucked sideways under one of the restraining hands. The cat within the rolled towel is held between the RANA's forearms. In this manner the scrotal area is exposed to the operator for local anaesthetic administration and surgery.

5. The unruly cat may also be restrained inside a towel for intravenous administration, the head and one leg being exposed. The "scruff" is grasped in the left hand and the head is turned upwards whilst the right hand extends the right foreleg and keeps the towel tight enough to restrain the other legs. Pressure is also exerted by the forearm holding the animal into the RANA's side.

The Difficult Cat

Restraint of a truly vicious cat can present the RANA with a considerable problem as the animal bites quickly and uses all four sets of claws. Even if she is able to grasp the animal by the "scruff" it will still contort itself and succeed in striking with the hindleg claws.

A cat that is proving difficult within a basket or cage, may often be restrained by crowding it into a corner with a thick blanket when it may then be grasped by a hand through the blanket. The use of thick garden pruning gloves has much to recommend it when handling the difficult patient. Occasions do arise when it becomes necessary to resort to the use of a catcher.

Whenever a difficult cat is being handled it is most important to ensure that it is kept well away from both the RANA's and the surgeon's face as the truly wild animal will always attempt to inflict injury to the eyes and face.

Resulting from the experience of the use of tongs for handling mink, various patterns have been developed and are now marketed for the catching and restraint of excited and vicious cats (Fig. 2.9). While holding the animals firmly they do not cause any injury or unwarranted distress.

Restraint by Medication

Within this section on restraint of the dog and cat, no attempt has been made to deal with restraint by drugs, nor has the administration of medicaments been covered as these points will be dealt with in the appropriate sections elsewhere.

Tranquillizers of various types are now being used more often than hitherto. The advent of the newer phenothiazine derivatives and morphine-like narcotics, that are safe for cats, has made it possible to subdue vicious and frightened dogs and cats without the necessity of prolonged forceful restraint. This is to be encouraged, but under no circumstances should the RANA take it on herself to administer such a tranquillizer without the expressed instructions of a veterinarian. Given to patients suffering from a particular stress or disease, these drugs can have grave consequences.

(b) MANAGEMENT AND HYGIENE

C. E. Woodrow, MRCVS

Introduction

"Though employment in kennels would not qualify for trainee registration under the scheme, intending trainees would find a period of practical work in kennels an advantage to them before taking up employment that could qualify for trainee registration." *Animal Nursing Auxiliaries Guide 1970*, published by the Royal College of Veterinary Surgeons, 32 Belgrave Square, London S.W.1.

This advice is reprinted here as the most fitting introduction to this section and to stress the benefit which can be gained by intending trainees who have not reached the entry age of 17 years by taking employment in good kennels, and for those who are still working for their three O-levels in the GCE (English Language, Physical or Biological Science or Mathematics, any other subject) by seeking temporary work in kennels during their holidays. They will learn a great deal of practical basic knowledge which they may not get a further opportunity of acquiring; such things as the handling of dogs, their feeding, exercise and grooming requirements, kennel hygiene and the recognition of the various breeds and their characteristics. They will also begin to recognize the signs of good health and to develop that invaluable sense, part experience and part instinct, of being able to spot the first indications of any departure from normal.

Housing

This may be conveniently divided into three sections, domestic, kennel and hospital.

DOMESTIC

A general knowledge of the optimum conditions for keeping domestic dogs is desirable as this is a subject on which advice is so often sought from lay staff. Primarily, both for the convenience of the owner and the contentment of the dog every house dog should have its own quarters or bed. Right from the start a puppy should be provided with such a bed and trained to go to it on command. It is due to the failure of the owner to provide such a bed or weakness in insisting on its use that so many dogs are found to be sleeping on chairs in the living rooms and on beds in the bedrooms. Such practice should be avoided at all times—it is to say the least unhygienic, frequently causes a stress relationship or even disruption between husband and wife, and is an imposition on visitors and friends. A dog must have its own bed in a fixed position to which it can be ordered to retire during meals, when visitors arrive and always at night. This bed may well be in the living room or kitchen. A dog is such a creature of habit and fundamentally requires to have a bed of its own for security that there should be no difficulty in the initial training. So many new owners start well, but fail to insist after a few days either through misplaced or mistaken sympathy or from sheer exasperation in coping with the noise a new puppy will always produce when left by itself at night. This problem is, of course, accentuated in urban areas and particularly in flats through fear of disturbing the neighbours. However, persistence is essential and there are some aids such as leaving a light on for a few nights, the presence of a loud ticking clock near the dog's bed, the giving of a dose of a soluble aspirin (e.g. Disprin) late in the evening and firmness in forcing the puppy into its bed continuously. Such measures usually have only to be continued for two or three nights. When such are insufficient it may be necessary to choose an inside room for a few nights when noise is less likely to carry through windows or doors.

A small puppy may be shut in a travelling basket at night, which is effective both in preventing scratching at doors and also in "house training", as even a newly weaned puppy will avoid soiling its own bed if possible.

The actual bed to be provided will depend on the size of the dog and its location, but ideally should be of the steel frame with stretched canvas type. Baskets make poor beds for any dog—impossible to clean thoroughly, a fine jungle for flea breeding, and a constant inducement to chewing and the encouragement of destructive habits. One folded blanket is all the cover required, which is easy to shake out, wash or replace. Such a blanket can be used for the larger dog either folded in a fixed corner of the floor area or in a low wooden box.

Obviously the location must be carefully chosen both for the owner's convenience, in a corner, under a table out of the way, and for freedom from draughts. When such a location is well chosen in living room or kitchen there is no need to provide any additional heating at night even in winter in a house without central heating.

KENNELS

To consider the full range and construction of kennelling would require a whole book to itself and it therefore presents a problem on the best presentation. The author has decided to consider in some detail what is perhaps the optimum so that the reader, be he student, nurse, lay or professional, may adopt from such a description methods of construction and management best suited to his own requirements and available space.

An excellent basic or starting point for such is to consider the requirements of the Ministry of Agriculture for the construction, maintenance and management of quarantine kennels. Most of these requirements are equally desirable in any other type of kennel whether boarding, breeding, research, greyhound, etc.

QUARANTINE KENNELS

Quarantine regulations are designed to ensure that every dog entering this country will be held for 6 calendar months in a kennel which is under the daily supervision of a veterinary surgeon (*sic*) and which is so constructed that it is quite unable to escape and that no nose or paw contact is possible at any time with any other dog either in quarantine or outside the quarantine compounds.

To satisfy these regulations the following are basic requirements:

(a) *Licences* for quarantine kennels are granted by the Ministry of Agriculture only to veterinary surgeons. Such veterinary surgeons may own the kennel or by contract be employed by a lay owner or company to visit the kennels every week-day. In the latter case he is still the only person recognized by the Ministry of Agriculture as being in charge and is solely responsible to the Ministry. Daily supervision of all dogs and the day-to-day management are thus assured and all required returns of arrivals, departures, health, etc., are his personal responsibility. While such close inspection is desirable for the early recognition of disease or errors in feeding and management, the Ministry of Agriculture is primarily interested in the early detection of any symptoms suspicious of rabies.

(b) *Escape-proof.* The only entrance to any block of quarantine kennels must be through a safety cage, i.e. a "lock" consisting of two doors both opening inwards and so arranged that one door may be closed before the second door is opened.

(c) *The exercise yards* within such a quarantine block or compound must be surrounded by a fence at least 10 ft high, or 6 ft if provided with a jumping guard at the top of the fence, sloping inwards at 45° from the vertical and at least 2 ft wide. This fence must either be of solid construction, i.e. breeze or concrete blocks or corrugated steel sheet, or if of wire mesh must be double with a space of 6–12 in. between the two fences. All doors or gates to these exercise yards must also be solid and must open inwards.

(d) *The individual kennels* must be constructed of "bite-proof" materials, e.g. cement, brick, rendered blocks of breeze or concrete or steel, closed in by the roof or netting over the top, and with doors or gates opening inwards, and so constructed that no dog can push his nose or paw through and so be at risk of such parts being bitten by any passing dog in the passage way. Earlier quarantine regulations specified that such doors should be solid to 3 ft 6 in. high but these are now modified to allow a suitably spaced and tough mesh to be used to floor level. A dog confined in a solid doored kennel and unable to see out is constantly jumping to look through the window or mesh in the upper part of the door. Extending the visibility to floor level keeps the inmates much happier and is now the usual construction in recent quarantine kennels. "The Ministry of Agriculture recommends certain sizes for the individual compartments or living quarters. In single-tiered compartments the height should be not less than 6 ft; width $1\frac{1}{2}$ times the length of the dog (the length of the dog to be measured from tip of nose to root of tail): length twice the length of the dog with minimum floor area of 12 ft^2 with no one dimension less than 3 ft. For toy breeds two-tiered compartments may be used of similar dimensions to those recommended for cats (see below under "Quarantine Catteries")."

Provided that such basic requirements as those outlined above are met in full a licence is issued by the Ministry of Agriculture to the veterinary surgeon in control and only to him, and such licence may be revoked at any time for breach of the regulations even by a lay owner or lay staff.

To pass on to construction and materials in more detail:

Inside floors. Here, the primary requirement is impermeability and ease of cleaning. Simplest and cheapest is concrete which, if properly laid and surface cured, is reasonably dust-proof, easily cleaned and will resist erosion from urine for 10 years. Modern surface finishes allow of colouring and can be sealed by the occasional application of suitable sealing compounds. More attractive, but at greater cost, are terrazzo finishes and exposed aggregate in which coloured stones are used in the surface level and the whole ground down after curing to expose the pleasant and varied colours of the aggregate.

One stage further is the covering of the concrete base with various tiles. It is unfortunate that no thermoplastic cork or rubber tile or its bonding can withstand the chemical action of urine and faeces. Quite pleasant concrete tiles are now available which are reasonably inexpensive, but suffer from the same eventual wearing and pitting as the cement floor. The only advantage, therefore, of a good appearance cannot be justified. Ceramic and quarry tiles are impervious, easily laid and are everlasting. The former, while having a better appearance, are ruled out by cost leaving the quarry tiles as the only satisfactory solution. They will resist all attacks by urine and faeces, are extremely hard wearing and are easily cleaned. Asphalt floors are one alternative to concrete but neither in cost or appearance show any real advantage. Composition floors such as magnesite are expensive and doubtful in their resistant properties, particularly in damp conditions.

Finally, wood floors are a thing of a past and nearly forgotten age, and should remain so!

Walls. Here the choice is greater and is largely governed by cost. Brick, rendered breeze or concrete blocks are, perhaps, the materials of choice. Reasonable in cost, the appearance is good and easily kept clean if the rendering is smooth and finally painted with emulsion paint. Asbestos cement panels are easily installed and cheap but are probably still too brittle. Partitions of walls made of plaster board with a float plaster finish are quickly and easily built but are a constant invitation to the dog which is bored by 6 months confinement to chew and gnaw, and once started impossible to stop, and are examples to any new inmate to follow.

Steel is used in some quarantine kennels but unless galvanized or of an inordinate thickness, rusts and erodes too rapidly. However, steel sheets in a variety of profiles are now available which are galvanized and plastic coated at the rolling mills. These coatings are very hard wearing and retain their surface and colour for a number of years. They are easily cleaned with suitable detergents and require no repainting. Complete prefabricated kennel units may shortly be available using such modern materials throughout.

Stainless steel and fibreglass are both excellent materials for the walls of kennels but must usually be ruled out from the question of cost.

Glass panels make a good wall, with good appearance, greatest ease of cleaning, freedom from any painting or maintenance and at a reasonable cost. Ample strength is available in the various wired cast glasses available and such sheets can be of any required size. They also give added light to kennels which, by their position in relation to available windows, would otherwise be too dark.

Doors. The earlier requirement of doors solid to 3 ft 6 in. having ceased, probably the best door is one of a welded steel angle frame covered with a suitable wire mesh. Any form of wire netting or chain link is either too weak or has too wide a mesh to be nose- and paw-proof. There are now available welded steel rectangular meshes of high tensile steel wires welded at every crossing point.

Wooden doors may be used if they are protected on the inside and to a reasonable height with sheet steel to prevent chewing. Such doors may have a panel of the welded rectangular mesh let into the lower half to ensure adequate ventilation and visibility for the dog inside to look out without jumping, and a glass panel above to give more light to the kennel and to enable attendants to see into the kennels. All doors must, of course, open inwards to lessen the chance of a dog bolting out when opened.

Benches. In spite of the constant wastage of wooden benches through chewing, they are probably the most economic and practicable. Dry and warm if raised a few inches from the floor they are easily removed for cleaning, repair or renewal, if necessary. Alternatives are canvas or moulded glass fibre beds with a blanket but much will depend on the type of heating—if any—installed in the kennels.

Exercise yards. These must be sited within the quarantine compound, i.e. within the double entrance gates. A minimum of 400 ft^2 is suggested and, while the ideal is one exercise yard to each individual kennel, considerations of cost and space usually make this impracticable. It is usual to find some four to six kennels sharing in turn one exercise yard. The fencing must be 10 ft high or 6 ft if provided with a jumping rail as explained above. The fence itself may be solid or of chain link. If the latter, it must be double with sufficient gap between the two to prevent any nose or paw access either to a dog in the next run or to any dog that may be outside the perimeter of the quarantine compound. In new construction and where space allows, the gap between a double fence should be wide enough to allow access for brushing down. Again, all doors or gates must open inwards and such an exercise yard is completely escape-proof.

Floors of exercise yards. As adequate hosing and washing down of any exercise yard which is shared by a number of dogs is a daily essential, only concrete or asphalt covering can be considered. Unfortunately, one of the most usual criticisms of quarantine kennels by owners is the bare concrete exercise yard, "the prison yard". They would, of course, prefer grass and so would the dog to scratch up. However it is easy to convince them of the erosion of such a grass plot—hopelessly insanitary and odiferous in summer, equally insanitary and a quagmire in winter! A compromise may be seen in some quarantine kennels where a small amount of grass is maintained in the centre of the run with a paved, concrete or asphalted path round the fences, where most dogs tend to empty themselves. Otherwise grass runs or paddocks must be sufficiently large to prevent the ground from becoming unduly fouled or trodden.

Drains. In older kennels, one still sees the practice inherited from stables of providing drains to the kennels inside the buildings, but such drains are not necessary and are not installed in most modern kennels. Cleaning does not involve hosing down which would make the floors too wet, but the use of mop-buckets. In the concreted runs, however, which should be hosed down daily the provision of drains is essential and the levels should be graded to a natural fall to each drain trap.

Quarantine Catteries

The Ministry of Agriculture in its "Welfare Standard for approved quarantine premises for canines and felines" recommend that the indoor cages should not be in more than two tiers. As regards size of cages where additional exercise areas are provided, they should have a minimum height of 3 ft, and a minimum floor area of 12 ft^2 with no one dimension less than 3 ft. Where exercise areas are not provided, the cage should have a minimum height of 6 ft, and a minimum floor area of 15 ft^2 with no one dimension less than 3 ft.

New Quarantine Regulations

As a result of the occurrence of rabies in three dogs during 1969 from one quarantine kennel, one of which developed rabies at Camberley shortly after its release at the end of 6 months quarantine, the Minister of Agriculture made an order on 4 December 1969 extending the quarantine period to 8 months. This was followed early in 1970 by a further case in a dog at Newmarket which had been released from quarantine 3 months earlier, i.e. after an incubation period of at least 9 months.

On 6 March 1970 the Minister set up a Committee of Inquiry under the chairmanship of Mr. Ronald Waterhouse, QC, with terms of reference "To enquire into the precautions and policy against rabies in Great Britain and to make recommendations". At the same time the quarantine period was extended to 12 months for all those dogs and cats undergoing quarantine and a complete ban was imposed on the further importation of dogs and cats.

On 17 August 1970 the Waterhouse Committee published its interim report to be followed 10 days later by a new set of regulations from the Ministry of Agriculture governing the importation and quarantining of dogs and cats.

(a) All dogs and cats in quarantine which had completed 9 months were released on 7 September 1970. The remainder were vaccinated against rabies and released when they had reached the 9-month period.

(b) On 16 September 1970 resumption of imports of dogs and cats were permitted.

(c) All new imports of dogs and cats must be vaccinated on arrival with an inactivated rabies vaccine with a further vaccination after 28 days.

(d) During the first 14 days after arrival, dogs and cats must occupy one group of kennels and have access only either to individual exercise yards or to one or two yards set aside exclusively for them.

(d) The quarantine period has now reverted to 6 months.

(e) There are numerous other changes affecting the daily routine within a quarantine kennel, such as the retention throughout the period of the same sleeping compartment and exercise yard by the same dog, the provision of washing-up facilities in each quarantine block for all bowls and utensils used in that block. Kennel staff are required to keep to one block throughout any one day and must wear protective clothing and boots and should wash or disinfect their hands before leaving that block using a non-irritating disinfectant such as Roccal. For general kennel disinfection, certain disinfectants are specified, i.e. those having maximum effect on the viruses, e.g. those which in suitable dilution will give 2% available chlorine.

(f) No boarders, either dogs or cats, may be allowed in quarantine blocks, and dogs and cats which have completed their 6 months' quarantine must be moved out at once. Where quarantine kennels also board dogs and cats, the boarding premises must be quite separate from the quarantine with their own kitchen utensils and ancillary services. As far as possible, kennel staff must be kept each day either on quarantine or on boarding.

These are the main changes at the time of going to press based on the interim report and there may well be further changes as a result of the final report. These changes are based on a premise which has been accepted by the Committee that there is a possibility, however remote, that rabies can also be carried by indirect or airborne infection, as well as the hitherto only known direct infection by bite or scratch. The vaccination on arrival and the complete isolation during the first 14 days is directed at ensuring that all animals entering quarantine shall be protected against such indirect infection during their stay. It seems unlikely therefore that there will be any change either in the duration of quarantine (6 months) or in the vaccination procedure. Any further radical alterations will be in the field of kennel construction to ensure more adequate isolation. If it were possible to rebuild all the forty-odd quarantine kennels, there is little doubt that they would have to be constructed on the principle of individual exercise yards to each sleeping compartment, but such a course is impracticable from the point of view of both cost and space. At least for a number of years some acceptable compromise will have to be attained.

BOARDING KENNELS

In general, the nearer the design of boarding kennels to the requirements described above for quarantine kennels the safer and more easily managed they will be, as, for example, the provision of double entrance gates and concrete exercise yards with jumping guards. The general specifications of floors, walls, exercise yards and drains should still apply. The high standards demanded for quarantine may be relaxed, however, in one or two ways. Nose- and paw-proof kennel fronts are unnecessary and inward-opening kennel doors, which are somewhat difficult to work in kennel cleaning, may now open outwards.

The Animal Boarding Establishments Act

This Act which came into force on 1 January 1964 makes all boarding kennels with certain exceptions subject to licensing by the local authority. The local authority is required to satisfy itself that certain conditions are fulfilled before granting or renewing such a licence. The conditions are set out below and following each is a summary of the interpretations suggested by the British Veterinary Association.

(a) Animals will at all times be kept in accommodation suitable in respect of construction, size of quarters, number of occupants, exercising facilities, temperature, lighting, ventilation and cleanliness.

It is not possible to lay down any exact dimensions as regards either sleeping quarters or exercise yards, as boarding establishments vary in their method of keeping dogs. Where wooden individual kennels are used, these kennels should be raised from the ground, be provided with a sloping roof which is completely waterproof, be of sufficient size for the dog to stand up and turn round comfortably, and should open on to an exercise area. If the dog has access to this exercise area at all times during the day there need be no window in such a kennel, but there should be adequate ventilation for such times as the kennel door is shut. Where, however, the dog does not have access at all times to an exercise area, there should be a window or door opening protected by bars or other form of strong mesh allowing the dog to look out during such time as it is shut in the kennel. Where kennels are constructed within a building there will not normally be continuous access to exercise areas, and here, either the kennel door shall be so constructed as to enable the dog to see out at all times, or a similar window opening provided. Partitions between kennels should be solid so as to prevent dogs from attempting to fight their neighbours and to lessen the spread of air-borne infection. Material used for kennel construction should, wherever possible, be capable of disinfection, and the physical construction of the kennels should be such that they are easily cleansed and have the minimum area for the lodgment of dust and dust particles where parasites may multiply.

Catteries. With regard to the provision of boarding cages for cats, these should be of such a size as to allow the cat to stretch full length both horizontally and vertically. The cages should have a height of not less than 1 ft 10 in. and should be separated from each other by solid partitions to lessen the spread of infectious disease. Such partitions and the floors (also constructed of impervious material) must be adequately maintained and readily cleanable. Each cage should be provided with a clean sanitary pan. There should be an exercise area available to each cage not less than 8 ft^2. This should be made escape proof and the building in which the cages are housed should be similarly escape proof through all doors, windows and other openings.

Number of occupants. This will be most difficult of interpretation, as during the height of the boarding season many boarding kennels double up their occupants or may house several dogs in one kennel. It is suggested that the local authority, in examination of the register required under section (e), should bear this in mind and satisfy itself that there is no overcrowding.

Lighting. Where kennels are constructed within a building it is suggested that there should be a minimum standard of natural daylight; but where this daylight is insufficient, adequate and suitable artificial light should be provided to allow the proper working and cleaning of the kennels. No suggestions can be made regarding temperature as experience has shown that even extreme cold will not seriously affect dogs or cats provided that they have a warm dry bed in a position free from draughts.

Ventilation. Provision should be made for the adequate ventilation of the individual kennels as well as the room in which they are contained, and there should be reasonable facilities for insulation so that the building and kennels can be kept reasonably cool in the summer and not too cold in the winter.

Cleanliness. It is suggested that the inspector should satisfy himself that both kennels and exercise yards are regularly cleaned every day including Sunday, and that bedding is changed at least once a week. Kennels should be disinfected at every change of occupant and new bedding provided. Adequate arrangements should be made for the disposal of excreta, sawdust and soiled bedding, preferably by burning. Kennels and exercise yards should be kept free from vermin, and the regular routine use of an efficient antiparasitic preparation is recommended.

(b) Animals will be adequately supplied with suitable food, drink and bedding material, adequately exercised and so far as necessary visited at suitable intervals.

Owing to the variation in feeding methods at boarding kennels, e.g. type of meat or offal used, raw or cooked, biscuits fed dry or soaked, tinned foods, etc., no standards can be laid down. This can be left only to the discretion and good sense of the inspector.

Storage of foods. Provision should be made for storage bins for dry food which are mouse- and rat-proof. As regards drink, it should be a minimum requirement that each kennel has a clean water bowl, scrubbed daily, and kept filled with clean water available to the dog at all times. Communal water bowls within exercise yards should not be permitted. Suitable washing-up arrangements should be provided for the daily cleansing of all feed bowls.

Bedding materials. During the summer months, or in kennels where heating is provided during the winter, canvas beds, blankets, sacks or newspaper are permissible, but during winter months where no heating is provided beds should be of deep straw or wood-wool.

Exercise. It is suggested that the inspector should satisfy himself that dogs are visited, and exercised either on a lead or within exercise yards twice daily.

(c) All reasonable precautions will be taken to prevent and control the spread among animals of infectious or contagious diseases, including the provision of adequate isolation facilities.

Many small boarding kennels are not in a position to prevent or control the spread of infectious or contagious diseases. The proprietors of such kennels often believe themselves to be adept at home treatment and do not seek the advice of a veterinary surgeon or practitioner. It is suggested that in determining whether a licence should be granted, the local authority should require the proprietor to make arrangements with a local veterinary surgeon or practitioner to attend the kennel if the proprietor has any suspicion of infectious or contagious disease among the inmates, and the onus should be placed on him to seek veterinary advice immediately. In this section the provision of adequate isolation facilities is included, although there was strong pressure during the course of the Bill through Parliament for the removal of the clause. Boarding being very much of a seasonal business it would be unreasonable to expect kennels to maintain separate isolation premises empty at all times, and even where such premises are provided it is certain that during the peak period they will be used for normal boarders. It is suggested, therefore, that it may be left to the visiting veterinary surgeon, when called to any case of suspected infectious or contagious disease, to arrange for certain isolated kennels to be used at that time.

(d) Appropriate steps will be taken for the protection of the animals in the case of fire or other emergency.

The local authority should insist on the provision of adequate fire extinguishers at points throughout the kennels where the fire risk is greatest, i.e. in wooden buildings. Such fire extinguishers should be kept in a position outside the buildings where they are immediately available to anyone working in the kennels, and these fire extinguishers should be regularly tested every year by manufacturers or their accredited agents and inspected from time to time by the Chief Fire Prevention Officer. Where no staff is resident immediately adjacent to the kennels a notice should be displayed in a prominent position stating where the keys are obtainable.

(e) A register will be kept containing a description of any animal received into the establishment, date of arrival and departure, and the name and address of owner, such register to be available for inspection at all times by an officer of the local authority, veterinary surgeon or veterinary practitioner authorized under this Act.

Where possible the inspector should arrange for frequent visits during the months of July, August and September, i.e. during the peak period, to check on overcrowding and the proper maintenance of the boarding register.

VENTILATION, LIGHTING AND HEATING

Here the problems are common to all types of kennels and may be considered together.

Ventilation and lighting. In view of the wide variety of kennel buildings it is not possible to lay down any clearly defined standards. One can only say that ventilation and lighting should be adequate. Theoretically, low inlets for fresh air with high outlets for stale air are desirable but most buildings will rely on the opening or closing of windows. Where such ventilation is insufficient to ensure clean air in the building, it may be possible to insert air bricks in the walls and air vents in the roof. Where these are impossible, an electric extractor fan placed in one of the windows is a reasonable and efficient means of improving the ventilation and is readily controllable to suit conditions of air temperature and freshness. Care should be taken to see that the position of fresh-air inlets will not cause draughts at floor level.

Much the same applies to natural lighting—it should be, but often is not, adequate to allow easy working of all floor areas even during winter months. It is usually a case of take it as you find it and it may only be possible to supplement insufficient natural lighting with artificial. However, the more frequent use of white paint within the kennels and on the face of any occluding outside walls will often make a surprising difference.

Artificial lighting. In view of the strange ideas many people seem to have of the cost of electric lighting it is necessary rather to overstress this matter—a single 100-watt bulb will burn for 10 hours for the consumption of one unit of electricity which in most areas now costs about 1p, or ten 100-watt bulbs will burn for 1 hour for the same consumption. Therefore, there is no reason to be "cheese-paring" in the provision of lighting—ensure adequate light for every part of the working area. Such lighting may be by the ordinary gas-filled bulbs or by fluorescent lighting. Although more expensive to install, the saving in running costs and the better distribution of light makes the use of fluorescent tubes in 4-ft or 5-ft lengths a sensible and practical investment.

Heating. Here we are on more difficult ground—always a controversial subject—fundamentally, because the standards of heating required by the owner are quite different from those required by the dog. Much of the heating installed in kennels is really for the benefit of the kennel owner and staff—and the owners of the dog inmates—and is unnecessary for the dog itself. It is a fact that no reasonable amount of cold will hurt a dog provided that it has a good bed in a dry position free from draughts. It is only rarely during an English winter that any heating is really necessary, but it is difficult to persuade the owners of a boarding dog of this, and the change from a central-heated flat to a non-heated boarding kennel is sometimes too drastic for the smaller dog.

Heating may best be dealt with under two headings.

1. Temporary heating which is only brought into use during cold spells.
2. Continuous "central" heating available throughout the year and contolled by air thermostats.

In the first category there is a wide choice of heaters.

(i) Electric radiant fires which are perhaps the least satisfactory because of the limited area warmed by radiation and the fire risk—too hot locally.

(ii) Electric convectors which produce a better distribution of heat and are safe to contact.

(iii) Electric blower heaters where convection is assisted by fans. These are probably the best solution for the rapid and widespread raising of the temperature in kennels as a temporary basis for extra cold weather.
(iv) Electric infra-red heaters usually installed near the roof but really more suitable for permanent installation than for emergency use.
(v) Oil convector heaters of many types. In spite of the obvious fire hazard the use of these heaters in kennels is probably more usual than of any other type. If their use is confined to cold spells, if these are of the modern type to British Standards specification and if they are placed in a position free from draughts and from any possibility of contact by dogs, they are allowable, cheap to install and run, and most efficient.

Central heating. As in this country the last few years has seen a rapid expansion in domestic central heating, so we shall see more kennels similarly equipped. The cost of installation and running has already reached a stage where it becomes an economical possibility and this has been largely brought about by two recent developments. The first is in the field of hot-water circulation from oil- or gas-fired or solid-fuel boilers where the use of a small electric circulating pump has reduced the size of pipes required to $\frac{1}{2}$–$\frac{3}{4}$ in. copper with no problems of gradients as in the use of large-bore pipes for natural circulation; easily installed they may be run unobtrusively on the surface. The second development is in the supply by the various electricity boards of cheap "off-peak" electricity. The off-peak electricity which is provided during the night hours has to be used for heating an area which will store the heat and release it slowly during the day. In new construction special heating wires can be laid in the concrete sub-floors. Sub-floor heating is reasonably cheap to install in new kennel floors and the running costs are competitive with other forms of heating. There are, however, some factors which need careful evaluation even in new constructions as between water-circulated central heating and electric sub-floor heating. There are problems of providing a sufficient area of sub-floor concrete to store sufficient heat to cope with a kennel building which requires good ventilation and doors which are constantly opened during working hours. Secondly, the heating cables should preferably be laid under the bed section of kennel only, to avoid the problem of the rapid drying and evaporation of urine during the night hours and the consequent ammoniacal smell, but such an arrangement may not provide sufficient storage area.

The latest development in storage heating is the appearance on the market of free-standing heaters which heat up during off-peak periods and release their stored heat slowly during the day. Such heating is more flexible than sub-floor heating and can be installed in existing buildings.

In a textbook of this sort one can only outline the methods available so that the reader is made aware of the possibilities and range, and has then sufficient general knowledge to discuss the subject intelligently with interested kennel owners or examiners.

Before leaving the subject of electric lighting and heating there is a warning which cannot be overstressed and which should be thoroughly appreciated by all who work in kennels or with any electric appliances in surgeries or hospitals. Electric supply is now universally at 230/240 volts and of the two wires, one is neutral at earth potential and the other live at 230/240 volts above. There is, therefore, a return path for the live main not only to neutral but also to earth through any earthed metal, e.g. water pipes or to the floor where this is made of concrete, tiles or any non-insulating material, most particularly when wet. There is, therefore, the possibility of a return path by contact with the live main through the body to the feet and so to earth and this may well be fatal. Hence the strict regulations laid down for the wiring of bathrooms and the provision of safe switches and outlet points. All electric appliances such as hairdriers, sterilizers, centrifuges, clippers, heaters, drills, etc., are today fitted with three wires, red for the live main, black for the neutral, and green for earthing the metal casing of the appliance. In the new wiring code following continental practice and now appearing in many electric appliances, these colours have been changed to brown for the live main, blue for neutral and green and yellow stripe for earth. No portable appliance should ever be joined up to a plug or used unless this third earth wire is connected—never use a two-pin plug. Then, in the event of a fault developing in the appliance which allows the live wire to touch the metal casing or frame, the fuse will blow instead of such casing becoming live to earth and a lethal weapon. However, there are exceptions to this rule in that a number of portable appliances are now supplied with double insulated high impact plastic cases which may be safely used on a two-wire system with no earth.

It follows from the above that all outlet points in kennels, surgeries, hospitals and work-rooms must be three-pin with an earthed connection and preferably shrouded. Where staff have to work in old or temporary premises where only two-pin points or even lamp-holder outlets are available, they should wear rubber boots on solid floors to insulate themselves from any earth return through the feet.

Bedding. For boarding or other kennels as distinct from hospital kennels the choice of bedding is limited to straw, wood-wool or blankets. Blankets are only suitable during summer or in central-heated kennels and the choice between wood-wool and straw is one of price. Only good clean wheat or oat straw should be used. During the warmer months a good bed can be made from sacks lightly stuffed with straw and then sewn up at the mouth. This makes a comfortable palliasse and saves much work in keeping the kennel clean.

Water supply. In spite of many arguments as to the cost of individual water bowls in kennels and the tendency to cause damp floors, experience has clearly shown that such individual bowls are one of the essential preventions of the spread of infection caused by common water troughs in the exercise yards. Each kennel should have its own bowl with a wide heavy base to avoid spilling, and these bowls must be regularly and thoroughly cleansed every day. No common bowls or troughs need or should then be provided in the exercise yards.

Feed bowls. Here, the same requirements of individual bowls which must be kept scrupulously clean, even if not sterilized, to avoid spread of disease. A great deal of time is taken up in a conscientious kennel in "washing-up" and much of this time and labour can be saved by the use of disposable dishes. These dishes which are made of waxed paper or compressed fibre are only economic in the smaller sizes, i.e. up to the size of terrier or Dachshund. Above this there is a disproportionate rise in cost and the usual enamelled or steel bowls must be used. Most plastic bowls are too brittle and can be a hazard to dogs chewing them and swallowing broken pieces. With the rapid developments in plastic, however, more bowls are becoming available in high impact plastics which are suitable for all but the confirmed chewer. The disposable bowls are burnt after use while the larger bowls may be sterilized sufficiently by washing in warm water with the inclusion of a suitable disinfectant detergent.

Cleaning of kennels and exercise yards. Exercise yards, which should be provided with a surface drain, are readily cleaned by daily hosing after the collection of all excreta (faeces) by spade and bucket.

Kennels are best cleaned by removing firstly any excreta, followed by brushing out if sawdust is used and finally mopping with a suitable disinfectant in the standard mop-bucket. Two points of importance should be noted here—firstly, that the disinfectant must not be too strong—adhere closely to the instructions or even use on the *weak* side. Kennelled dogs seem particularly susceptible to most disinfectant solutions and soon show a mild to moderate conjunctivitis if at all strong. Secondly, great care must be taken in mopping the kennel floor as dry as possible—some kennels even go as far as dusting out with sawdust and a final brushing out to absorb the very last of the disinfectant and leave the floor almost dry.

Bed boards should be lifted every day and the floor below swept. Straw or wood-wool bedding should be changed completely once a week and shaken out well every day.

HOSPITAL KENNELS

The requirements here are somewhat different from those of boarding kennels in that they are occupied for a short time only and the primary consideration, therefore, is ease of cleaning rather than space. Modern hospital or holding kennels are usually made of glazed tiles, stainless steel or fibreglass with doors of steel mesh. These are all readily cleaned by scrubbing down with detergent or soap and are entirely reliable for post-operative asepsis.

Bedding for these "cages" are blankets or newspaper. Heating is essential here and may well be by electric convector or infra-red heaters. Such holding or hospital cages are often, through limitations of space, installed in small rooms or basements and ample artificial lighting, preferably by fluorescent tubes, should be provided. Adequate air circulation and ventilation can best be assured by electric extractor fans.

KENNEL HYGIENE

Cleaning. The cleaning of kennels, exercise yards and feeding bowls has been dealt with earlier and it remains to consider the care of kitchen, cooking, disposal of refuse, and the special cases of infectious disease and parasitic infection.

Kitchen and cooking. The section on the feeding of dogs will show the desirability of feeding cooked foods and the kennel kitchen should therefore be provided not only with sink and hot water but also with suitable cooking arrangements for dealing with bulk meat. The ideal kitchen should have a refrigerator or deep-freeze to store the fresh meat, a cutting block and sharp carving knives, an electric or gas boiler and a power mincer.

The meat should only be lightly cooked and the hot stock used for soaking the meal or broken biscuit. While this is soaking, the meat can be minced and the whole feed well mixed and blended. It should be fed at once so that the warm meaty smell whets the appetite of the more choosy feeders. No such mixed food should be fed the next day as it soon sours and it is important, therefore, that the "cook" learns to assess the right amount for the whole of the kennel inmates. Except for the slow or "over-night" feeder, all left-overs should be cleaned up after the usual afternoon feed and before closing the kennels down for the night. Such waste food can be fed to poultry or pigs. The feed bowls must also be washed up immediately after feeding when it is much easier to clean them thoroughly than to leave them to the next day when the biscuit has set and is well and truly glued to the bowl. Finally, the kitchen should be cleaned down, not forgetting the mincer and boiler, so that all is ready for a fresh clean start the next morning.

Disposal of refuse. Whenever possible a fire should be kept going to burn all old bedding, sawdust, disposable food bowls and faeces. It is most important that no such waste should be allowed to accumulate at any time to attract rats, mice and flies. Such a fire may be an open bonfire or incinerator in the country, but may have to be a more elaborate brick-built incinerator with chimney in large kennels or in populated districts where the smoke must be carried well up into the air.

MEDICAL PROBLEMS

Distemper

Some years ago the greatest problem facing the proprietor of any boarding or quarantine kennel was, of course, distemper. It is some tribute to the research workers on distemper immunity, and to the manufacturers of distemper vaccine, that this has now become the least of his worries. The present level of some 75–80% of the dog population in this country which is now vaccinated means that the great majority of dogs for which boarding facilities are required have, in fact, already been immunised. It is now the normal practice of all well-run kennels to request proof by sight of the vaccination certificate of distemper inoculation, and if there is any doubt on this question to insist that the dog should be revaccinated before admission.

The position is a little more complicated in quarantine kennels in that it is not possible to assess the efficacy of distemper vaccine given abroad, either by reason of the use of unknown vaccines or, where British vaccines have been used, doubt of the potency of such vaccines when shipped abroad and stored in unknown circumstances. At a meeting a few years ago of the Quarantine Group of the BSAVA it was decided that all dogs entering quarantine should be vaccinated on admission. It is usually possible to convince the owner of a previously vaccinated dog that the cost of such a booster is a small price to pay as insurance against distemper.

Gastro-enteritis and diarrhoea

Both in practice and in kennels this condition seems to assume an ever increasing incidence and importance. Some workers believe that this is due to a specific pathogenic *Escherichia coli*; others incriminate an unknown virus. Yet others believe that this is not an infection at all, but a "home-produced" allergy such as purpura. The syndrome may be divided roughly into three types:

(a) Hyper-acute: in this there is frequent vomition early, followed at once by diarrhoea rapidly assuming a haemorrhagic type with haemorrhage throughout the whole intestinal tract. This is rapidly fatal if untreated, but if suitable treatment is initiated immediately the mortality is low. An intravenous drip of glucose-saline in large quantities should be set up at once and while this drip is proceeding an intravenous injection should be given through the tube of the maximum dose of oxytetracycline* according to weight. A concomitant subcutaneous injection of adrenoxyl should be given in very severe cases. In most cases a single such treatment will suffice.

(b) Acute: in this there is again vomition followed by persistent watery diarrhoea with varying amounts of blood. This form is readily controlled by subcutaneous injections of penicillin† combined with adequate dosage of sulphadimidine‡ by mouth.

(c) Subacute: in all kennels the frequent occurrence of an uncomplicated diarrhoea is well known. The aetiology is obscure, but the condition responds readily to simple oral administration of sulphadimidine.

Kennel cough or infectious laryngotracheitis

This still remains a serious problem to any large community of dogs such as occur in kennels or stray dogs' homes. Until 2 years ago the cause was unknown, but was usually ascribed to a throat infection with *Bacillus bronchisepticus*. However, recent work in Canada has shown that this condition is caused by an adeno-virus. There is no prophylaxis or adequate treatment, although serious symptoms are rare. The owner is, however, understandably annoyed that a dog who is fit on admission leaves the kennels with a cough which continues for some weeks afterwards. There is rarely any temperature and lung involvement is absent. This infection seems to have periods of exacerbation and remission, and 1963 was a particularly bad year. It affects dogs of

* Terramycin.
† Orbenin: Beecham Laboratories Ltd.
‡ Sulphamezathine.

all ages, and once it has broken out in a kennel it is extremely difficult to eradicate. In lost dogs' homes, where there is a continuous influx of new dogs throughout the year, kennel cough remains a perennial problem; but in boarding kennels with a lower admission rate it usually dies out after 2 to 3 months. Being a viral infection it is insensitive to most antibiotics, but chloramphenicol relieves the worst of the cough in most cases. Erythromycin has also been helpful.

Endoparasites

In boarding kennels where dogs are admitted only for a short period it is not usual to deal with endoparasites, but in quarantine kennels, owing to the various exotic worms which admissions may bring with them from overseas, it is standard practice to take faecal samples on admission and to treat them with the specific remedies indicated by laboratory tests. For example, a proportion of dogs entering this country are shown to be affected with hook-worm, but this does not spread under quarantine conditions. Moreover, it is now possible to deal effectively with hookworm infestation with Ancaris.*

During the summer months, when there is a high flea population in kennels, the concomitant problem of *Dipylidium caninum* also occurs. This worm is notoriously difficult to eradicate without very severe purgation, but Yomesan† has proved most effective in the elimination of the worm and its scolex without the anxiety of violent purgation.

Ectoparasites

In the years before the war sarcoptic mange was considered one of the hazards of the boarding dog, but with the introduction of the modern parasiticides, this too has ceased to be a problem. The old treatment of close-shaving the dog and the daily application of sulphur tar and oil required a nice discretion to decide when the mange infestation ended and the sulphur dermatitis began. Now two or three baths of the unclipped dog in gammexane is all that is required.

The inevitable population of fleas and lice which occur in boarding and quarantine kennels is also easily dealt with, preferably by suitable medicated baths. The problem here is rather one of recognition than of treatment. Kennel staff should be trained to recognize the symptoms of flea and louse infestation and to make a regular skin examination of the dogs in their care.

Non-specific skin diseases

There is no difference between the incidence of these conditions as between the boarding and the domestic dog, and the treament is the same. There may, however, be a higher incidence of some conditions in long-term boarders or quarantine dogs, such as the dry scurfy skin which may be due to overheating of the kennels, inade-

* Thenium and piperazine.
† Niclosamide.

quate ventilation, or be dietary in origin due to lack of fat in the diet. Pedal eczema is another condition frequently caused by damp kennel floors and perpetuated by the constant licking of a bored dog.

Feline panleukopenia (feline infectious enteritis)

This highly infectious and fatal disease was, until recently, responsible for heavy losses in quarantine and boarding catteries. Fortunately, vaccination has gone a long way towards controlling this problem and it has now become standard practice for quarantine catteries to insist on a booster vaccination on admission. Many of the better boarding catteries also insist on the productior of a current certificate of vaccination before acceptance.

Feline pneumonitis

In the absence of any satisfactory vaccine against the "snuffles", this highly infectious and recurrent disease still poses major problems. Fortunately, with good nursing the mortality rate is very low. The only adequate method of control really depends on the construction of the cattery. There must be a complete physical barrier between every cat cage to prevent spread by sneezed droplets and preferably the only wired openings should be to the outside of the building. Equally important is the maintenance of good hygiene in the retention of individual feeding bowls, beds and sanitary pans to each cage and their thorough cleansing.

(Medical Problems abstracted from BVA Paper presented at 82nd Annual Congress of the Association, September 1964. By the author.)

(c) THE FEEDING OF ANIMALS

I. General Principles and the Nutrition of the Dog

J. T. ABRAMS, MA, MSc, PhD

FOODS

Foods may be defined initially as those substances which animals, including dogs, will normally eat both voluntarily and repeatedly and which, taken in sufficient quantities, will maintain the beasts in good health subject only to (a) accidental injury, (b) attacks by the vectors of disease and (c) the apparently inevitable disabilities attending old age. Clearly, such a definition rests upon the meaning of the word, health. Here we need look only at the more obvious aspects of health, such as alertness, brightness of eye and of coat, soundness and straightness of limb, correct weight for age—neither fat nor too thin—and, in the adult, ability to produce healthy young with a good capacity for rapid growth.

From a variety of foods, a given animal tends to select food in relation to its species and age. Thus, dogs beyond the suckling stage prefer meat and fish to foods of vegetable origin, yet, for unknown reasons, both wild and domesticated dogs at times will freely eat *small* amounts of vegetable matter.

Now the capacity to live on largely vegetable diets requires a beast to possess (a) teeth that are capable of thoroughly grinding such foods and (b) an alimentary canal of such large size as to house enormous numbers of bacteria to share in the digestion of the food. But, as indicated earlier (Chapter 1), the dog's teeth are suited to cutting and tearing, not for grinding, while its short, relatively straight and simple gut offers no sufficient cul-de-sac for housing large colonies of bacteria. It seems logical, therefore, that the feeding of the dog should be based upon two main principles: either to give the animal that kind of food for which the processes of evolution have shaped it, or to take advantage of modern technology and nutritional knowledge in such a way as to enable the animal to derive nourishment from foods that it would not naturally consume in appreciable amounts. There is no reason why the two principles should not be used together. On these grounds, dogs are given cooked rather than raw vegetables and cooked flour rather than the raw grains fed to most farm animals. And since there is one component of plants, namely, crude fibre (see below), which is not digested at all by the alimentary secretions of mammals or birds, it is common sense to exclude from the canine diet those foods or the by-products of foods, such as plant stems, husks and seed-coats, that are relatively rich in crude fibre.

Whilst the dog has a natural liking for meat, its fondness is not restricted to the red muscle, e.g. steak, so much preferred by man, but includes what are best described as butcher's offals, such as liver, kidney, heart and stomach (tripe). Nor should it be forgotten that dogs will crush and swallow bones of a suitable size and shape. Indeed, when the diet of the dog is limited entirely to red meat, it eventually becomes ill as a direct result of the restriction. Apart from this the presence of a fair amount of fat in the food is also necessary.

Appetite

When their last meal has been largely digested, so that the gut is relatively empty, healthy adult dogs—like men—will go in search of food, their restlessness being temporarily allayed when the stomach is again filled. By this and other means appetite is alternately stimulated and depressed, so that the wild dog, which needs to work to obtain its food before it may eat, normally maintains a fairly constant weight. Since, however, any animal consumes many times its own weight in food during a year, the maintenance of a constant body weight requires quite accurate physiological control, and small but regular reductions or increases, below or above the amount of food which would lead to constancy of weight, can affect the dog very markedly. In the former instance, the end-result is a lean and hungry hound, whilst in the latter the dog becomes obese and even ill; indeed obesity in the house dog is a problem of some importance. So, whilst there are general rules for guidance in the feeding of dogs, they usually need to be modified slightly to fit the individual animal, which should be rather slim and sleek—not thin!—than fat and sluggish. The instinct of the healthy dog is to eat whenever food presents itself, since opportunities for the wild dog to feed are relatively few and usually have to be worked for: the house dog retains that instinct in face, too often, of a constant supply of food. Dog owners must be made to realize this risk.

When dogs are sick, and especially when there is a rise of bodily temperature, appetite may fail partially or completely. There is a like result if the animals are in pain or are frightened, as by fireworks on 5 November. In such circumstances, there is little point in trying to force the dog to eat. On the other hand, when the stress has been removed, the desire for food usually returns: in the convalescent animal it may be hastened by the presentation of dietary items the dog is known to enjoy or simply by giving it a normal, complete diet.

There are times when dogs show very unusual appetites. They will then eat earth, stones, rank grass, or even the dung of other animals. Such unusual appetites are given the name, pica. And, whilst one cannot impose human dietary habits on creatures of other species, for dogs evidently enjoy smells and tastes foreign to man, the regular exhibition of pica in a dog should call for some examination of the origin of the habit. It may indeed be due to poor feeding but, especially where the animal eats dung and other filth, the action inevitably introduces the risk of parasitic or other infection from other beasts.

The Proximate Analysis of Foods

The number of different foods, even of those which the dog will accept avidly, is large: the number of diets into which those foods may be blended is almost limitless. Clearly any attempt to systematize the feeding of dogs must first be an effort to reduce all foods to simpler common denominators. Whilst no really simple system is yet known or is likely to appear, a century-old method of analysis, still in everyday use, serves remarkably well. This is the scheme of proximate analysis, which describes the amounts of six different components, namely, water, fats, protein, crude fibre, ash (inorganic elements) and soluble carbohydrate, as percentages of the fresh weight of the food. The sixth figure is merely 100 less the sum of the first five. Table 2.1 shows the outline of the method of assessment, the technical chemical details of which are of no present importance.

The significant question is now this: what is the effect on the health of a dog if continually it is fed nothing but diets lacking in any of the six components? If one uses the most searching test of all, namely, the ability to maintain successful reproduction generation after generation, then water, fats, protein and inorganic elements are each essential. Without water the dog survives a few days: without protein, the major organic component of muscles and organs, its span of life can be measured in weeks. Whilst, for reasons which are made clear on page 138, the course of events is more difficult to predict in the instance of fats, since the survival of an individual will depend upon his previous history, there is also no doubt of the ultimate outcome.

TABLE 2.1

THE PROXIMATE ANALYSIS AND COMPOSITION OF FOOD

(1) *Proximate components*					(2) *Chemical equivalents*
Food	**Water**				Water
	Dry matter	**Ash** (inorganic elements)			Sodium, potassium, chlorine, calcium, phosphorus, etc.
		Organic matter	**Fats**		Glycerides (Fat-soluble vitamins)
			Non-fatty matter	**Protein**	Protein, amino-acids (Vitamin B-complex)
				Crude fibre	....
				Soluble carb.	Starch, cane and milk sugars, glucose

For dogs, crude fibre has no positive value, though a little of it may be useful as a stimulant to the movements of the intestine. Again, whilst it may be possible to keep dogs in health on diets affording very little soluble-carbohydrate, this is not important under modern conditions, when such material is just about the most abundant and cheapest dietary component.

The Composition of Foods

Full details about the composition of foods must be sought in the reference books listed at the end of this section, but a brief survey here is necessary.

Excluding water itself, foods of high water-content (75–90%) include fresh fruits, roots and green vegetables. Cow's milk is 87% water, and fresh, lean meat or fish contains over 70%. Cereal grains, e.g. wheat, and dried legumes, e.g. peas, contain about 10%, as do biscuits.

As for fatty foods, lard, mutton and beef tallows, margarine, butter, and olive, groundnut and maize oils contain 85% or more of fat. Even the leanest of meat contains a little fat, whilst, calculated on the dry-matter basis, there is more than 30% in cow's milk.

Rich, natural sources of protein are rare; indeed, proteins seem to be the world's least abundant kind of food, so that they are expensive and should consequently be used with skill and economy, in the feeding of both man and beast. No cereal grain contains more than an average of about 10% of protein. For dried peas and beans the content is around 20%, for nuts of various kinds 15–20%, for *fresh* lean meat and fish 25%, and for the solid types of cheese 25–35%. Fresh fruits, roots and green vegetables can be dismissed as suitable protein sources for the dog, no matter how good some of them may be for herbivorous animals. Dried fish and dried meat, provided that they are acceptable on hygienic grounds, contain 65–80% of protein and, other factors being suitable (see below), can be valuable foods for dogs.

When we come to consider the ash which different foods leave behind after the burning of the organic matter, it is necessary to distinguish that which is really a part of the food and that which is adventitious, such as blown sand or adherent soil. Very few of the foods suitable for feeding to livestock provide more than 1–4% of ash: on the other hand, amongst the exceptions are to be found valuable dietary ingredients, such as common salt, clean raw bone, sterilized bone-flour, calcium phosphate and ground limestone. Save for the first these exceptions are valuable sources of *calcium*. Furthermore, with the exceptions of both first and last, they provide an abundance of *phosphorus*. These two elements are major components of bone (ash). On a dry-matter basis, diets should contain about 0·6% of calcium and about 0·5% of phosphorus (see below). There is no virtue in diets which contain more than such amounts, whereas their absence will lead to poor teeth, badly shaped or diseased bones, anaemia and other ills.

Where other foods contain more than 5% of inorganic matter, they should be viewed with suspicion: they are probably dirty or have been mishandled or both.

The large amount of ash may not necessarily include poisonous substances, but it may also be sand, which has no positive value for the dog, whilst the careless handling which causes such high proportions of inorganic matter in the food can result in contamination of food with bacteria and other disease-producing organisms.

THE DIGESTION OF FOODS

Before we consider in more detail the changes undergone by foods as they pass through the canine digestive tract, it is perhaps as well to pause and to ask another pertinent question, namely, whether a diet, shown by proximate analysis to contain all six of the components, will sustain life and health in dogs. The only answer to this question is a firm negative. Tables of proximate analysis are invaluable, but they are too incomplete and too uninformative to be used in such a way.

That the science of nutrition involves a *relationship* between animal and food, and cannot be adequately described in terms of either alone, is obvious to anyone who watches attentively the behaviour of animals to their food.

For a normal cow good, clean, sweet-smelling grass is an attractive food, but it is not a palatable food for the healthy dog, save in odd whisps. It is true, of course, that all animals are less fastidious in their choices as they become increasingly hungry, so that, during the winter scarcity of flesh, wild dogs will eat small quantities of berries that are normally unattractive to the species. Even soil or inflated balloons in the gut help to allay the pangs of extreme hunger!

Again, dogs will eat very dry food, such as hard biscuit, provided that its physical texture is right, i.e. that it is in pieces of suitable size and is not finely powdered or gritty. In such instances the information provided by proximate analysis is quite clearly insufficient.

Finally, such simple analytical schemes say nothing of two powerful stimulants to appetite, canine and otherwise, namely, the taste and smell of food. This is one good reason why the small volume of liquid, i.e. gravy, in which food has been cooked and in which much of the taste and smell now may reside, should not be thrown away.

The salivary secretions with which the normal hungry adult dog meets the sight or smell of food is quite easily visible if the beast is kept waiting briefly before it is able to eat, since drops of rather thick saliva may fall from the corners of the mouth. Such salivation is necessary if swallowing is to be facilitated, but the simultaneous secretion of other essential digestive fluids further along the digestive tract is not seen under ordinary conditions. One should remember always that secretion tends to stop when the animal is severely ill, or especially if it is in pain or is frightened. In other words, the satisfactory digestion of food involves the whole animal and not simply its mouth and gut. Moreover, digestion in the very young, suckling puppy is different from that in the older animal; the pup at first can only deal with its dam's milk.

Food passing along the canine stomach and intestine encounters two types of secretion. From the walls of the stomach there flows hydrochloric acid, together with the enzyme, pepsin, whereas the cells lining the intestine secrete an alkaline fluid, together with other enzymes. At this stage, therefore, we need to consider the functions of such secretions, particularly with reference to the components of proximate analysis.

The Digestion of Fats

Under the action of gastric juice, fat is little changed, but the secretions and movements of the small intestine have two effects, provided that the melting point of the fat is below about 45°C. Firstly, the insoluble fat particles are broken down into smaller globules, so that eventually they are small indeed; secondly, the fats are chemically attacked by the enzymes of the intestinal secretions, during which process the subdivision of the fat particles is enhanced, until, when they have reached a certain size, the tiny fat droplets can pass through the wall of the intestine and are then, for the first time, really inside the canine body. Although this is essentially what occurs, the details of the process are complex and further details must be sought in more advanced books on biochemistry.

At this stage, reference to the *fat-soluble vitamins* is advisable. Four kinds of vitamin dissolve more easily in fats than in water: these are the fat-soluble vitamins A (scientific name: *retinol*), D (*calciferol*), E (*tocopherol*) and K. Different dietary fats vary greatly in the proportions of the different vitamins they contain, although even the richest contain much less than 1% by weight. Thus, cod-liver oil and halibut oil are both relatively rich sources of vitamins A and D, whilst good sources of tocopherol are to be found in the fats of the cereal grains. On the other hand, fat which has been exposed often and extensively to the action of atmospheric oxygen (as in cod-liver oil kept for months in a half-empty, poorly sealed vessel) becomes rancid and it is then highly probable that its fat-soluble vitamins will have been destroyed. Now this is highly important, since the presence of the fat-soluble vitamins in the diet is necessary for health and life. Whilst it is true that one can give in a single dose enough vitamin A to last a dog for several months, there is no doubt that the better and safer practice is to have the very small but necessary amounts of the vitamins in each day's food.

Our system of proximate analysis tells us nothing about the minute amounts of fat-soluble vitamins in different dietary fats: indeed, their separate determinations can be both laborious and expensive. The average dog-owner or dog-handler will be better occupied in seeing that the diet is so variously selected as to contain sufficient amounts of the vitamins A, D, E and K, rather than to think about their measurement in the diets he has formulated.

Finally, one further reason for introducing this necessary group of nutrients at this stage is that their absorption through the intestinal wall requires the simultaneous presence of the rest of the fat.

The Digestion of Protein

As a useful analogy to the process of protein digestion, which begins in the stomach and ends in the small intestine, one may compare the proteins derived from different foods to long strings of beads. The strings may consist of very large numbers of beads, indeed, several hundreds or even a few thousands being by no means unusual. Furthermore, there are only about twenty-five kinds of bead (*amino acid*) from which to choose, whilst the proportions to be found in particular strings vary greatly. Nevertheless, the proteins from the muscles of fish, amphibia, mammals and birds are all rather similar in kind and, since the greater part of the organic matter of the healthy body consists of such protein, this is a matter of importance.

So far as present evidence goes, only single amino acids (beads) can pass through the wall of the gut into the body. If, therefore, the gastric juices cannot accomplish this liberation, then since the movements of the bowel propel the ingested food steadily on towards the rectum and anus, i.e. beyond the sites where amino acids can be absorbed, such undigested material is lost to the dog and thus becomes part of the dung. Most soft fish or meat protein is readily digested and absorbed, as is that of milk or cheese: the proteins of horn, hair, skin and sinew are very much more resistant to digestion. Simple cooking, especially where the food is kept moist, may even make protein more digestible than in the raw state, but the use of high temperatures in dry ovens is disadvantageous, save for very brief times. Proteins of vegetable origin are also easily digested, provided that the digestive juices gain access to them (see section on Crude Fibre below).

Finally, just as fats may carry fat-soluble vitamins with them, the water-soluble vitamins of the *vitamin B complex* tend to be associated with the protein fraction of foods. This group of about ten vitamins is also necessary for life and health: it is not accounted for in the scheme of proximate analysis, save that natural foods of high protein-content tend to be rich in the vitamins B, although foods of animal origin alone can be regarded as good sources of *vitamin* B_{12} (*cobalamin*).

The Digestion of Crude Fibre

The minute cells that form the structures of plants consist essentially of crude fibre: within the cells lie fats, proteins and other useful nutrients. Since, as indicated earlier, digestive juices secreted by mammals cannot break down crude fibre, this store of nourishment remains untapped unless it is first liberated by rupture of the cell walls. The teeth of herbivora can do this; those of the dog cannot. On the other hand, the swelling of the cell contents during the cooking of food bursts open the cell walls. If they are to have any value to the animal, other than simple filling of the gut or stimulation to defaecation, vegetable foods for dogs should thus be adequately cooked. If the foods are in small pieces, about 15 minutes at boiling point should be enough. Not only is prolonged cooking unnecessary, but it can lead to partial or complete destruction of one or two members of the vitamin B family, notably *thiamine* (vitamin B_1).

The Digestion of Ash or Inorganic Matter

Inorganic matter which is already capable of dissolving in the aqueous contents of the digestive tract is then in a state in which it may pass into the body: this is true of common salt. Substances such as bone-flour or limestone may be absorbed to the extent that they are dissolved in the acid secretions of the stomach: the particles must not be too large, however, otherwise they will move past the site of absorption, i.e. the small intestine, before complete solution has occurred.

An important component of foods of vegetable origin, especially cereal grains—and hence flour—is *phytic acid*. This is a derivative of phosphoric acid, which tends to pass unabsorbed through the gut of the dog, carrying with it, as phytates, some of the calcium and magnesium that may be present in the food. One may thus discount most of the vegetable phosphorus in the diets of dogs and, with it, an equivalent amount of calcium.

The Digestion of Carbohydrate

The soluble carbohydrate of foods such as are fit for dogs consists very largely of starch: thus, the cereal grains may contain 60% or more of it. Although the starch is present in the uncooked cereals in the form of distinct grains, varying in size according to the kind of cereal, these grains are ruptured during cooking and the starch is altered physically, becoming translucent and more easily dissolved in water and in aqueous fluids. Due to the action of the intestinal secretions such starch is converted into a simple sugar, glucose, prior to its absorption into the body.

Carbohydrate occurs in small amounts in animal tissues in the form of glycogen, a substance comparable to starch. Thus, the natural dog probably never encounters large amounts of carbohydrate and is perhaps better adapted to using fat than this class of nutrient. Furthermore, whilst it is necessary to use some carbohydrate in modern canine dietaries, it seems important not to feed it to excess.

Nutrients

The nutrients may loosely be defined as those substances which pass through the intestinal wall and are then capable of being used by the organism for the maintenance of life and health. They include glucose, the amino acids, fats (glycerides), fat-soluble and water-soluble vitamins, and inorganic ions and complexes.

REQUIREMENTS FOR FOOD AND NUTRIENTS

The Animal as a Machine for Combustion

Life in animals is dependent upon oxidation processes and the energy they release. Nutrients, especially sugar and fat, are burned in the body more slowly but more efficiently than they would be in the domestic fire. Clearly, very fine control of the process is necessary if constancy of bodily temperature, amongst other essential biological characteristics, is to be achieved. Amongst the substances that help to regulate the whole process are the members of the vitamin B complex and some of the inorganic elements. It is the burning of the major nutrients, namely glucose, fats and amino acids, which produces most of the required energy, but since protein is scarce and since, in the form of muscles and organs, it is part of the structure of the body itself, to use protein as fuel is a waste of valuable material. So, whilst some amounts of carbohydrate and fat, as well as inorganic elements, also comprise part of the structure of the organism, we should try to use as little protein as possible for fuel purposes.

If, then, life in part is a process of slow combustion, can we say that the bigger the organism, the bigger the fire and the more fuel it needs? To give a precise answer to the question, we need to frame the question itself more carefully. First, for what purposes does the living body require the energy it derives from oxidation? Briefly, it needs energy (a) as heat for the maintenance of the bodily temperature, (b) for processes invisible to the eye, such as the work of the kidneys, (c) for the work done by muscles, and (d) for the growth or repair of the tissues. Now muscular work may be of several kinds and includes, for example, such vital movements as those of the heart and respiratory system, which are unceasing save for very brief intervals indeed. The whole digestive tract is muscular, too, and for its work food energy needs to be provided, but, since the larger mammals do not starve to death in an hour or even in days, there is not the immediate urgency here that there is for the heart and lungs. Finally, the large muscles of the neck, trunk and limbs require a corresponding energy provision when they are used. As we know, however, the body can be kept very still—as in people who are paralysed—for very long periods of time, certainly for many days.

Just as we can use a calorimeter to measure the heat produced by the burning of a given weight of coal, or wood, or starch, so, though with more complicated calorimeters, we can tell how much heat a dog produces in 24 hours. If the dog lies at rest in a warm chamber whilst the measurement is being made, then it is clearly not using energy for the muscles of its limbs; neither is it burning fuel to keep up its bodily temperature, as it would have to do were the chamber a cold one. Furthermore, when the dog has been given no food for the previous day or so, there will be no work of digestion going on. One can thus say that the animal's fuel usage is that which is consistent with the really vital activities of the body; those, and those only. Under such conditions the animal's metabolism is said to be basal, whilst its daily heat production is called its basal metabolic rate. If one studies normal adult dogs one finds that the larger the beast, the greater is its basal metabolic rate (BMR). However, the relationship of basal metabolic rate to weight is not a simple arithmetical one, as Table 2.2 shows. It should be clear that if we fed a dog of the toy-breeds, weighing 5 lb, the same amount of food *per pound of weight* as a St. Bernard, weighing 200 lb, the small dog would probably starve, other circumstances being the same.

TABLE 2.2

APPROXIMATE BASAL METABOLIC RATES OF ADULT DOGS IN KILOCALORIES PER DAY

Weight of dog (lb)	BMR (kilocal/day)	BMR (kilocal/day/lb weight)
200	1900	9·5
150	1550	10·3
100	1150	11·5
80	980	12·2
60	800	13·3
40	590	14·8
20	360	18·0
10	215	21·5
5	130	26·0

What quantities of digestible nutrients do these figures signify? For normal purposes one can assume that the calorific values of carbohydrate, protein and fat are 4, 4 and 9 kcal/g respectively, i.e. the full burning of 1 g of these substances gives rise to the heat productions indicated. An 80-lb dog would thus satisfy its needs by burning either 245 g of digestible starch, or protein (980/4), or about 110 g of *digestible* fat (980/9). On the other hand, provided that the dog is not being fed appreciable amounts of crude fibre, the correction for indigestible matter is a small one.

Feeding for Maintenance

When the dog is released from its chamber and comes out to eat so as to maintain its weight, and to move around quietly—and little else!—by what factor is its need for energy increased? If it is a house dog and is not being used for breeding, then its total *maintenance* needs will be about twice those of basal metabolism and feeding may be begun on that assumption, with the food intake being reduced slightly if the dog shows signs of becoming fat (it should be weighed regularly), or increased if it is too thin.

The balance of the diet

One may ask next what proportions of carbohydrate, fat and protein should be given to the animal, in order to yield the estimated amount of maintenance energy?

Since the animal loses hair, abraded skin, and, in the dung, bacteria, cells from the wall of the intestine and incompletely recovered digestive secretions, all of which contain protein, some dietary protein is essential. Now different food proteins contain different proportions of amino acids, from which the dog must attempt to extract such quantities as it needs. However, whilst the dog, given a simple source of fat or carbohydrate and of nitrogen, can make about fifteen of the amino acids for itself, should any one of them be lacking from the diet, there remain ten essential amino acids which must be supplied preformed in the diet. Whilst foods of animal origin are better generally able to supply the required balance of essential amino acids than are the vegetable proteins, the line of separation between the two classes is not sharp. If the dog receives 20% of its digestible energy in the form of mixed protein, then its requirements for protein and essential amino acids are more than likely to be met. In practice this implies that the diet must consist of a blend of cooked cereals, together with some fat, and fish, meat, milk or cheese. If the diet is of low fat-content, then this means that about 20% of the digestible dry-matter should consist of mixed protein, whereas a diet providing most of its non-protein calories in the form of fat would have to provide more nearly 35% by weight of protein.

Under experimental conditions, dogs may have been kept in apparent health on diets of lower protein content than those described above, but the ordinary dog-owner would not be advised to try to pursue such a course, since the protein-rich foods are the ones that normally carry good amounts of the vitamins B, which are needed for the proper utilization of fat, carbohydrate and protein alike. For similar reasons it is not a good plan to stick to a rigid dietary regime: there should, for example, be an alternation of tripe, liver, kidney, heart or other offals with ordinary red (muscle) meat.

Whilst the dog may be given a level teaspoonful of steamed bone-flour for every half-pound of dry food, a better alternative is to provide clean sheep ribs about twice weekly, unconsumed bone being removed at the end of the day and disposed of.

During the cooking of food a little common salt may be used, as in ordinary domestic cooking, whilst cod-liver oil should also be given daily. A 4-oz bottle of cod-liver oil, either BP or Veterinary Codex grade, is sufficient for 1 month for a dog weighing about 60 lb, e.g. Labrador or Boxer; the needs of other dogs are in proportion to their weights.

The healthy adult dog will do quite well on a single daily feed, given in the evening; rejected food should also be thrown away and not left around to become sour or to attract flies or vermin.

The Feeding of Breeding Stock

The stud dog needs little better food than that described above. It is worthwhile making sure that foods such as liver, which are useful sources of iron, copper and the vitamin B complex as well as protein, appear regularly on the menu. Apart from this the rule should be simply that of "feeding according to condition".

This also applies to the bitch up to the time of mating. Although the evidence is far from conclusive, most animal breeders think that fat beasts do not breed well. Whether this is rigorously true or not is of no importance, since sleek animals certainly do tend to breed well.

For about the 1st month after conception the bitch will not require much more food than she received before; thus, an increase of 5% (average) will suffice. At 4 weeks, however, food intake may then be up by 20% compared with normal maintenance requirements, whilst for the 5th and 6th weeks it may be as high as 66%. This rather abrupt increase is due to the growth of the pups within the womb, a growth which then increases steadily up to the time of whelping. For the last 2 weeks, however, food consumption may fall from its previous high level, perhaps because there is not the room in the one small body for large feeds and for several relatively big pups. The owner of the bitch may allow the animal a little more "meat" than before, although this should not be necessary if the diet is of the kind described on page 143.

At parturition the bitch may go off feed for a day: if all is otherwise well, this is no cause for alarm, provided that, *as for all dogs*, there is constant free access to clean water.

Feeding during Lactation

Once the pups are in the world, it should be clear that their dam has to meet even higher demands for nourishment than before, for the increasing size of the pups means that their food requirements for growth (see below) are also greater, whilst each small body, previously sheltered, now has to meet the conditions of the environment. For the latter reason, among others, the bitch and her litter should be in a clean, draught-proof and warm place.

Depending upon the number of pups to be fed, the requirements of the bitch may rise from about double those of normal maintenance during the 1st week of lactation to three times from the 4th to the 7th weeks, after which the strain should lessen. This is because the pups should be beginning to take solid food themselves.

The amount of food allowed to the bitch should then be regulated to her condition. If she has lost weight during lactation, the chance should be given to put back her reserves, but she should not be allowed to become fat.

Feeding Puppies

For the newly-born puppy there is no food so good as its dam's milk, which contains (a) a high proportion of good protein, (b) a relatively high amount of energy because of its large fat-content and (c) the bone-forming elements, calcium and phosphorus, in good amount and in correct proportions. Furthermore, it is clean, i.e. free from bacteria, it is warm, and it can be taken in a number of small feeds rather than one big, disturbing "blow-out". Lastly, if the bitch is still in the same house where she conceived, her milk will contain antibodies, serving to protect the pups against some of the diseases in the surroundings. These antibodies are in the protein fraction of the milk secreted just after parturition *only*.

Young animals grow, firstly, by increasing the size of the bones and, secondly, by development of the organs and muscles; the sequence is important. Thus, the first food offered to pups should be finely minced and should contain good sources of calcium and phosphorus, together with vitamin D, without which the utilization of these inorganic elements is seriously impaired. It should also be rich in protein (20–25% on the dry-matter basis, see page 143). Useful foods are milk, fresh or dried, cheese, cooked meat or fish (bones removed) and cooked peas or beans. If the two last named are given, then the dried legumes, cooked until they are very soft, may be mixed with a preponderance of meat or fish. A little cod-liver oil should also be given. The aim should be to allow as rapid growth as possible; there is no justification or even economy in the production of rachitic or weakly animals.

At first a little feed may be given to the pups whilst they are still suckling, but the bitch should be kept away from this more expensive kind of feed. When lactation has ceased, five daily feeds may be given to the pups of as much food as can be cleaned up in about 5 minutes, uneaten food being removed each time and rejected, so that there is some need to try to gauge the appetite of the animals and not to increase wastage. The first 8 weeks of such feeding are very important and should see a substantial growth of the puppies, which *at first* can be expected to require about twice as much food as would adult dogs of the same weight.

By observing the height of the dog at the shoulder, as well as by regular weighing, one may judge the progress of the animals. As they grow the number of feeds can be reduced, until morning and evening feeds alone are being given, by which time the dogs should be somewhere near their expected mature weights. They should be sleek and vigorous but not fat, their food intakes having also been gradually reduced with the approach of maturity.

The difficulties of rearing orphan pups depends upon the age at which the dam has been lost; the younger they are, the more skill is needed.

Such pups need warmth and good hygiene, together with several daily feeds of a milk substitute given from a clean, i.e. sterile, miniature feeding bottle or from an eye dropper. Swedish workers have claimed success with a mixture made from 800 ml of whole, cow's milk, 200 ml of single cream and one egg yolk. Into the mixture is carefully stirred 6 g of sterilized bone-flour and 4 g of citric acid, in that order. The food, which will keep in the refrigerator for a few days only, is removed in small amounts for feeding, being slowly warmed to 100°F. Initially, the daily amount of such food should be about 15–20% of the weight of the pup, rising gradually to 35%. From 3 weeks of age feeding from a shallow saucer may be tried.

The Feeding of Working Dogs

Working dogs are of two chief kinds, racing Greyhounds, which move very quickly but do not race for more than minutes, and other breeds, including Sheep-dogs, police dogs, guide dogs, and hounds, which may need to keep up a steady pace for hours on end. In every case, of course, it is the voluntary muscles of the limbs that require extra energy above that needed for simple bodily maintenance, although the heart and respiratory system also have to increase their rate of work.

What kind of food, to supplement that for simple maintenance, should be given to such dogs? Protein *can* be used, if there is no other food available, but it is certainly not necessary, since either fat or carbohydrate can be used successfully, provided that the supply of the vitamin B complex increases correspondingly. It is also true that the daily amount of extra food needed is proportional both to the severity of the work and to its duration, for which reason Greyhounds in training may be kept fit on diets providing a little more than simple maintenance requirements, whereas Sheep-dogs, working solidly for 10 or more hours daily, may require three times as much.

It is very difficult to measure work output, save in the artificial surroundings of a laboratory. We can, however, take cognizance of data such as those just quoted and feed dogs according to their condition, allowing them to eat more food if they show signs of becoming thin or, if they can eat no more, giving them less work. Where they show signs of becoming fat, their allowance should be reduced.

For heavy rates of work there is much to commend the use of foods of high fat-content, one of the cheapest of which, on the dry-matter basis, is cheese, but cheap meat, with adherent fat, is also good. In place of high-fat foods, biscuit and other starchy material can be used. Where there is doubt as to the vitamin B-content of the diet, a weight of dried, unextracted brewer's yeast equal to about 2% of the dry matter in the diet is very useful.

The feeding of working dogs is also a matter of management. Beasts in good condition can work for hours without food, but their efficiency falls by as much as 50% if they do not have free access to water. The time when food is given is important; if one feed only per day is given, then it is best offered in the evening when work is done. Perhaps a better system for the constantly hard-working dog is a small morning feed—say, one-quarter of its daily quantity—about 1 hour before it begins work, with the rest of the feed after work is over for the day. For such animals easily digested diets are necessary. It is also a point of some significance that a small feed, given just before the performance of work, does not improve the immediate efficiency of the well-nourished dog; in other words, one gives hard-working dogs two daily feeds just because it may be difficult to give it all in one large meal.

The Feeding of Sick and Convalescent Dogs

Animals that are acutely ill should, as at all times, have water freely available. If they will accept food, which is usually not the case, small feeds of lightly cooked meat may be offered; if they are not disposed to eat, it is doubtful whether the effort to persuade them to do so is justified.

With the passage of a crisis and the emergence of convalescence, however, one may then try persuasion, though what is to be done will depend upon the nature of the disease and the advice given by the veterinary surgeon in charge of the animal. Where the kidneys have been damaged, for example, it may be necessary to feed diets of low protein-content for a while (10% or so on the dry-matter basis). Such foods tend to lack the vitamin B complex, one member of which, namely thiamine, is closely linked with good appetite. Dried yeast, as indicated, is a good source of this complex; a more potent one, which dissolves easily to make a "gravy", is the proprietary product, "Marmite". Members of the vitamin B complex give a stimulating smell and taste to food.

During illness, both man and beast tend to burn up their own tissues, perhaps to save the "work of digestion". Whatever the reason, the result is a loss of bodily weight and substance, so that the muscles may look weak and flabby. The restoration of such a loss can be accomplished by the more generous allocation of protein-rich foods, always provided, as indicated above, that the condition of the dog permits this.

Proprietary Foods

Proprietary foods are as good as the care that is taken in their manufacture. Biscuits, dehydrated foods and canned products can have the virtues of convenience, cleanliness and careful blending. Many such products can be fed to dogs as their sole item of diet for long periods of time without the animals losing condition. Quite clearly, however, one cannot give unqualified approval to such products without knowing in any given instance what the ingredients were that entered into their preparation. There is no doubt, however, that the first step towards approval can be taken only where the composition of the product is given without ambiguity, i.e. proximate analysis at the very least.

Further Reading

ABRAMS, J. T. (1962) *The Feeding of Dogs*, Green & Co., Edinburgh.

McCAY, C. (1949) *Nutrition of the Dog*, Comstock Publishing Co., New York.

WIDDOWSON, E. M. and McCANCE, R. A. (1960) *The Composition of Foods*, H.M. Stationery Office, London.

Note: Although data concerning calorific values and compositions of different foods are given in all of the texts listed above, the Medical Research Council Report of Widdowson and McCance (above) contains analyses of all foods likely to be encountered in canine nutrition, with the natural exception of proprietary foods.

II. Nutrition of the Cat

R. S. ANDERSON, BVMS, PhD, MRCVS

Since much of the material in the preceding chapter is referable to the cat as well as the dog, the main purpose of the present section is to highlight certain aspects of nutrition which are particularly relevant to the cat.

Before embarking on specific aspects of feline nutrition, there is, however, a useful general concept which merits some further consideration; this is the concept of an animal being in nutritional balance. Many find, not without reason, that nutrition is rather a diffuse subject and this concept often helps to integrate the relationship between the animal and its food.

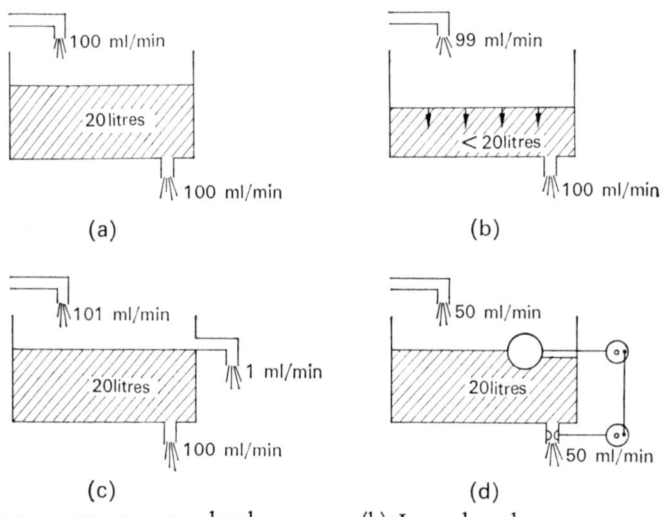

Fig. 2.10. (a) Input = output; water level constant. (b) Input less than output; water level falls. (c) Increase in water level compensated by overflow; water level constant. (d) Servo-mechanism controlling outflow in relation to water level; decreased inflow compensated by restricted outflow; water level constant.

BALANCE

An animal is said to be in nutritional balance for a particular nutrient when the measured intake of that material in food and water is equal to the measured output in faeces, urine, expired air, fur and (in the case of the nursing female) milk.

The balance concept is commonly illustrated by drawing a comparison between the animal and a tank of water. Nutrient intake is represented by the inflow of water from the supply pipe and output by the outflow of water from the tank (Fig. 2.10a).

The water level in the tank and its fluctuations up or down represent the nutritional status of the animal (i.e. deficiency or superfluity) in relation to the nutrient.

It is obvious that, in order to maintain a constant water level in the tank, water outflow must be equalled precisely by water inflow. The slightest deviation from precise equality in inflow and outflow will result in a progressive alteration in the level of water in the tank. Thus, assuming the tank normally contained 20 litres and inflow and outflow were normally 100 ml/min, a decrease in input from 100 to 99 ml/min would cause a deficit of 7·2% in 24 hours and the tank would be dry in 2 weeks (Fig. 2.10b). Similarly an increase in the rate of outflow or the development of a leak would also cause a progressive decrease in the water level. Clearly such a system is highly susceptible to variation in water supply or to sudden increases in rate of outflow and in practice can have some safety factors built in. To prevent excessive filling of the tank in the event of a decrease in outflow or an increase in inflow, the simplest control is to install an overflow pipe (Fig. 2.10c); however, more precise control over variations in input can be obtained by a servo-mechanism designed to restrict the rate of outflow when the water level falls and increase it when the level rises (Fig. 2.10d). It is possible to evolve further complex control systems for our water tank but the present examples are sufficient to illustrate the balance concept.

In an animal a parallel situation exists—only the servo-mechanisms are rather more complex. The easiest example to use initially is water—substituting an animal for the water tank. The intake and output of water which contribute to normal balance are shown in Table 2.3.

TABLE 2.3

WATER BALANCE

Input	Output
Drinking water	Urine
Water in the food	Faeces
"Metabolic" water*	Expiratory water
	Perspired water
	Milk

* Water arising from the metabolism of carbohydrate, protein and fat.

A decrease in input may result from an inadequate supply of drinking water, whereas an increase may result in certain disease states or when the food itself contains a high water content (e.g. milk). Increased water output occurs in hot weather (expired and perspired water), pneumonia (expired water), diarrhoea (faeces) and diabetes or kidney disease (urine).

If intake is decreased or output increased without compensatory mechanisms coming into operation then inevitably the "water level" in the animal falls and it becomes dehydrated. Imbalance of water, however, is usually partially or totally compensated by a physiological servo-mechanism. Thus, in response to dehydration due to reduced intake or increased output in diarrhoea, urinary water output is decreased thus reducing the rate of water loss, whereas increased intake is compensated by increased urinary output (diuresis). By the use of the balance technique an animal's nutritional status in relation to nutrients such as protein, calcium, phosphorus, magnesium, sodium and potassium may be assessed. A simple balance technique cannot be used with carbohydrate, fat and vitamins since these are changed to other substances in the body; the use of isotope labelling, however, has permitted detailed study of the fate of materials such as these.

STORAGE OF NUTRIENTS IN THE BODY

Just as in the water-tank analogy, the susceptibility of an animal to nutrient deficiency is dependent on the relationship between the amount stored in the body and the rate of intake and output (or turnover) of the nutrient. If turnover is high and stores are low then deficiency is much more likely than when turnover is low and stores are high. There is, for instance, relatively little storage of the vitamins of the B complex in the body, thus the onset of vitamin B deficiency is relatively rapid if a deficient diet is fed. On the other hand, clinical evidence of calcium deficiency in non-reproductive adults takes a long time to develop even when a deficient diet is fed because calcium turnover is low and large amounts are stored in the skeleton; whereas, when turnover is increased during growth or lactation, calcium deficiency may develop rapidly.

SPECIFIC FEATURES OF FELINE NUTRITION

Protein

The high nutritional requirement of the cat for protein is constantly reiterated and there is no doubt that most cats, if fed a diet containing less than 32% protein (dry weight) or 29% of the total calories as protein, will go off their food, lose weight, and show a negative protein ($N_2 \times 6{\cdot}25$) balance. The effect of lowering the protein content in reducing the acceptability of the food, however, makes assessment of protein requirements rather difficult. Thus high levels of animal protein of high biological value are necessary to make the food sufficiently acceptable to maintain adequate intake not only of protein but also all the other nutrients. The importance of using highly acceptable protein was demonstrated by a recent experiment in which steady growth and good health were obtained in kittens receiving a diet containing only 12% of the total calories as protein but ensuring high acceptability.

Protein Calories

As pointed out in the previous chapter in which the animal was described as "a machine for combustion (of energy containing foods)", protein, fat and carbohydrate when totally oxidised in the body release energy to the extent of 4, 9 and 4 kcal/g respectively. Thus, if the proximate analysis (see p. 135) is known, then the theoretical calorie content can be calculated as shown in the two examples in Table 2.4.

TABLE 2.4

	Food A		Food B	
	g/100 g	kcal/100 g	g/100 g	kcal/100 g
Protein	10	10 × 4 = 40	10	10 × 4 = 40
Fat	5	5 × 9 = 45	8	8 × 9 = 72
Carbohydrate	4	4 × 4 = 16	22	22 × 4 = 88
		101		200
Percentage of total calories supplied by protein =		$\frac{40 \times 100}{101}$	=	$\frac{40 \times 100}{200}$
	=	40%	=	20%

The difference between protein content (g/100 g) and protein calories is illustrated by the values obtained from the proximate analysis of the above two hypothetical foods in which, although the protein levels by analysis are identical, the percentage of the calories supplied by protein in B is approximately half of that in A. The nutritional significance of this difference is shown in the following example:

Calorie requirement of a cat = 250 kcal/day.

Amount of food (g) required to provide 250 kcal.

Food A (101 kcal/100 g)	Food B (200 kcal/100 g)
$100 \times \frac{250}{101}$	$100 \times \frac{250}{200}$
= 248 g	= 125 g

Since appetite is controlled primarily by the need for calories the cat would need much less of the high calorie Food B to satisfy its appetite than of Food A, thus the protein intake when Food A is fed would be $10 \times \frac{248}{100} = 24{\cdot}8$ g day, whereas if Food B were fed the protein intake would be $10 \times \frac{125}{100} = 12{\cdot}5$ g day.

The above calculation is important when comparing foods of two different types such as a moist meaty food and a dry biscuity food, although calculation of protein percentage for both foods on a dry weight basis also gives useful comparative data.

Fat

Kittens in particular appear to benefit from diets having a high fat content. In moist foods containing less than 100 kcal 100 g, improved growth rate has been obtained by the addition of up to 8% of fat as lard. The presence of fat in the diet is important in the absorption of the fat soluble vitamins and added fat may improve the absorption and utilization of Vitamin A for which the kitten has an exceptionally high requirement.

Carbohydrate

There is no known requirement for carbohydrate and, although it is a cheap energy source, cats and particularly kittens appear to utilize fat more efficiently than carbohydrate. The addition of large amounts of carbohydrate will certainly reduce acceptance of moist foods and may limit the growth rate of kittens.

Vitamins

Vitamin A. Cats cannot convert the vitamin A precursor carotene to vitamin A in their intestines, thus they are dependent on the vitamin A which has been preformed in the bodies of other animals. Liver and milk are rich sources of vitamin A and if included at moderate levels in the daily feed should prevent deficiency occurring. Where these constituents are not included in the diet, $\frac{1}{2}$ oz of cod liver oil per week will meet requirements.

Vitamin A requirement of the cat is very high in relation to that of other animals (1600 to 2000 i.u. of the preformed vitamin per day for a cat, whereas the recommended intake for a 10-year old child is only 2000 i.u./day). Excessive intake of vitamin A, such as may occur when the diet is made up exclusively of liver, or after prolonged over-dosage with cod liver oil, may cause severe irreversible bone disease characterized by abnormalities of the spine and long bones.

Vitamin D. In contrast with the previous vitamin, the requirement for vitamin D is small (50–100 i.u. per day) and the cat probably obtains most of its requirement by licking its own fur from which it obtains cholecalciferol from an irradiated sterol, 7-dehydrocholesterol. Rickets has been produced experimentally in growing kittens when diets deficient in vitamin D have been fed, but in practice vitamin D deficiency is unlikely.

Vitamin E. Vitamin E deficiency or "yellow fat disease" occurs when diets high in polyunsaturated fats and low in vitamin E are fed to cats. The field cases have usually occurred when the polyunsaturated fatty acids have been derived from fish, particularly red tuna fish. Kittens become inappetent, lethargic and appear to find movement painful. At post-mortem examination, body fat is a browny orange colour instead of the normal creamy white colour. The disease, however, is not readily reproduced under experimental conditions, and one group of workers concluded that the most prominent feature of their studies was the relative resistance of cats to gross signs of vitamin E deficiency. The condition if suspected is readily reversed by changing the suspect diet and supplementing with vitamin E.

Vitamin B. Thiamine (B_1) deficiency in cats has been described in several reports. The thiamine requirement of cats has somewhat arbitrarily been set at a high level (0·4 mg/day or 0·1 mg for each 50 kcal consumed) but there is little doubt that severe symptoms of deficiency occur when diets low in thiamine are fed. Since over 50% of the thiamine in food may be destroyed by heating or cooking, canned food is usually supplemented with thiamine to offset processing losses. When food is prepared in the kitchen, the fact that substantial amounts of the vitamin may be lost in the cooking water should be borne in mind. Some fish contain a specific thiaminase which inactivates naturally occurring thiamine and thiamine deficiency in foxes fed on raw fish has occurred.

Early signs of deficiency in the cat are anorexia, listlessness and weight loss but the disease progresses to predominantly nervous signs including ataxia, ventroflexion of the head, dilatation of the pupils and abnormal postural reflexes. The condition responds to vitamin B therapy but residual ataxia may persist for several weeks.

Thiamine is readily administered orally to the cat in the form of yeast tablets.

Minerals

Calcium. The kitten, like all growing animals, has a large requirement for dietary calcium for bone formation and other metabolic functions. Likewise, the lactating queen must replenish her own body stores of calcium which are transferred to her kittens during their intra-uterine life and through her milk during lactation. The absorption of calcium is closely associated with the amount of phosphorus and vitamin D in the diet. Optimum absorption occurs when the Ca/P ratio is between 0·9 and 1·1; when the Ca/P ratio is outside this range, adequate supplies of vitamin D are beneficial in promoting calcium absorption.

The Ca/P ratio in muscle meat (0·04) is such that kittens fed on solely raw heart develop severe bone disease including spontaneous fractures, misshapen bones and paralysis due to collapse of the vertebrae and consequent damage to the spinal cord. Approximately 5 g of calcium carbonate must be added to every kg of meat in order to bring the Ca/P ratio to the correct level for optimum calcium absorption and to provide sufficient calcium to support normal bone formation.

Milk is a useful supplementary source of dietary calcium when meat is fed, but calcium should not be added to processed foods unless there is evidence that the Ca/P ratio is incorrect, since the Ca/P ratio is usually corrected by the manufacturer in the feed formulation.

Iodine. Deficiency of iodine has been produced by feeding raw-meat diets to growing kittens and there appears to be some interaction between the metabolism of calcium and iodine in the cat. Fish and fish liver oil are good sources of dietary iodine.

Sodium, potassium, phosphorus, copper, cobalt, magnesium, manganese and zinc. All these elements are undoubtedly essential in the diet of the cat, but there is no documented evidence of field cases of deficiency and since all are contained in sufficient quantity in most of the foods commonly fed to cats, deficiency seems unlikely.

ENERGY REQUIREMENT, APPETITE AND FREQUENCY OF FEEDING

The energy requirement of the young growing animal is very high in relation to its body weight. Beagle puppies aged 7 weeks and weighing about 2 kg consume about 300 kcal kg body weight and the figure usually quoted for kittens is about 250 kcal/kg body weight. Thus, assuming that a 42-day-old kitten weighs 500 g, calorie requirement is 125 kcal/day. Using a proprietary cat food containing 125 kcal/100 g, the required intake of food is 100 g/day or 20% of the total body weight. This relationship between energy and food requirement of the kitten and body weight underlines the necessity of feeding the young kitten at frequent intervals—at least 4 times a day in the 6–12 week range, 3 times a day from 12 to 24 weeks and twice a day from 24 to 40 weeks. The alternative course is to have food constantly available at an early age, but if this procedure is used it is essential that food be replaced regularly with fresh supplies.

The calorie requirement per kg body weight decreases as the young cat grows and adult requirements vary between 60 and 90 kcal/kg body weight depending on exercise. In terms of commercial canned products, a lethargic 3-kg cat should have its requirements met by one small can of a product containing about 80 kcal/100 g, whereas an active cat of the same weight would require a small can of a food containing about 120 kcal/100 g. The "all-meat" type of commercial food falls into the first category and the "complete" or meat and cereal or "loaf" type of product is in the second category.

Pregnancy and Lactation

Food intake of the pregnant queen may show a slight increase during the second half of pregnancy, but may in fact decrease during the last week due to distension of the abdominal cavity by the uterus and its contents and the consequent restriction of gastric filling. The effect of this reduction on alimentary capacity may be offset by offering food on two or three occasions during the day and also offering fresh milk frequently. If the queen has received a balanced diet prior to pregnancy, then her additional requirements during pregnancy should be met from the increase in food intake. The provision of fresh milk should ensure adequate supplies of vitamin A and calcium. Cats which will not drink milk should receive vitamin A supplementation as cod or halibut liver oil and a calcium supplement.

Nutritional requirements during pregnancy depend on the number of kittens in the litter, but where four to six kittens are being nursed, the queen will require up to three times her normal food intake. It is desirable to continue to offer food on several occasions during the day as her requirement may be much greater than can be satisfied at a single meal. Milk and/or water should be regularly available. The alternative system is to leave food constantly available, but the importance of replacing stale with fresh food must be stressed.

It is particularly important to watch for any sign of a sudden decrease in food intake during lactation as this may be the first sign of illness such as an infected mammary gland. Decreased food intake is rapidly followed by a fall in milk production with disastrous results for the litter. If there is no evidence of illness, alternative foods should be offered; yeast tablets may also be effective in stimulating a jaded appetite. During the suckling period supplementation with cod liver oil may well be beneficial if milk intake is low.

Processed vs. Fresh Foods

Opinions vary on the relative merits of cooked and uncooked foods for cats, but it is clearly unrealistic to place all cooked foods into one classification and all raw foods into another.

Both raw and cooked foods will be nutritionally inadequate if the appropriate nutrients or supplements are omitted. Conversely, there is abundant evidence that excellent growth and reproduction can be achieved with either raw, cooked or processed proprietary foods. Because of the wide range of proprietary foods available, however, it is advisable to ascertain from the manufacturer as much information as possible in relation to the suitability of a particular food for maintenance, growth or reproduction.

(d) CAGE BIRDS

D. K. Blackmore, BSc, PhD, FRCVS

Introduction

It is not often appreciated that the total number of cage and aviary birds kept in this country far outnumbers the combined total of cats and dogs. Although in the past relatively few bird-owners sought veterinary advice, the veterinary profession is now taking a much greater interest in birds, with the result that the practitioner is seeing many avian patients, and the techniques of nursing birds are becoming of increasing importance.

There are approximately 8650 species of bird in the world, many of which may be kept in cages or aviaries, so that although some generalities can be made about the class aves, as can be made about the class mammalia, it must be remembered that each genus has different characteristics and may be affected by different patterns of disease, and require different systems of management and nutrition. The budgerigar is as different from the canary as is the cat from the dog.

Apart from the differences between the species of bird, the conditions and systems of management under which they are kept profoundly affect them. The pet bird kept individually in a cage shows a very different pattern of disease from the same species kept in an outdoor aviary and allowed to breed. For instance, a much higher incidence of neoplasia is seen in the longer-living pet budgerigar compared with the breeding bird owned by the fancier. The very common vice of self-inflicted feather plucking seems to be associated with the single bird allowed little activity much more than its more active relation housed in an aviary.

Space does not permit more than a somewhat cursory discussion of some of the problems associated with the veterinary aspects of nursing cage birds, and the reader who wishes to study the problems in greater detail is recommended *Diseases of Cage and Aviary Birds*, edited by Dr. M. L. Petrak, and published by Lea and Febiger of Philadelphia, but easily available in this country.

General Characteristics of Birds

Obviously space does not permit detailed discussions of avian anatomy and physiology, but discussion of some of those features which particularly differ from mammals is worth while.

Birds evolved from reptilian ancestors during the Mesozoic period over 150 million years ago, and the earliest known fossilized bird is Archaeopteryx. From this time onwards, birds successfully populated the environment, and were probably most numerous between a quarter and half a million years ago, since which time their numbers have been slightly declining. Even today, birds show several reptilian characteristics and suffer from some conditions which also occur in reptiles.

One of the most obvious characteristics of birds are their feathers, which are of two distinct types: the body feathers, which are important in insulating the bird and maintaining the body temperature, and the flight feathers, occurring on the wings and tail, which are of course necessary for flight. The normal body temperature varies considerably between species, usually the smaller the bird the higher the temperature, that of a small finch being 45°C (109°F).

Although birds have no sweat glands, there is a preen or uropygial gland at the base of the tail, which produces an oily secretion used by the bird when preening.

The legs of most species of bird are unfeathered and covered in reptilian-like scales. They have four toes with claws, and in most species three point forward and one backward, although in owls, psittacines and some other species, two toes point forward and two back.

The musculo-skeletal system of birds shows many special features, which will influence their care and treatment. The bones are light and rather fragile, and many of the long bones are pneumatic and actually communicate with the respiratory tract, so that it is possible for direct respiratory infection to follow amputation, unless precautions are taken. The sternum is particularly large, to provide attachment for the massive pectoral muscles, and extends rather far backwards, making abdominal palpation less easy than in mammals. Many bones of the vertebral column and limbs are fused together in birds. In the legs, the upper row of tarsals is fused with the tibia to form the tibio-tarsal, and the lower row of tarsals is fused with a single metatarsal to form the tarso-metatarsal bone.

Birds have no diaphragm, resulting in a combined abdominal and thoracic cavity, a feature which profoundly affects the signs and symptoms of disease.

The nostrils or nares are situated at the base of the beak, and in birds such as the budgerigar, they are in a fleshy unfeathered structure termed the cere. The trachea is relatively similar to that of mammals in most species, but voice production is mainly from the syrinx, a structure at the base of the trachea and within the thoracic cavity.

The primary bronchi enter the lungs, which are relatively small structures closely applied to the vertebral column. These primary bronchi divide into secondary and tertiary bronchi within the lung, the latter forming an anastamosing network of airways. The primary bronchi also pass directly through the lungs to communicate with a series of thin-walled air sacs, the majority of which are paired. These air sacs are situated in the abdominal and thoracic cavities, and in some of the long bones and the lower cervical region. The normal respiratory rate of small birds such as the canary is extremely rapid compared with mammals, and is between 100 and 120 per minute.

A special feature of the cardio-vascular system is a renal portal system, which occurs in addition to the hepatic portal system present in both mammals and birds. The blood itself shows several differences from that of mammals; the red blood cells are large, oval and nucleated, instead of platelets birds have small nucleated cells termed thrombocytes, and the neutrophyl is represented by a cell known as the heterophil, which at first glance could be confused with the mammalian eosinophil. The blood of birds also contains eosinophils, basophils, lymphocytes and monocytes. Birds do not have discrete lymph nodes except for tissue in the cloaca known as the bursa of fabricus.

The digestive tract varies considerably amongst different species, but usually the oesophagus contains a special dilation or storage organ, known as the crop. The true stomach, or proventriculus, is rather similar to the stomach of mammals, but most birds also possess a grinding organ known as the gizzard. The intestine is rather short and simple, and some species of bird have paired caeca. There is a common external opening from the uro-genital tract and colon, known as the cloaca.

The kidneys are relatively large trilobed structures, closely applied to the vertebral column, and rather primitive in structure, with no sharp distinction between cortex and medulla. The urine is a rather thick white material, and most of the nitrogenous waste is in the form of uric acid. Urea, the main form of nitrogen excretion in mammals, is only produced in small quantities. Urine is, therefore, voided at the same time as faeces, producing droppings of typical brown and white appearance.

The paired testes are always intra-abdominal and are situated ventral to the anterior pole of each kidney. In most species, only the left ovary is present, which sheds its extruded ova into a single left oviduct. The oviduct is a complex glandular and muscular organ which produces both the albumin and shell for the egg that is finally laid, and opens on the dorsal surface of the cloaca near the openings of the ureters.

SEXING AND AGEING BIRDS

Although the male and female adults of some species of bird, such as the cockatiel, have different plumage, in many other species both sexes appear identical. In budgerigars, the colour of the cere often denotes the sex, being blue in males and brownish in females, but the white and yellow varieties have a similar flesh-coloured cere. It is, therefore, important to ask the owner the age and sex of the bird presented. In the case of the fancier or aviculturist such information is likely to be accurate, but many pet-owners often have a bird where the sex is opposite to that which they believe.

Although it is usually possible to recognize a young bird by its immature plumage, there is no accurate way of assessing the age of most adult birds. Young budgerigars less than 10 weeks of age usually have horizontal lines of darker feathers on their foreheads, and the young of most species give the impression of having larger darker eyes than the adults. Young finches also tend to have yellow rather fleshy commisures to their beaks. The scales on the legs of rather older birds often tend to show signs of wear and tear, and have a more scaly appearance.

General Problems of Feeding and Management

The most popular pet birds are not surprisingly those whose management and feeding are comparatively simple. The psittacines, a group which includes the budgerigar and other parakeets, lovebirds, true parrots, cockatoos and macaws, are at present the most common of the pet birds in this country. The passerrines, which include the canaries and various finches, are also quite popular, although the numbers of canaries kept as pets have declined rapidly since the last war. Both these groups of birds are essentially seed eaters, and therefore simple to feed. Although a wide variety of commercially available seeds are theoretically suitable for these birds, they can become conditioned to certain types of seed and may refuse apparently suitable alternatives. The most common types of food for these birds are canary, millet and sunflower seed, maize and peanuts, depending on the size of the bird. It is, therefore, important when keeping a bird for treatment or observation for a few days to find out from the owner exactly the type of food that is normally offered. This is particularly important with the more exotic species, especially those which are omniverous, such as the mynahs, or those which are insectivorous or nectar feeders. In these latter cases, it is advisable to ask the owner to provide the staple diet when the bird is admitted.

It is important to remember that the more conventional seed-eating birds can die of starvation in less than 48 hours. A continual source of seed should always be available, and the husks which the bird removes should be blown off the surface of the food pot each day so that it can reach the seed underneath. Fresh water should always be available, and suitable vitamins and mineral supplements according to the specific dietry requirements of the species.

There are no special requirements for food and water containers, but for smaller birds the plastic "flomatic" container are probably ideal for both purposes.

Probably the most useful type of cage for keeping smaller birds admitted for treatment or observation is a conventional budgerigar breeding cage, which is essentially an open-fronted box measuring approximately 24 in. long, 12 in. high and 10 in. deep, with a wire front containing a large door, and a dropping tray. Such a semi-enclosed cage prevents smaller birds from becoming frightened by movements in the room, apart from those directly in front of it. Some of the larger psittacines have powerful beaks, and require large cages with strongly constructed bars.

If birds are to be admitted regularly, a special bird room with wire-covered windows and a safety wire mesh door to prevent escapes is obviously desirable.

Most of the popular pet birds require perches, which should be situated at either end of the cage, and as high as possible. The diameter of these perches should be such that the birds' claws can grip them without excessive contraction of the toes.

Associated with the high body temperature and metabolic rate of birds, an important part of the treatment of any sick bird, or one recovering from anaesthesia and surgery, is the provision of extra warmth. Special hospital cages with thermostatically controlled heaters are produced commercially, but an infra-red heater, the distance of which from the cage can be regulated according to the temperature required, is a useful alternative. An ambient temperature within the cage of between 85°F and 100°F is usually indicated, and a thermometer in the cage is necessary to ensure the correct temperature is maintained.

Catching and Handling Birds

Whenever an attempt is being made to catch and handle a bird, it should be made certain that all windows and doors are closed, and any other openings such as fireplaces are covered. If a bird is being removed from a cage, all perches and other accessories should also be removed, to facilitate the operation and prevent the bird damaging itself on any of these obstructions. It should be grasped firmly but gently, with the hand completely enclosing the bird so that the wings are immobilized.

Most birds will not move in the dark, and can therefore be much more easily caught if the lights are turned off or the cage taken into a darkened room or cupboard. Small birds should not be handled longer than necessary, but if a bird has to be kept out of its cage for a period of time, it can be put in a small dark cloth bag with a draw string opening, where it will remain quiet and be easily recaptured without the stress of being constantly handled. Birds may also be weighed while in such a bag, or while rolled in a paper towel or piece of cloth.

Larger psittacines can inflict quite serious injuries if not handled carefully, and budgerigars, especially hens, will give quite painful nips, although most small finches will cause a handler no damage. If smaller birds are held in the palm of the hand with the head between the thumb and forefinger, such bites will be avoided. For the larger psittacines, leather gauntlets are usually recommended, but they tend to restrict one's movements, and in certain circumstances it may be easier to drop a towel over the bird, attempting to grasp the back of the head through the towel with one hand, while holding the body with the other. This technique reduces the fear of injury to the handler, but great care must be taken to avoid injury to the bird while covered with the cloth.

In spite of taking every reasonable precaution, birds will sometimes escape and have to be caught while flying free in a room. A large net with a well padded rim is invaluable for catching them, and is an essential piece of equipment.

Administration of Medicaments

(A) ORAL DOSAGE

The method of oral dosage depends very much on the type of bird concerned, its water and food requirements and the palatibility of the drug. With a bird such as a mynah, medication of food or water may be perfectly acceptable, but obviously water medication can only be satisfactory if the daily water consumption is known, so that an accurate dosage can be achieved. On the other hand, the pet budgerigar kept in a small cage drinks a very small and variable quantity of water, and always dehusks its food. Medicaments in the water may therefore be rejected, and if mixed with the seed it will be discarded with the husks. Birds kept in aviaries tend to have a higher water consumption; aviary-housed budgerigars drink approximately 1·2 ml of water each day.

If the patient has a crop distended with seed, a drug can be injected directly into the upper digestive tract via the crop by means of a hypodermic syringe and appropriate needle. Frequently birds require medication when the crop is almost empty, which makes such direct injection difficult. In such cases, medicaments can be given via a tube that can be passed from the pharynx directly into the crop. In small birds, the beak can be held open by a pair of forceps, used as a gag. In the case of budgerigars and other small parakeets, a small blob of solder on the lower arm of the forceps, which fits the concavity of the lower mandible, prevents the gag from slipping out of position. A length of narrow-gauge polythene tube with one end pushed over a 15-gauge hypodermic needle with its point removed can now easily be passed into the crop by pushing it over the back of the tongue in a slightly oblique direction from the left to the right of the bird's pharynx. The other end of the tube can now be attached to a syringe by means of the needle, and, in the case of a budgerigar, up to 1 ml of solution injected. A very similar technique can be used for birds as large as a macaw, but using a more robust gag. An ideal instrument for such purposes can be made from a tapered metal rod approximately nine inches in length, $\frac{3}{4}$ in. in diameter at its thickest point, with a horizontal slit through its length, and a handle at one end. If one of the larger psittacines is approached, it will almost invariably bite the rod at a point dependent on the size of its open mandibles. As soon as the rod has been grasped by the bird, it can be held firmly in place and rotated until a tube can be passed through the slit into the bird's oesophagus in a manner similar to that already described.

Medicated seeds, the kernels of which are impregnated with various drugs, are commercially available. Although these can be most useful, the range of drug-impregnated seeds is rather limited, and they are only suitable for the smaller species of seed-eating birds.

(B) PARENTERAL INJECTIONS

(i) Subcutaneous

Subcutaneous injections may be given on the side of the chest, under the wing, or on the dorsal surface of the neck. Care must be taken to ensure the tip of the needle is directed downwards and away from the actual site of the injection in order to prevent seepage from the puncture wound in the rather inelastic avian skin. Up to 1 ml of fluid may be given to the smaller species by this method.

(ii) Intraperitoneal injection

When administering an intraperitoneal injection to a bird, care must be taken to avoid entering the abdominal air sacs. A short needle should be used, and inserted in the midline in the posterior part of the abdomen.

(iii) Intramuscular injection

Intramuscular injections are best made directly into the pectoral muscles, but the plunger of the syringe should be slightly withdrawn before administration of the drug, to ensure that a blood-vessel plexus, which occurs in this region, has not been inadvertently penetrated.

iv) Intravenous injections

In larger birds, the median vein on the ventral aspect of the humero-radial joint is probably the most accessible point for an intravenous injection. In smaller birds, the right jugular vein, approached from the dorsal surface of the neck, is more suitable. Both techniques are facilitated by plucking away the feathers overlying the point of the injection. The veins of smaller birds are rather fragile, and serious haematomas or subcutaneous haemorrhages can occur unless great care is taken.

Superficial Dressings and Limb Immobilization

The majority of the smaller pet birds are rather light, the weight of canaries varying between 12 and 50 g, and that of budgerigars between 30 and 60 g. It is therefore important that any superficial dressing or bandage is not too bulky and heavy, or the whole balance of the bird will be altered and it may be unable to move about the cage and feed. Probably the most useful material for superficial dressings is thin adhesive tape or Sellotape.

Fractures of the tarsometarsus are particularly common, and in larger birds they can be fixed and immobilized by intramedullary pins. In small birds, many fractures of the legs can be satisfactorily splinted with three layers of adhesive tape as the only supporting material, which should be left in position for 2 or 3 weeks. Sellotape can be used for splinting the toes of smaller birds.

In fractures of the wings, it is important that the wings are taped to the body in a normal position. The weight of the tape around the anterior portion of the body may unbalance the bird, and it may also be necessary to tape the wing tips together, which will both aid immobilization and act as a counterweight.

With birds of over 100 g, such as the larger parakeets and mynahs, other splinting materials, including matchsticks, quills and fine-gauge wire, may be incorporated in the dressing. With the exception of the psittacines, the patients do not usually interfere with the dressing applied. In these powerfully hook-billed species, an "Elizabethan collar" may be required, which can be made from thin card for a bird the size of a budgerigar; a discarded playing card is ideal. A circular disc of card, 2–3 in. in diameter, is cut out with a central hole for the neck approximately $\frac{1}{2}$ in. in diameter. The radial split necessary to fix the collar round the bird's neck can be closed with Sellotape after it is placed in position. For medium-sized parakeets, a similar collar can be made by cutting the top off a plastic detergent bottle. A leather collar will be needed for the larger parrots and macaws.

With the exception of the chronic granuloma of birds' feet known as "bumble foot", purulent skin infections of birds are relatively uncommon. If skin lacerations are present, or surgery is to be carried out, the feathers around the site should be plucked out, so that the area can be cleaned and treated appropriately. Plucking feathers from the area of skin to be exposed is more satisfactory than clipping or shaving.

Anaesthesia

In spite of the special avian anatomical and physiological features which obviously affect inhalation anaesthesia, the majority of the techniques used for mammals are also applicable to birds. Perhaps the most important factor to be considered is the birds' high body temperatures and less efficient homiothermic regulator processes, which make them more susceptible to chilling when subjected to a general anaesthetic. Factors particularly associated with avian anaesthetic failures include excessive haemorrhage during a surgical procedure; excessive heat loss; prolonged abnormal postures, particularly those involving extreme abduction of the limbs; a sudden drop in abdominal pressure, such as that associated with the removal of a large neoplasm; too deep a plane of anaesthesia; obesity; the inadvertent introduction of fluid into an air sac; and excessive excitement of the bird immediately prior to the administration of the anaesthetic.

(A) LOCAL ANAESTHETICS

Local anaesthetics should be used with caution, as the stress of handling a conscious bird may be greater than administering a general anaesthetic. It should also be remembered that all procaine derivatives can be extremely toxic to small birds and some small mammals. Ethyl chloride sprays have been used successfully for minor procedures of short duration.

(B) GENERAL ANAESTHESIA

(i) Volatile agents

The majority of the volatile anaesthetic agents used in veterinary practice are suitable for cage birds, and halothane is particularly popular. Such agents are usually given by an open-circuit method for obvious technical reasons. A small transparent plastic box connected to the anaesthetic apparatus can be a useful method for the induction of an anaesthetic, after which the bird can be removed from the box and a face mask improvised from a variety of materials. Often the end of the elephant tubing from the gas machine is adequate as a face mask without any further attachments. It is also possible to intubate most species of bird. The author, who makes no pretension of being an anaesthetist, still finds ether on a cotton-wool pad in a glass jar a most useful anaesthetic for operations of comparatively short duration.

(ii) Non-volatile anaesthetics

Many veterinary surgeons prefer the intramuscular injection of non-volatile agents, especially barbiturates, for general anaesthetic purposes; 0·05 mg of sodium pentobarbitone per gram of body weight given by the intramuscular route is still a most reliable method. Equi-Thesin* is another agent favoured by certain avian specialists, which is also given by the intramuscular route.

The success of the parenteral administration of an anaesthetic is very much dependent on the accuracy of administering the computed dose. Injections should, therefore, be given using a tuberculin or microlitre syringe. Readers are referred to

* Jensen-Salsberry Laboratories. Each 500 ml contains 21·3 g chloral hydrate, 4.8 g pentobarbitone and 10·6 g of magnesium sulphate.

the 1960 report of the AAHA on Drugs and Dosage in Budgerigars, published on page 27 of Volume 4 of the *Journal of Small Animal Practice.*

Conclusions

A healthy bird usually has sleek plumage, appears bright and alert and holds its wings close to its body. The consistency of the droppings will vary according to the species of bird and its diet, but should consist of two distinct parts. The faecal part is usually brown or black, and the urine should be white and semi-solid. Any deviation from these broad parameters should lead one to suspect some ailment, but obviously during the moulting period the plumage will be less sleek.

On the whole, infectious diseases are less common in the individually housed pet bird than in the colony-housed aviary bird, which may have direct contact with wild bird vectors of disease. As a wide generalization, the psittacines are less susceptible to infectious diseases than most other orders of birds.

Many of the more common epidemic diseases are difficult to diagnose on clinical criteria, and autopsy facilities are an important facet in the diagnosis of diseases of cage birds.

Obviously, to give a complete description of even a few of the more common diseases of cage and aviary birds would be an immense task and beyond the scope of this section. For those who wish to study the subject in greater detail, a list of further reading is provided.

Further Reading

Arnall, L. (1961) Further experiences with cage birds. *Vet. Rec.* **73,** 1148–54.

Arnall, L. (1965) Conditions of the beak and claws of budgerigars. *J. Small Anim. Pract.* **6,** 135–44.

Beach, J. E. (1962) Diseases of budgerigars and other cage birds. *Vet. Rec.* **74,** 10–14, 63–68, 136–9.

Blackmore, D. K. (1963) The incidence and aetiology of thyroid dysplasia in budgerigars. *Vet. Rec.* **75,** 1063–72.

Blackmore, D. K. (1965) The pathology and incidence of neoplasia in budgerigars. *J. Small. Anim. Pract.* **6,** 217–33.

Dall, J. A. (1965) The administration and dosage of drugs to budgerigars. *J. Small Anim. Pract.* **6,** 21–25.

Drugs and dosages in budgerigars (1963). Report of A.A.H.A. Committee on Avian Medicine and Surgery. *J. Small Anim. Pract.* **4,** 27–36.

Frost, R. C. (1961) Experiences with pet budgerigars. *Vet. Rec.* **73,** 621–6.

Keymer, I. F. (1958) The diagnosis and treatment of common psittacine diseases. *Mod. Vet. Pract.* **39** (21) 22–30.

Keymer, I. F. (1959). The diagnosis and treatment of some diseases of seed-eating passerine birds. *Mod. Vet. Pract.* **40** (7) 30–37.

Keymer, I. F. (1959). Specific disease of the canary and other seed-eating passerine birds. *Mod. Vet. Pract.* **40** (17) 32–35, (18) 45–48.

Keymer, I. F. (1961) The post-mortem examination of pet birds. *Mod. Vet. Pract.* **42** (23) 35–38, (24) 47–51.

Petrak, M. L. (1969) *Diseases of Cage and Aviary Birds.* Lea & Febiger, Philadelphia.

Taylor, T. G. (1965) The nutrient requirements of the budgerigar. *J. Small Anim. Pract.* **6,** 11–13.

(e) SMALLER MAMMALS

D. K. BLACKMORE, BSc, PhD, FRCVS and ANNE KEELEY, RANA, AIAT

Introduction

It is impossible in one chapter to give comprehensive details on the veterinary aspects of nursing the host of different species of small rodents, lagomorphs (rabbits and hares) and small carnivores, which are kept as pets, especially by children. However, the most important factor in the successful treatment of any animal, or giving advice to its owner, is an understanding of the nutrition, husbandry and reproductive physiology of the normal healthy individual. The main part of this section therefore consists of a table giving brief details of certain normal characteristics of some of the more common smaller pets. To avoid overcomplexity, only approximations are listed, and certain individuals may show some slight deviation from these average values.

Brief sections are also included on topics such as sex determination, feeding and special disease considerations, but these sections are rather cursory, and anyone requiring further details should consult a textbook on the particular species concerned. The UFAW *Handbook on the Care and Management of Laboratory Animals*, published by Livingstone Press, and parts of the IAT (Institute of Animal Technicians) *Manual of Laboratory Animal Practice and Techniques*, by Crosby Lockwood & Sons Ltd., are particularly recommended.

General Considerations

It is important to avoid any undue stress when handling a small animal, particularly if it is already sick. When approaching the cage, no sudden movement or noise should be made, and if in spite of such precautions the animal is still extremely excited, it should be allowed to calm down before being handled.

Mice, rats and gerbils may be picked up by the base of the tail, other small rodents in "cupped hands", and rabbits by the scruff of the neck and with support under the buttocks. If rabbits become frightened and struggle excessively, they can easily damage or fracture their spine, and can inflict serious scratches with their hind feet. Tame ferrets can be picked up by a hand around the chest and neck, but even tame ferrets quickly sense a nervous handler and can inflict painful bites. Mink should never be handled without gauntlets and catching tongs, and it is sensible to ask the owner to catch and restrain such animals.

Many of these small animals become particularly excitable if placed on a smooth slippery surface, and are much more easily examined if placed on a tea towel or similar non-slip material.

As the rodents tend to rely rather more on their powers of hearing and smell than on their sight and tend to have rather high body temperatures, warmth and quiet are essential factors in their successful nursing.

Many of these small animals can be quite aggressive amongst themselves, and this is particularly true of hamsters, the males of which can be badly bitten by the females. Such fighting amongst the sexes is often lessened if hamsters are kept together from weaning onwards, and not introduced to each other when already adult.

Table 2.5 gives some facts on the breeding cycles of various small pets, but it should also be appreciated that the majority exhibit a post-partum oestrus, and if the male is kept with the pregnant female, mating will occur within a few hours of the birth of the litter, and another pregnancy will immediately ensue perhaps to the detriment of both animal and owner.

Environmental Temperatures

Laboratory animals are kept in simple wire-topped boxes without separate nest boxes, and great care is therefore taken to control the temperature and humidity of an animal room, within fairly precise limits. When these animals are kept as pets, more elaborate cages with nest boxes are usually provided, and advice to owners concerning temperatures at which the animals should be kept will be influenced by the type of cage in which the animal is housed. As a general rule, mice, rats, hamsters, lemmings and gerbils require some extra heat in the winter, and should be kept indoors or in a heated shed, so that within the nest the temperature is in the region of 22°C (70°F). Lemmings particularly require a nest box containing loose litter in which they can burrow. A sudden drop in room temperature during the winter may cause golden hamsters to hibernate, a state easily mistaken for illness or death. The animal will be curled up and feel cold and stiff, with a very slow respiratory rate and heart beat. Gradual warmth will revive the animal, but alternating periods of hibernation can cause adverse physiological effects.

Rabbits, guinea-pigs and chinchillas can be kept out of doors throughout the year as long as well-constructed hutches shield them from the prevailing wind and nesting compartments with plenty of nesting material are provided. The temperature in such nest boxes should not fall below 16°C (60°F).

Mink and ferrets are well suited to outdoor cages and pens, as long as such accommodation is well constructed and weather-proof. The quality of mink pelts will suffer if the animals are not housed outside, in open-sided sheds.

Feeding

Any veterinary establishment that is likely to keep any of these smaller pets for observation or treatment should have available a supply of suitable diets. Although pet shops sell a variety of packaged foods, these are often of doubtful nutritional value. Commercially prepared and standardized cubed diets are easily available for laboratory animals and are therefore ideally suited for these domestic pets. To simplify the problem, the table indicates only four rations, for all the species listed.

DIET A

For mice and rats, cubed diets known as FFG, 41B, 86 PRM, etc., are the only

source of food necessary, and can be obtained from the usual animal foodstuff compounders.

DIET B

For the remainder of the small rodents, the basic ration can consist of mouse and rat pellets supplemented with greenfood, roots and possibly sunflower seed. Lemmings and gerbils will probably completely satisfy their water requirements from these fresh vegetables. Hamsters should not be fed oats or similar grain, which might damage the mucous membrane of the cheek pouches.

DIET C

The basic diet of rabbits, guinea-pigs and chinchillas can again consist of commercially available pellets known as RGP or SG1. Such a diet for guinea-pigs must be supplemented with greenfood or other source of vitamin C. An extra source of roughage in the form of good-quality hay is also imperative for all three species.

DIET D

Ferrets and mink are carnivores, and their staple diet is usually fresh meat or fish. Obviously, care must be taken when feeding raw meat to ensure that the diet is not deficient in vitamins or minerals, particularly calcium, and that feeding utensils are regularly cleaned. If such animals are to be kept under observation, it would be wise to find out what is normally fed to them.

Sex Determination

It is usually relatively easy to determine the sex of adult animals with well-developed genitalia. Young animals, particularly just after weaning, when they are usually purchased, may provide more of a problem. In most species, one of the most useful criteria is a comparison of the relative distance between the anus and the uro-genital opening, which is greater in the male than in the female.

The scrotal sac is fairly obvious in hamsters, so that the females appear to have a more rounded rump than the males when viewed from the ventral surface. Mice and rats, if frightened, often retract their testes, which may cause confusion when sexing these animals. The sex of young mice is determined by the distance between uro-genital opening and anus, and the shape of the uro-genital opening, which tends to be rather cone-shaped in females and more spade-shaped or square in males. Guinea-pigs can be rather difficult to sex, but the penis can be extruded by gentle pressure just anterior to the uro-genital opening. This opening in the female has a distinctive Y-shape. Similarly, the penis of rabbits can be extruded, and the vulva is rather slit-shaped, with the labia extending backwards almost to the anus. In adult males, the testes are found either side of the prepuce.

Ferrets have a limited breeding season, and out of season the testes are retracted, and the penis tends to be small and situated rather anteriorly. During the breeding season, the vulval lips of the female become obviously enlarged and elongated, which on cursory examination could be mistaken for two scrotal sacs.

Some Disease Considerations

It would be impossible, within the limits of a few pages, to summarize all the different diseases to which the animals listed in Table 2.5 are susceptible. Such detailed information can only be obtained from specialist publications. However, there are a few broad concepts, which can be briefly discussed and are relevant to the nursing of such species.

Although every group of animals is susceptible to certain specific diseases—for instance, ectromelia or mouse pox only affects mice and myxomatosis is entirely confined to rabbits—rodents and lagomorphs can all be affected with conditions associated with their continually growing incisor teeth. Associated with either insufficient wear on these teeth, due to inadequate exercise or improper food, or to developmental defects, overgrown incisors and malocclusion defects are relatively common. Similarly, overgrown and distorted claws occur quite frequently, especially in rabbits.

Neoplasia is a relatively common condition of mice, but the type of tumour and the organ affected varies considerably amongst different strains. Rats are particularly susceptible to infectious respiratory disease which although probably is primarily of virus origin is always associated with mycoplasma infections. Rabbits, guinea-pigs and chinchillas are particularly susceptibly to pseudotuberculosis and bacterial respiratory conditions. Organisms associated with these latter respiratory infections include species of *Pasteurella*, *Bordatella* and *pneumococci*. Although intestinal coccidiosis can affect most of these smaller pets, it can be a particular problem in rabbits which can frequently be affected by a variety of enteric disorders. The soiled perineum which can result from such diseases or following back injuries from incorrect handling can be a major problem, if the region is not cleaned and treated properly. Flagellates can also cause enteric syndromes in most species and chinchillas are particularly susceptible to infection with Giardia species. Although ectoparasites frequently infect most of these species the main problem seen clinically will be ear mange of the rabbit.

Both ferrets and mink are highly susceptible to the canine distemper/hard pad complex, and mink are also susceptible to infectious feline viral enteritis (panleucopenia). Great care must therefore be taken to separate such animals from cats or dogs, if being kept in hospital for treatment or observation.

(f) GENETICS AND ANIMAL BREEDING

JOHN E. COX, BVet Med, BSc, MRCVS

Genetics is the science of heredity, the study of how qualities of all kinds are transmitted from parent to offspring, both in plants and animals. Any explanation of inheritance must account both for the tendency for individuals related by descent to resemble one another, and for the tendency for related individuals to differ from each other (vaiiability). This chapter explains how this can occur.

Cell Division

To understand genetics it is necessary first to study the way in which a cell divides. Each animal is the result of the fusion of two cells (the sperm and the ovum) at fertilization into one cell, the egg (see Chapter 1). The individual develops from the egg by its division into a multitude of cells which become specialized for different purposes, some as skin cells, others as nerve cells, others as liver cells, etc.

From the genetical point of view, some of the most important structures in the cell are the chromosomes. These bodies are condensations of nucleoplasm which are only readily seen in cells which are dividing. Each chromosome consists of a pair of elongated rod-like structures, the chromatids, which are joined together at some point along their length by a body called the centromere. In the dog there are seventy-eight chromosomes altogether and they occur in thirty-nine pairs. In thirty-eight of the pairs the partners resemble each other in shape. These pairs are said to consist of homologous chromosomes. In the other pair, one chromosome is always shorter than its partner in the male animal although in the female this pair resembles one another. This pair of chromosomes are called the sex chromosomes, the small one being called the Y chromosome and its partner the X chromosome. A female mammal always has two X chromosomes and a male mammal one X and one Y.

Cells normally divide by a process of mitosis (Fig. 2.11). It begins with the disappearance of the nuclear membrane. The chromatid pairs then split up, one member going to one side of the cell and the other in the opposite direction. The cell begins to divide so that each half contains one chromatid from each original chromosome. The nuclear membrane reforms round each collection of chromatids and the cell completes its division into two. The chromatids reproduce themselves so that each chromosome is again represented by a pair of chromatids.

A different type of cell division occurs in the testicles and ovaries when the germ cells or gametes are formed, i.e. the spermatozoa and the ova. This particular type of cell division is called meiosis (Fig. 2.12). It begins with the appearance of chromatids as in mitosis. However, before the chromatids move apart to different parts of the cell, the four chromatids of a pair of chromosomes come together and exchange

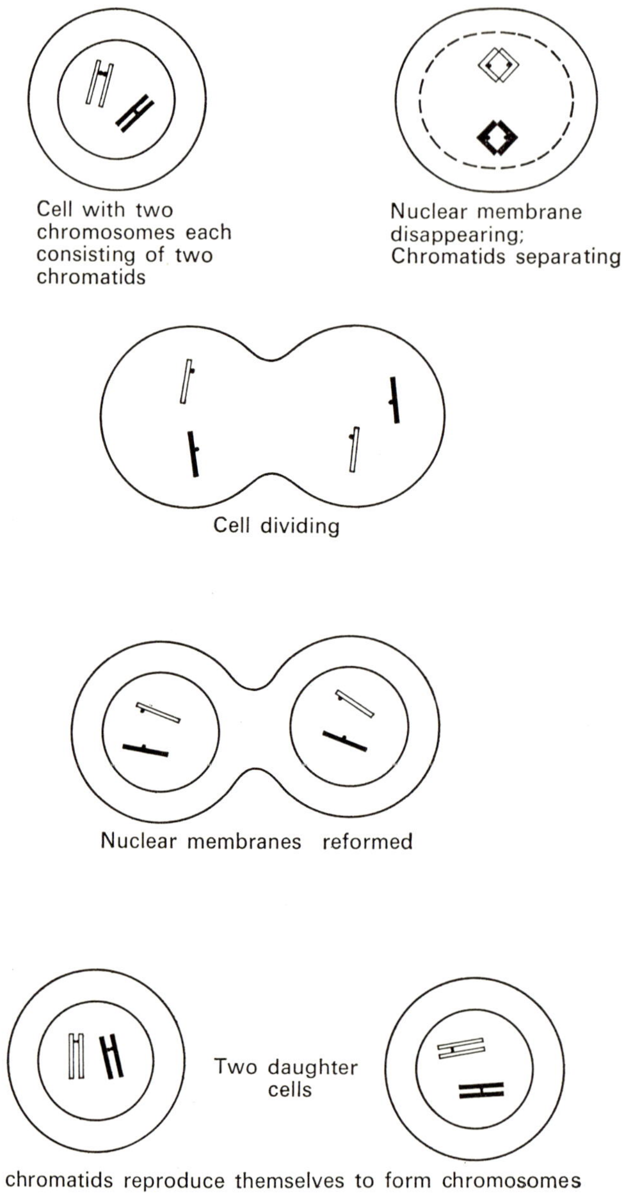

Fig. 2.11.

parts of chromosome material with each other. This peculiar phenomenon is called "crossing-over" (Fig. 2.12). Crossing over may occur at any point along the length of a chromosome, at more than one point along the length, and between any homologous pair of chromatids. Once "crossing-over" is complete, the chromosomes

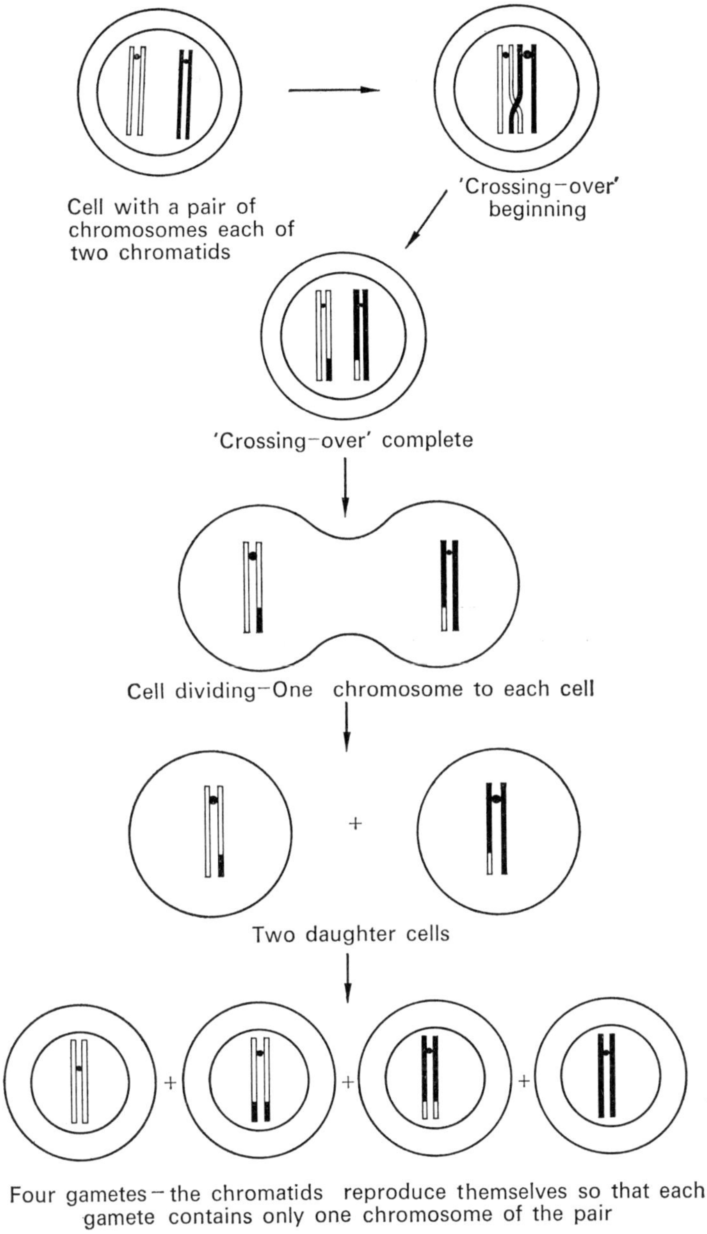

Fig. 2.12.

move apart and the cell divides, each new cell now having only one chromosome of each pair of chromosomes. Immediately afterwards each nucleus and cell divides again taking with it only one of the chromatids. The chromatids reproduce themselves so that each chromosome is represented by a pair of chromatids. These granddaughter cells of the original cell now constitute the sperm or ova. Their chromosome number is only one-half that of an ordinary body cell and they have only one chromosome of each of the pairs that are present in the ordinary body cell. When a sperm meets and fertilizes an ovum the resulting egg (called a zygote) acquires the full complement of chromosomes and begins to undergo division by mitosis.

The Inheritance of a Pair of Genes

The most satisfactory explanation of genetics results from the work of Gregor Mendel, a monk who lived in Brno in Czechoslovakia at the end of the last century. The experiments on which he based his explanations were performed on peas but the principles discovered by Mendel are applicable to animals. What Mendel discovered can best be illustrated by an example of a breeding experiment in the Dalmatian dog.

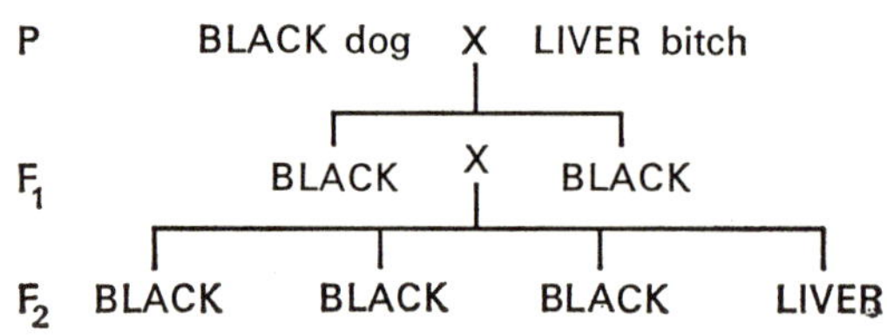

Fig. 2.13.

If a black-spotted dog from a family which has always bred black-spotted, i.e. has bred true, were mated to a liver-spotted bitch who similarly came from a family which has always bred liver-spotted, then all the puppies born to the bitch would grow up into black-spotted Dalmatians. If these black-spotted Dalmatians were now allowed to mate with each other, one in four of the puppies would develop into liver-spotted animals, the other three of every four into black-spotted animals.* This is represented diagrammatically in Fig. 2.13. P stands for "parent generation", F_1 for the "first filial generation from P" (i.e. the children) and F_2 for the "second filial generation from P" (i.e. the grandchildren).

The experiment shows that some particle or factor is transmitted from the parents (P) to the grandchildren (F_2) which causes the dog to become liver-spotted, and is masked but not eliminated in the children (F_1) because they can pass this factor on to their children (F_2). These particles are called genes, and the experiment can best be explained if it is assumed that genes occur in pairs, and that a parent transmits one, and only one, of a pair of genes to its offspring. Thus, each individual obtains one gene of a pair from its mother and one from its father. The gene which causes a black-spotted coat to develop may be represented by B, and since the black-spotted

* In practice, it would require large numbers of animals to be used in such a breeding experiment to obtain exactly a 1:3 ratio. With only four puppies it is only a chance, not a certainty, of one of them being liver-spotted. For simplicity these considerations of chance are omitted.

dog in Fig. 2.13 has two genes (they occur in pairs) he can be represented by B B. Any animal having this pair of genes will be black-spotted. The gene for liver-spotting we can represent by b and so the bitch can be represented by b b. Any animal having this pair of genes will be liver-spotted. The gene b is unable to make the spots liver-coloured in the presence of gene B. The gene b is said to be recessive to the gene B and gene B is dominant to b. Usually recessive genes are represented by the small letter corresponding to the capital letter used for the dominant genes. Both dog and bitch transmit only one of the genes they possess to each of their offspring, i.e. B from the dog, and b from the bitch, and the offspring (F_1) can, therefore, be represented as B b. Animals having this particular pair of genes will be black-spotted. When the offspring (F_1) are mated with each other, each one may give either gene B or gene b to their offspring. Their offspring (F_2) may, therefore,

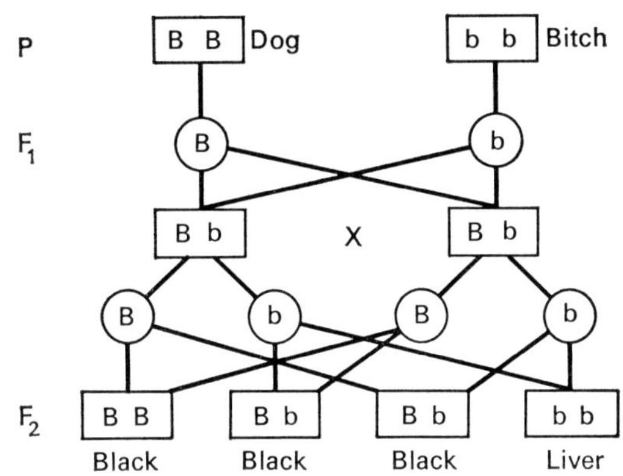

Fig. 2.14.

receive two B's (one from father, one from mother) or one B and one b, or two b's. All this can be represented in a modification of Fig. 2.13 (Fig. 2.14).

This shows how the idea of genes or particles transmitted from one generation to another, one of which dominates the other, explains how liver-spotting survives through the F_1 generation.

The correspondence of the division of meiosis which results in a reduction of the number of chromosomes by a half and the recombination of ovum and sperm at fertilization restoring the full chromosome number, with the behaviour of the genes, whose pairs split and then recombine in the next generation is no coincidence. The genes are, in fact, strung along the chromosomes like beads on a string. It has been estimated that each gene is about 0·000030 mm^3 and that a human being has 100,000 genes. Each gamete contains only half the number of genes as well as only half the number of chromosomes that an ordinary body or somatic cell contains. Fusion of the gametes into a zygote results in a restoration of the number of genes and of chromosomes to the normal level.

It is now possible to state the *First Law of Genetics*. Genes exist which influence character and which retain their identity from generation to generation. They occur in pairs in individuals and in the formation of gametes, each gene separates from the other member of the pair so that each gamete has only one of each kind of gene.

At this point it is also necessary to define certain new genetical terms.

Allelomorph. Allelomorphs are a group of genes which affect the same character in the body, e.g. those genes, such as B and b in the example, which affect coat colour. Allelomorphs occupy the same locus (i.e. the same corresponding place) on a chromosome.

Dominant genes. Those genes which have the property of suppressing the effect of their allelomorphic partner, e.g. B.

Recessive genes. Those genes, e.g. b, whose effects are masked by their allelomorphic partner unless they are inherited as a pair, as, for example, b b.

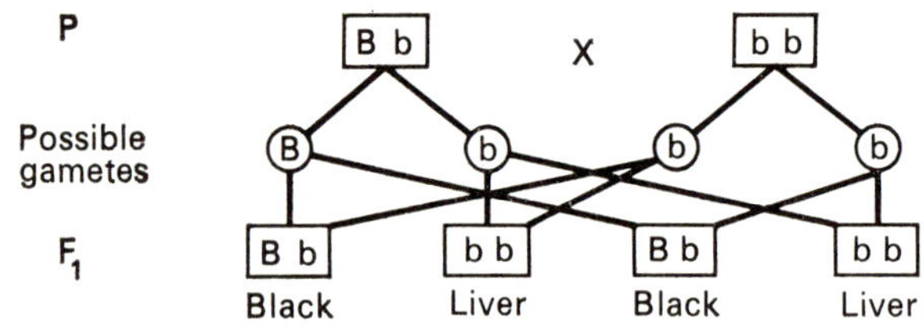

Fig. 2.15.

Homozygous. An allelomorphic gene pair, the two members of which are identical, e.g. b b or B B.

Heterozygous. An allelomorphic gene pair, the two members of which are dissimilar, e.g. B b.

Genotype. The genetical constitution that an animal receives from its parents, e.g. b b, B b or B B.

Phenotype. The appearance of an individual—liver-spotted or black-spotted. The importance of this distinction is discussed later on p. 184.

"BACK-CROSS" TO THE RECESSIVE

Animals homozygous for a particular pair of genes always breed true. Phenotypically black-spotted Dalmatians which are genotypically B B, will always have black-spotted offspring. A similar statement can be made about liver-spotted Dalmatians. However, phenotypically black-spotted Dalmatians which are genotypically B b, i.e. heterozygous, will always have some genotypically mixed offspring as well as genotypically homozygous offspring. Figure 2.15 gives a diagrammatic representation of what happens if we mate a phenotypically black-spotted Dalmatian who was genotypically heterozygous (i.e. B b) with a liver-spotted bitch.

This type of mating is known as the "back-cross to the recessive". It is being successfully used to eliminate progressive retinal atrophy (PRA) from Irish Setters.

PRA is caused by a recessive gene represented by s which is the allelomorph of a gene for sight S. Dogs with S S and S s are phenotypically normal (but, of course, dogs genotypically S s are carriers of the gene for the disease); dogs with s s are phenotypically blind. The PRA scheme as run by the Irish Setter breeders aims at eliminating the gene s from the population. Dogs or bitches carrying the gene s are identified by mating them with a homozygous blind animal (genotypically s s) kept for this purpose. A litter of six or more puppies are retained until the age when early symptoms of the disease appear about 8 weeks of age. If the litter contained no affected puppies the dog or bitch was assumed to be free of the disease (Fig. 2.16).

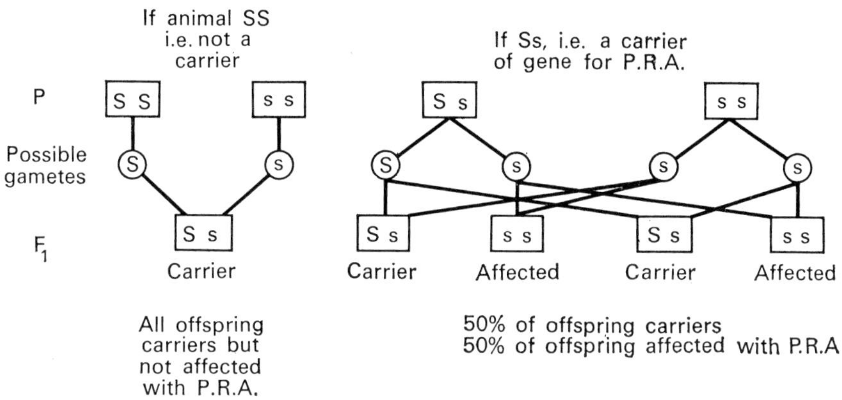

Fig. 2.16.

SEX-LINKED INHERITANCE

In both of the two situations described above the sex of the animal has been immaterial. In Fig. 2.13, for example the sexes could have been reversed and a black-spotted bitch mated with a liver-spotted dog and the result would have been the same. What happens, however, when the genes are carried on the sex chromosomes X and Y? Very, very few genes are carried on the Y chromosome so most examples are based on genes on the X chromosome. Normally, therefore, the female, with two X chromosomes, has both allelomorphs, but the male, with only one X chromosome, can have only one of the two genes of the allelomorphic pair.

An important disease both in dogs and mankind is inherited in this sex-linked fashion. The disease is haemophilia, characterized by very poor clotting of the blood so that even a minor wound can result in a fatal haemorrhage. The normal gene, H, is located on the X chromosome and its allele, the gene causing haemophilia, h, is recessive to H. Provided there is one H gene present clotting will be normal. There is no corresponding gene on the Y chromosome and thus a male who is X^hY will suffer from haemophilia since he has no H gene which allows normal clotting. Figure 2.17 shows what happens when a carrier female X^HX^h is mated with a normal male X^HY.

Problem 1

What happens if a male haemophiliac dog lives long enough to be mated to (a) a female carrier and (b) a normal female? What will be the genotype and phenotype of the offspring?

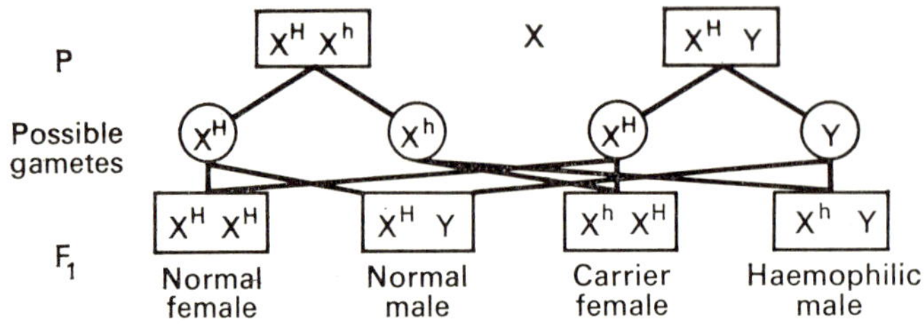

Fig. 2.17.

INCOMPLETE DOMINANCE

We must now consider a situation where a pair of genes cannot be differentiated into dominant and recessive but both have equal power of expression. The completely dominant and completely recessive pair of genes is, in fact, much less common than is often supposed. In Shorthorn cattle allelomorphic genes exist for red coat colour (C^R) and for white coat colour (C^W), but an animal which possesses gene C^R on one chromosome and C^W on the other of the pair is roan, i.e. has a mixture of red and white hairs irregularly over its body. Figure 2.18 represents the P and F_1 generations.

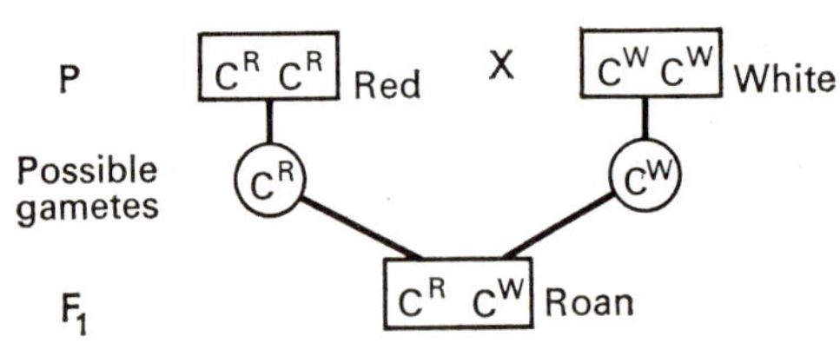

Fig. 2.18.

Problem 2

Work out the phenotype and genotype of the F_2 generation, the generation which results from crossing the F_1 generation with itself.

A special type of incomplete dominance occurs in the Kerry breed of cattle where an allelomorphic pair of genes exist, one of which allows normal growth to occur (K^N) and the other of which produces stunting of growth (K^D). Dexter cattle, which are a short-legged variety of Kerry, are heterozygous for this pair of genes, i.e. they are genotypically $K^N K^D$. If two Dexter cattle are mated, Fig. 2.19 represents the possible gametes and genotypes of the F_1 generation.

Animals (2) and (3) are normal Dexter cattle. Animal (1) is a normal specimen of the Kerry breed since it has the two genes for normal growth. Animal (4), which has the gene for stunted growth in double dose, is a very severely stunted animal and is known as a "bulldog" calf. It is often so severely deformed that it dies during development or during birth. Clearly Dexter cattle cannot breed true—on average only 50% of the pregnancies which result from Dexter/Dexter matings will result in Dexter cattle.

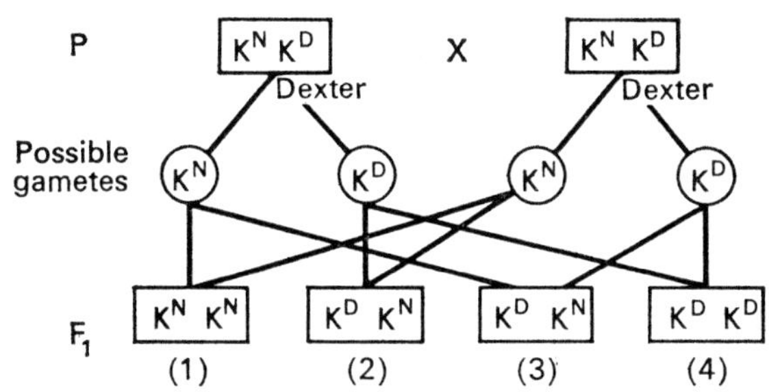

Fig. 2.19.

This situation is an example of a lethal homozygous combination of genes. In this case the gene combination only becomes lethal late in the intra-uterine life of the animal. It is possible that gene combinations exist which become lethal much earlier in pregnancy and some people believe that the infertility which arises when closely related dogs are mated is due to the occurrence of lethal homozygous combinations.

ALLELOMORPHIC GROUPS

So far we have dealt only with allelomorphic pairs but allelomorphs may exist in a series, i.e. a number of genes may exist which could occupy the same locus on a chromosome, but, of course, only two members of a series can be present in any one animal.

The most well-known sorts of allelomorphic series are those which form blood groups. In cattle at least five different types of a serum protein called Transferrin are known. The five common ones are Tf^A, Tf^B, Tf^D, Tf^E and Tf^F. They can be distinguished by separating them from one another by starch gel electrophoresis. It has been discovered that Tf^A, Tf^D and Tf^E are only found in European cattle whilst Tf^B and Tf^F are found in Zebu cattle. Blood groups are useful for checking parentage of animals. Suppose, for example, it is required to know whether a bull which is $Tf^A Tf^D$ was the sire of a calf born to a cow $Tf^A Tf^A$. If the calf were $Tf^D Tf^A$ or $Tf^A Tf^A$ then the bull could be the sire. (This test does not prove that he is the sire, only that he could be the sire.) If, on the other hand, the calf is any other combination of transferrin groups, the bull cannot be his sire. Prove this for yourself by setting out the possibilities as in Figs. 2.18 or 2.19.

The Inheritance of Two Pairs of Genes

So far situations where a single pair of genes is involved have been considered. What happens when the inheritance of two pairs of genes together is considered. In pigs there are animals with flop ears or erect ears and with black coats or red coats. It is a simple matter to show that the condition of erect ears is dominant to that for flop ears and the condition of black coat is dominant to that for red coat. Let E stand for the gene for erect ears and e for the gene for flop ears and Bl for the gene

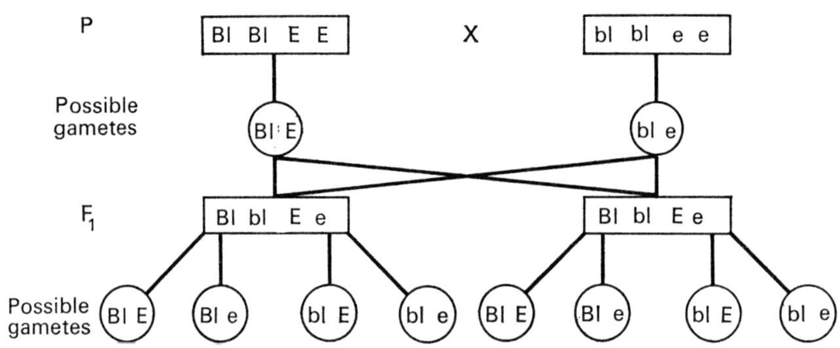

Fig. 2.20.

for black coat and bl for the gene for red coat. A pig which comes from a line which breeds true for black coat and erect ears will be genotypically Bl Bl E E and a pig which comes from a line of pigs which breeds true for red coat and for flop ears will be genotypically bl bl e e. Figure 2.20 shows what happens if we mate two such pigs. Each pig of the F_1 generation can produce four different sorts of gametes since in the reduction division of meiosis there is an equal chance of any combination of genes occurring, but every gamete must have one of each pair of genes. The possible combinations of genotype and phenotype which would occur if two F_1 pigs were mated are set out in Fig. 2.21.

The ratio of phenotypes in the F_2 generation is nine black-coated, erect-eared pigs to three black-coated, flop-eared pigs to three red-coated, erect-eared pigs to one red-coated, flop-eared pig. The ratio of black-coated to red-coated pigs is 12 to 4, i.e. 3 to 1, and the ratio of erect-eared to flop-eared pigs is also 12 to 4, i.e. 3 to 1. The conclusion is that considering two pairs of allelomorphic genes together has not affected the way in which they are inherited individually. This finding leads to a statement of the Second Law of Genetics, the *Law of Independent Assortment.* This states that when two or more pairs of genes are concerned, each pair separates independently of every other pair.

Its importance is that it provides an opportunity for genes which were originally separate to come together and be passed together to successive generations without interfering with each other. It is of particular value to livestock breeders since it allows good points possessed by different individuals to be brought together into one animal by selective matings. The example above, for instance, began with one animal with black coat but erect ears and a second animal with red coat and flop ears. Suppose a line of pigs with black coat and flop ears were wanted. The two original lines are bred up to the F_2 generation and the three animals phenotypically black-coated and

	(Bl E)	(Bl e)	(bl E)	(bl e)
(Bl E)	Bl Bl E E Black erect	Bl Bl e E Black erect	bl Bl E E Black erect	bl Bl e E Black erect
(Bl e)	Bl Bl E e Black erect	Bl Bl e e Black flop	bl Bl E e Black erect	bl Bl e e Black flop
(bl E)	Bl bl E E Black erect	Bl bl e E Black erect	bl bl E E Red erect	bl bl e E Red erect
(bl e)	Bl bl E e Black erect	Bl bl e e Black flop	bl bl E e Red erect	bl bl e e Red flop

Fig. 2.21.

flop-eared are picked out. Breeding from these will produce animals that are generally black-coated and flop-eared—selection has been exercised to breed a line of pigs with two characters we want from two lines of pigs, each one of which had one of two characters we wanted. In Australia, for example, the hardiness, good fertility and satisfactory meat quality of Merino sheep have been combined with the good mutton qualities of Border Leicester, Romney Marsh and Dorset Horn sheep. Most modern chickens are genetic combinations of breeds of animals that have had different desirable characteristics, now combined in the hybrid.

Problem 3

In the example of the pigs, notice that only one-third of the F_2 will breed true for black coat but all three will breed true for flop ears. How could you breed these three animals to find out which of them were genotypically homozygous for black?

Exceptions to the Second Law of Genetics

Unfortunately exceptions to the Second Law are very common but they form an important part of genetics because they are mostly responsible for the variation that occurs between related individuals.

LINKAGE

Two pairs of genes are said to be "linked" when they occur on the same chromosome. At meiosis such genes tend to move together so that they do not assort independently.

Figure 2.22 shows in diagrammatic form the inheritance of two pairs of genes

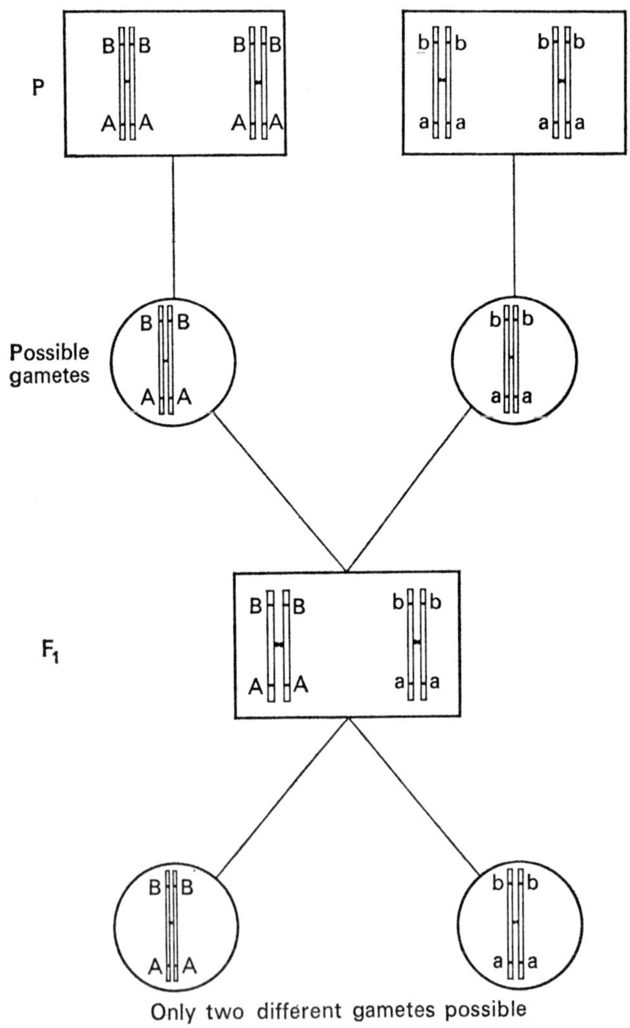

Fig. 2.22.

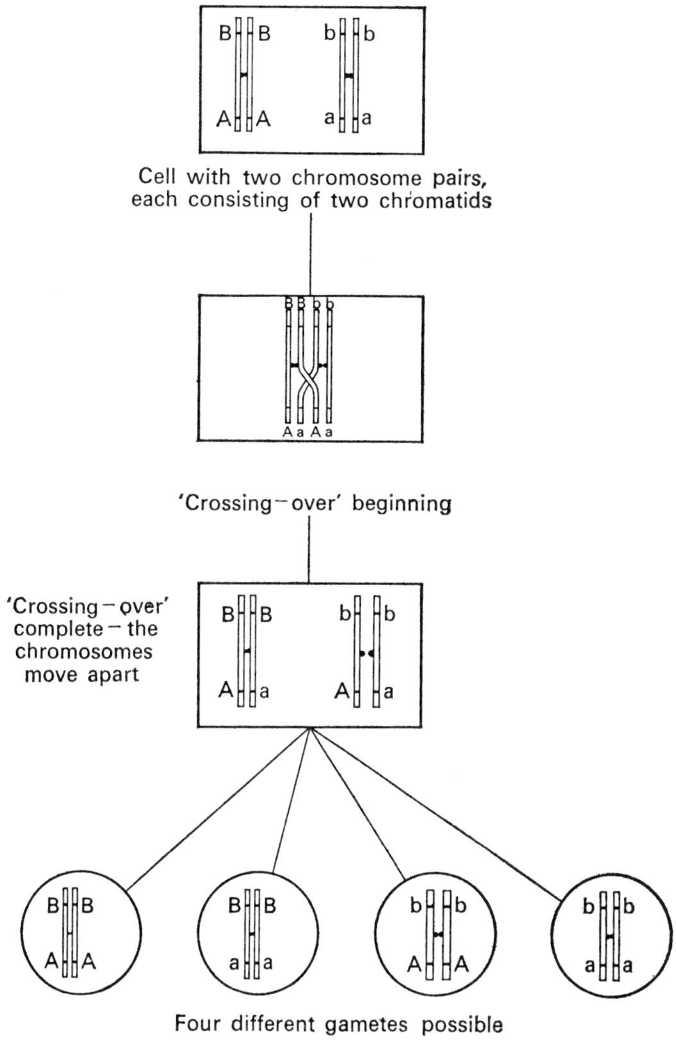

Fig. 2.23.

represented by the letters A, a, B, and b on the same chromosome assuming that "crossing-over" does not occur. It shows that where genes are on the same chromosome they are inherited together and in this situation the chromosomes are the unit of inheritance, not the genes. Given the characteristics P (the parent generation) it would be impossible for an animal ever to acquire both gene A and gene b on it no matter now many times the animals were bred. An animal would inherit chromosomes just as they had existed in either sire or dam, and, further back in time, in one or other of its grandparents. This would be a very restricting situation on inheritance. Fortunately, however, two things mitigate this otherwise constricting phenomenon.

The first thing is the phenomenon of "crossing-over". This was described on p. 170 and was a process by which chromatids exchanged parts during meiosis. Figure 2.23 shows how the phenomenon of crossing-over modifies what was described in Fig. 2.22. It can be shown that "crossing-over" is a random phenomenon, i.e. the same pattern of "crossing-over" probably never occurs twice. Genes close together on the same chromosome are less likely to be separated by "crossing-over" than that at different ends of the chromosome and since crossing-over may occur at any point along the length of a chromosome, at more than one point along the length, and between any homologous pair of chromatids (since we have to represent in two dimensions on paper what actually occurs in three dimensions), its effects are very far reaching. It ensures that no two products of meiosis, no two gametes are exactly alike. It allows new combinations of genes to arise in the gametes and, therefore, in the egg also. New combinations of genes, i.e. new genotypes, mean that new phenotypes can occur. "Crossing-over", therefore, is a very important source of the variation that occurs between individuals, between parent and offspring or even between members of the same litter.

The second factor which reduces the significance of linkage is that most animals have more than one chromosome so that many pairs of genes are not linked together. In the dog there are seventy-eight chromosomes altogether, with thirty-nine pairs so that linkage is a comparatively rare phenomenon. In a fly called *Drosophila*, which is used for a great amount of genetical research, there are only four pairs of chromosomes so linkage is fairly common in this species.

EPISTASIS

There is another special case of the inheritance of two pairs of genes. In the example of the pigs, the factors for black or red coat and erect or flop ears did not interfere with each other, either in the segregation at meiosis, or during the development of the young. Sometimes, however, two pairs of genes occur which do not interfere with each other at segregation in meiosis but do interact with one another and influence one another during development.

This can occur when the two pairs of alleles involved both control the same character. A good example is given by the genes for coat colour in rats. Rats have a gene C which allows coat colour to develop and a recessive gene c which prevents the coat from being coloured under any circumstances. Animals genotypically C C or C c, therefore, have normal coat colour but animals genotypically c c are albinos with white coats and pink eyes whatever other genes for coat colour they possess. Rats also have a gene called R for coat colour which gives a black coat and a recessive allele r, which gives a cream coat. Figure 2.24 shows what happens if a rat heterozygous for both R and C genes is mated to an albino rat which is heterozygous for gene R. The genes C and c segregate independently of R and r at meiosis but during development any rat having both genes c c will fail to develop a normal coat colour, and will be an albino.

Multiple Factor Inheritance and Environmental Variation

All the phenotypes described before have been distinct from one another, e.g. black-spotted Dalmatians *or* liver-spotted Dalmatians; red *or* roan *or* white Shorthorn cattle. Many of the characters, however, which animals possess do not exist in distinct or discrete forms like these. One example would be the height of adult human beings which may vary, in general, between 160 cm and 210 cm with every possible size existing in between; a second example would be the weight of adult Labrador dogs which might vary from 25 kg to 35 kg and, again, at least one dog could be found for every weight between these limits.

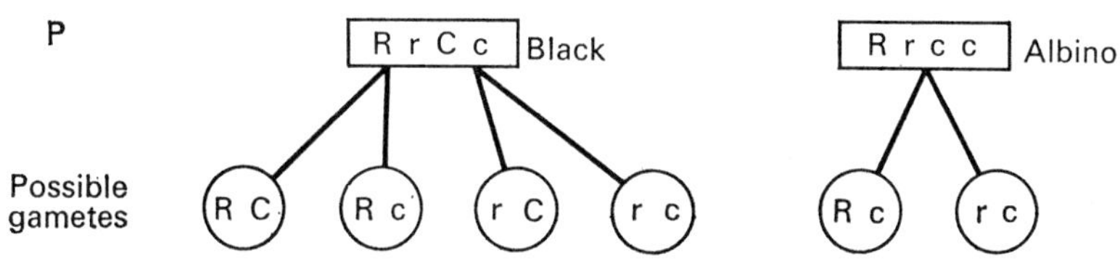

F_1 Genotypes and Phenotypes

	R C	R c	r C	r c
R c	R R C c Black	R R c c Albino	R r C c Black	R r c c Albino
r c	R r C c Black	R r c c Albino	r r C c Cream	r r c c Albino

Fig. 2.24.

There are two genetical explanations for this phenomenon. The first, "multiple factor inheritance", is an extension of the idea of blending inheritance, illustrated above by Shorthorn cattle. In that example only one pair of allelomophic genes were involved. If more than one pair of allelomorphic genes all controlling the same factor were considered, we would increase the possible number of genotypes the more pairs we took. It can be shown that with two pairs of genes, nine possible gentotypes exist and with three pairs of genes, eighty-one possible genotypes!

One possible explanation of skin colour in whites and negroes is based on the idea that two pairs of genes are involved. The pairs are S and C, S^D and C^D producing a dark skin colour and S^L and C^L producing a light colour. The more D-type genes a person has the darker he or she is and the more L-type genes, the lighter he or she is. The various gene combinations and phenotypes are shown in Fig. 2.25.

A number of pairs of genes controlling one factor can, therefore, produce quite a large number of genotypes and phenotypes. This is one explanation for continuous variation.

The second explanation is based on the fact that every gene exerts its effect in an environment over which it may have no control. A gene causes an animal to form in a certain way only because the environment in which the embryo is growing allows the gene to act in that way. In some cases, e.g. spotting in Dalmatians, coat colour in Shorthorn cattle, the environment is relatively unimportant; the gene causes the character to develop whatever the environment. But many genes are dependent on the environment and their effects can be modified by non-genetical factors.

Genotype	Phenotype
$s^Ds^Dc^Dc^D$	Negro
$s^Ds^Dc^Dc^L$ $s^Ds^Lc^Dc^D$	Dark brown
$s^Ds^Lc^Dc^L$ $s^Ls^Lc^Dc^D$ $s^Ds^Dc^Lc^L$	Medium brown
$s^Ds^Lc^Lc^L$ $s^Ls^Lc^Dc^L$	Light brown
$s^Ls^Lc^Lc^L$	White

Fig. 2.25.

Thus, it is not always true that two individuals with the same genotype will develop the same phenotype if brought up in a different environment. Different strains of Labrador may tend to differ in body size, one strain producing smaller dogs than another strain. This variation is inherited but no two Labradors will receive exactly the same food or the same exercise at the same stage of their life. This will produce dogs of different weights and this variation is due to the environment. No two people receive exactly the same amount of sunlight so that the skin colour of an individual depends both upon the genes he possesses and the environment in which he lives.

Mutation

The first law of genetics stated that genes "retain their identity from generation to generation". By that was meant that they remained the same and did not alter in any way. For the great majority of cases this is true but occasionally a gene does change its nature when being passed from one generation to another and produces a different effect in the new generation. This change in the gene is called a mutation and is a fairly rare occurrence. Even though a new gene has been formed by mutation it will behave from then on as an ordinary gene and will be subject to the rules of genetics which have been described. The majority of mutations are lethal, i.e. they are incompatible with the normal development of an individual. A small minority are beneficial, i.e. they allow the animal to survive better than animals without this particular gene, or they are useful to the stock-breeder. Most exotic breeds of dog that we now know are probably descended from dogs in which peculiar mutations occurred, which the breeders then selected. Mutations are important because they give us yet another possible source of variation between offspring and parents.

From the point of view of the veterinary nurse, it is also important to realize that the number of mutations which occur can be greatly increased by exposure to external influences such as X-rays. Thus, the person who has been exposed to large doses of radiation may suffer genetically in one of two ways. Firstly, new mutant genes may be induced in the ordinary cells of the body and these new mutant cells may start to grow in peculiar ways such as tumours, or may stop growing at all leading to stunted finger ends if that was the part exposed. Secondly, if the ovaries receive doses of radiation, the genes in the cells which are going to change there by meiosis into ova may mutate. These mutations may show themselves in the offspring in the form of deformities.

Summary

At the beginning of the chapter the statement was made that any account of inheritance must explain both how individuals related by descent resemble each other and how related individuals differ from each other. The gene and chromosome theory does this.

The concept of genes which are transferred without change from one generation to another via the gametes and which bring about development in a particular and predictable way explains why related individuals are similar. Clearly related individuals have a large number of genes in common and might, therefore, be expected to resemble each other.

Variation between individuals arises for several reasons.

Because of crossing-over during gamete formation and because of the occurrence of mutations, no two individuals inherit exactly the same genes from their parents (except in the case of identical twins). Each individual, therefore, is genotypically unique.

New gene combinations can result in variation for genetic reasons, such as blending inheritance and epistasis and multiple factor inheritance. New gene combinations can also result in variation because the environment of each individual is unique.

Further Reading

FRANKLING, ELEANOR, *Popular Dog Breeding and Genetics* (Popular Dogs).

Solutions to Problems

Problem 1 (a)

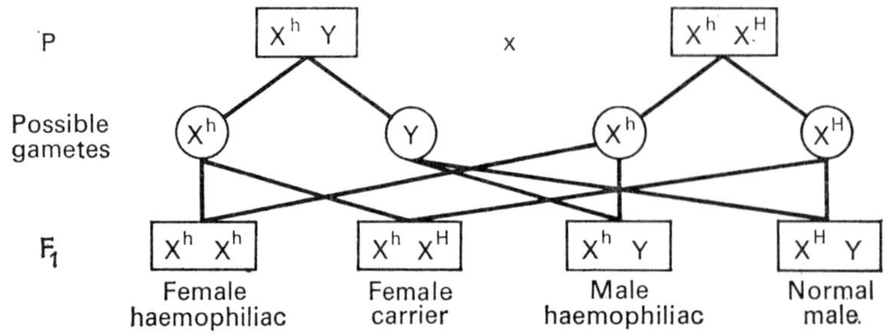

Two affected offspring (one male, one female) and one female carrier

Problem 1 (b)

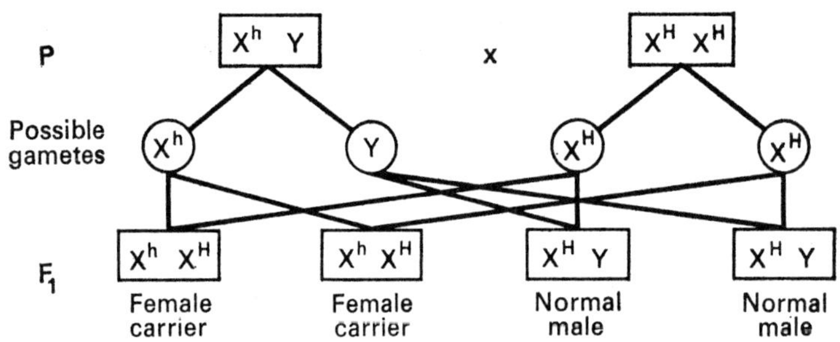

No affected offspring but two female carriers

Problem 2

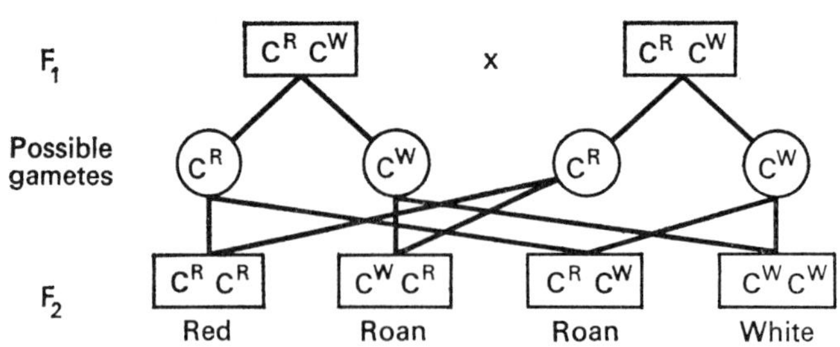

Problem 3

Mate the pigs to red-coated pigs, i.e. those homozygous for the recessive. Those black-coated pigs which have any red-coated offspring must have been heterozygous for black. Those which have only black-coated offspring will be homozygous for black. This is another example of the "back-cross to the recessive" (p. 174).

CHAPTER 3

First Aid

F. G. Startup, PhD, BSc, MRCVS

General Principles

First aid is a branch of veterinary science which provides for the immediate treatment of animals who are suffering from the effects of accidents and sudden illness.

It is the duty of the veterinary surgeon to cure injuries or disease—the purpose of first aid is to fulfil certain objects, of which the most important is to preserve the health and strength of the animal until there is a chance of obtaining professional assistance.

Animal nursing auxiliaries will be concerned mainly with the emergency case brought to the surgery, when no veterinary surgeon is immediately available. The majority of such emergency cases will be street accidents; others will be associated with bites, burns and scalds, wounds, fits, heart attacks, poisoning, foreign bodies or parturition.

The objects of first aid are to preserve life, to alleviate suffering, to promote recovery and to prevent the aggravation of the abnormal condition until the arrival of the veterinary surgeon. Pending professional treatment, or humane destruction, or during transport of the patient to hospital, the greatest possible degree of calm and comfort must be ensured.

The administration of first aid requires a sound knowledge of the recognized methods of approach to and handling of the various species of animals, together with a knowledge of normal structure and function of the animal body, and an understanding of abnormal conditions.

CASE-TAKING

An accurate history of the case is of the utmost importance. Notes should be made of all relevant details, and these notes should be made available to the veterinary surgeon who attends the case. Telephone messages concerning an emergency case, particularly a street accident, should include the following information: the whereabouts of the animal concerned, the name and address of the owner, the name and address of the person reporting the case, the nature and extent of the abnormal condition, and details of the breed, sex and age of the patient. Owners should be advised not to give anything orally, to keep the patient warm and to apply clean dressings to areas of extensive wounding or haemorrhage.

On arrival at the surgery, the following principles will apply:

1. Whenever possible, remove the cause of injury.
2. Regardless of other injuries, severe haemorrhage must receive immediate attention.
3. The air passages must be free from obstruction, and any equipment fastened too tightly around the neck must be loosened. The patient must be in a position in which breathing is as easy as possible.
4. The patient must be kept warm.
5. The patient will usually assume the position in which it is most comfortable. This should not be altered unnecessarily. Injured parts should be supported to help prevent further damage, and the animal should be made as comfortable as possible on a bed or rug.
6. Wounds should be covered with a clean dressing.
7. The patient should be carried in such a way as to support injured parts and avoid pressure. Injured limbs should be kept uppermost.
8. Small amounts of water may be given to drink, provided there are no signs of serious injury.
9. Provision should be made for professional attendance at the earliest possible moment.

DIAGNOSIS

It will be appreciated that, whenever possible, a diagnosis—that is, the discovery of the injuries that have been sustained—should be made before undertaking treatment. This, in first aid, is usually possible in a large proportion of cases.

In accident cases, the diagnosis must always be provisional and subject to amendment at a later stage. It is important to appreciate the most serious injuries first, and to deal with them accordingly. At a later stage, when the opportunity arises, the case may be considered more thoroughly.

A diagnosis is made by considering the history and the physical signs. *Symptoms* are subjective, that is, feelings experienced by the patient, and, as such, are not applicable to veterinary medicine.

The history is a description of the events preceding the illness or accident, and the manner in which the illness manifested itself or in which the accident took place. This history will be obtained from the person presenting the animal for treatment. Inquiries should be made into the former health of the patient. Failure to take a history may lead to the wrong conclusion.

Physical signs are the objective signs of disease, that is, the unusual features that will be noticed by the observer. They are described as general or local. General physical signs include changes in the colour of the mucous membranes of the mouth or eye, the temperature of the body, the condition of the breathing and the general attitude of the patient. Local physical signs, such as swelling or deformity, are confined to the injured part of the body. Physical signs are detected by examination, which will consist of observation and feel. Comparison with the opposite side is often useful to detect swellings or deformities.

ROUTINE EXAMINATION

Each individual part of the body is examined, beginning at the head and working backwards.

Eyes. The lids should be lifted and the eyes inspected.

Nose. The escape of blood should be noted.

Ears. Each ear should be similarly examined.

Mouth. When possible, the mouth should be opened, and the origin of any bleeding determined. The odour of the breath should be noted.

Head. Any deformity of the bones of the skull will be noted.

Ribs and sternum. These should be examined for any swelling or deformity.

Forelimb. Every bone in the forelimbs should be examined, and any wounds noticed. If there is no evidence of fracture the joints may be tested for movement.

Spine. The spine should be felt throughout its length, together with the pelvis.

Hindlimb. Every bone in the hindlimbs should be examined.

Body. Wounds on the abdominal surface will be noted. Abdominal palpation should not be undertaken. Haemorrhage from the urinary passages or bowel should also be noted.

Multiple injuries. Several injuries may be caused by the same accident, and failure to make a routine examination may result in injuries being undetected.

In the case of doubtful diagnosis, the most serious injuries must be considered possible and treated as such until a veterinary surgeon is available.

TRANSPORT OF INJURED ANIMALS

The methods used to transport injured dogs and cats will depend on several factors, such as the size of the animal and its temperament, the nature and extent of its injuries, the help available and the distance to be travelled.

Whatever method is adopted, the position of the injured animal should not be unnecessarily altered, and the animal should not be alarmed more than is absolutely necessary. During transport, it is important to watch the positioning of any dressings or tourniquets that have been applied.

Injured small animals may be transported either by carrying in the arms, by using a suitable box or basket, by means of a stretcher or in wheeled transport.

Carrying in the arms. Small dogs may be carried in the following manner. The animal is lifted by placing the right hand round the body and under the breastbone. The left hand is placed on the collar or the scruff of the neck. A small dog may be lifted in this way and tucked under the right arm. This method should not be used if spinal injury is present.

Larger dogs may be lifted by placing the forearm which is nearest the tail-end of the dog across the back of the dog's buttocks, turning the hand forward and inward to reach the area of the stifle joint. At the same time, the forearm nearest the head-end of the dog is placed across the front of the dog, turning the hand backward and inward to contact the area of the dog's elbow. The person carrying the dog then presses the body of the dog against his own, and, in rising, carries the fore-end of the dog slightly higher than the tail-end, so that the bulk of the weight is thrown on to the animal's buttocks resting on the carrier's forearm. If only one side of the dog is injured, this side should be carried next to the carrier. Suitable methods of restraint may have to be applied before lifting.

Boxes and baskets. This is a suitable method for cats and very small dogs. The most convenient article is the fibreglass or wicker basket made especially for the purpose. In an emergency, strong boxes, or even sacks, may be used for cats, care being taken that adequate ventilation is provided.

Stretchers. Special stretchers have been designed for the transport of large and medium-sized dogs. These are based on the human pattern of two parallel poles, kept apart with wooden strips with a piece of canvas stretched between them in the central portion. Around the canvas, a wooden rectangular box, with a hinged lid and side, is constructed, the floor being formed by the canvas. In use, the stretcher is placed on the ground, with the top and side open, the injured animal is lifted on to the canvas, and the box is closed.

Improvised stretchers may be made from sacks, rugs, blankets or coats.

Wheeled transport. This includes motor cars, hand-carts and special ambulances.

Haemorrhage

Haemorrhage—bleeding from any part of the body—is usually caused by injury, but may also occur in cases of illness when blood vessels are affected by disease. It must always be regarded as serious, for a sudden and severe loss of blood may result in death, and even a slight haemorrhage, over a long period, may mean such loss of blood as to jeopardize the life of the patient.

Haemorrhage is usually classified under two main headings—*primary* and *secondary*.

PRIMARY HAEMORRHAGE

This includes the bleeding that occurs as a result of the wounding of a blood vessel, or begins suddenly during the course of an illness.

(a) *External*—bleeding on the surface, where it can be seen. This will occur from wounds, and may be arterial, venous, capillary or mixed; and also from special regions of the body, such as mouth, nose, ear, stomach, lungs, bowels, urinary tract or uterus.

(b) *Internal*—concealed haemorrhage into the tissues or into a cavity, such as the chest or abdominal cavity, either as the result of disease, or from injury to an organ such as the liver, spleen or lungs.

General Signs

The general signs will vary according to the amount of blood lost, and the rate at which the loss has occurred. The immediate effects are those of shock.

In cases of severe haemorrhage, there is pallor of the visible mucous membranes—the gums, inside the lips and the conjunctiva of the eye are pale, and, in the severest case, almost white. The patient is dull and listless, and will sometimes show a desire for water; the pulse is rapid and feeble; the skin of the legs is cold; the temperature falls below normal; and there is increased rate of respiration. Further loss of blood resulting in anaemia of the brain, will result in extreme restlessness, gasping breath, staggering gait, and, finally, convulsions, collapse and death.

Local Signs

These will depend on the type of blood vessel that has been severed, and the region of the body affected.

The Natural Arrest of Haemorrhage

Three factors tend to stop the initial bleeding. These are:

(a) *The retraction of the cut ends of the vessel*, due to the elastic nature of the artery wall. This reduces the size of the aperture through which blood is flowing, thus lessening the flow of blood and hastening the formation of a clot in the vessel itself.

(b) *Reduced circulation*. Loss of blood will result in a lowering of blood pressure, so that less blood reaches the affected vessel.

(c) *The clotting of the blood*. Clotting takes place both in the wound and within the cut end of the vessel. The clot acts as a plug and prevents the further loss of blood.

When the haemorrhage has been arrested by the above methods, repair may take place in the cut vessel, so that it is restored. If this is not possible, then the vessel will become permanently sealed. The flow of blood will be diverted via other branches, which will become enlarged to carry the increased supply, and new vessels will develop to re-establish the natural circulation.

SECONDARY HAEMORRHAGE

This is bleeding which commences 7–10 days after the injury, and is due to the presence of germs around the injured blood vessel which destroy both the blood clot and the new repair tissue that is being formed.

Arterial Haemorrhage

Blood from an artery is bright red in colour, and issues from the wound in spurts which synchronize with the beats of the heart; the force behind each spurt will depend on the size of the artery that has been severed. If the wound is large the blood issues from the side of the wound nearest the heart. Usually, a definite bleeding point can be detected.

Venous Haemorrhage

Blood from a vein is dark red in colour and issues from the wound as a continuous steady stream, the force varying with the size of the vessel damaged; the force, however, will never be as great as with arterial haemorrhage. In the case of a large wound, the blood will issue from the side farthest from the heart. A definite bleeding point is usually visible.

Capillary Haemorrhage

This is the type of bleeding that occurs after scratches, cuts and minor wounds. The blood is red and oozes from the wound with very little force. No definite bleeding points are visible.

Mixed Haemorrhage

The arteries and veins lie close to one another and often all three types of blood vessel are injured at the same time. Capillary haemorrhage is always present when there is either arterial or venous haemorrhage, and is present, to some extent, in all wounds. When both an artery and a vein are severed at the same time the haemorrhage may be so great that the characteristic features of arterial haemorrhage are not detectable.

TREATMENT OF HAEMORRHAGE

A number of methods can be employed to stop bleeding; these are as follows:

(a) *Direct digital pressure.* Direct pressure on a wound, particularly over the bleeding point, using the finger or thumb is both effective and quick. If possible, to prevent the introduction of germs, the hands should be washed or a piece of clean material placed over the wound before pressure is applied. Care must be taken, if the presence of a foreign body is suspected, not to push this deeper into the wound; in the presence of fractures, care must be taken not to cause further displacement of the fragments.

(b) *Pad and bandage pressure.* A pad of gauze or cotton wool, applied over a wound dressing, is bandaged firmly in position. If the bleeding continues, a second pad may be bandaged over the first; it is best not to remove the first dressing, or the blood clots will be disturbed. Deep wounds may have to be packed with sterile gauze before the pressure pad is applied.

(c) *Pressure points.* A site in the body where it is possible to press an artery against a bone is called a pressure point. The point selected should be as near as possible to the wound on the heart side. The pressure of the artery against the bone prevents the flow of blood along the vessel. This method is limited, in the dog and cat, to three points:

1. The brachial artery as it passes obliquely over the inner aspect of the lower third of the humerus, 1–$1\frac{1}{2}$ in. above the elbow joint. Pressure at this point will arrest haemorrhage from below the elbow.
2. The femoral artery as it passes obliquely over the femur on the inside of the thigh. Pressure at this point arrests haemorrhage from below the stifle joint.
3. The coccygeal artery as it passes backwards along the underside of the tail. Pressure at the root will arrest haemorrhage from the rest of the tail.

(d) *Tourniquet.* This appliance stops bleeding by constricting the main arteries supplying blood to the wound. Correct application is essential, and a tourniquet should only be used in cases where there is severe haemorrhage that cannot be controlled by other methods and for limbs that have been severed.

Many forms of tourniquet are available, the usual one consisting of a flat rubber bandage with a fastening clip. It can be fixed firmly round a limb, a few inches above the wound. It should be adjusted so that the pressure is only just sufficient to stop the haemorrhage, and should never be left in position for longer than 15 minutes. When removed, it should be slackened off slowly, and any further bleeding controlled, if possible, by pressure bandages. If it is found necessary to reapply the tourniquet, it should be applied a little further towards the wound, to allow the tissues at the original site to recover from the effects of the constriction. At no time should a tourniquet be covered with a dressing, and no animal should be returned to a kennel with a tourniquet applied.

(e) *Observation of the patient.* A patient that has been treated for haemorrhage must be carefully observed in case of recurrence; dressings should be inspected at frequent intervals. On occasion, within 12 hours of the injury, the blood pressure will increase, and this may displace clots that have formed in the vessels.

Following haemorrhage, the animal should be kept quiet, in a confined space, and supplied with warmth, in the form of blankets, hot-water bottles, electric blankets or infrared heater. Provided there are no other contraindications, fluids should be allowed, but no stimulants, such as brandy, should be given because of their effect of dilating blood vessels.

Wounds

A wound is an injury in which there is a forcible break in the continuity of soft tissues. In first aid, this will usually mean a break in the skin or mucous membrane, but the term may also be applied to an injury to a tissue or organ within the body.

INCISED WOUNDS

An incised wound, usually caused by sharp cutting instruments such as knives or broken glass, is one in which the edges are clean cut and well defined. The edges of such a wound will usually gape, especially on movement, but small incised wounds may remain closed. Incised wounds usually bleed freely, but tend to heal quickly, leaving little scar.

LACERATED WOUNDS

These are the commonest type of wound encountered in small animals, caused, in most cases, by car accidents, bites, kicks, gunshot, barbed wire and blows from blunt instruments.

A lacerated wound is irregular in shape, with jagged edges and, sometimes, considerable loss of skin. They vary considerably in severity, but often the underlying muscles, fat and other tissues will also be irregularly torn. Haemorrhage, even from large wounds of this type, is often surprisingly little, as the ragged tearing of blood vessels favours rapid arrest of bleeding by clotting. Wounds of this type carry a considerable risk of infection, and will tend to heal slowly, with considerable scar formation.

PUNCTURED WOUNDS

These are produced by blows from sharp-pointed instruments such as nails, stakes, thorns, fish-hooks, bullets and also, commonly, from bites. The actual skin wound may be quite small, but this will lead to a long, narrow track, often deep in the tissues. Infection of such wounds is common, for germs may be carried deep into the tissues, hidden under the skin.

Bleeding from punctured wounds is often very small, and such wounds are liable to be overlooked in animals with hairy coats. In some cases, the cause of the wound may be seen projecting from the surface, but in others the damaging instrument may be hidden below the surface. Bullets may penetrate right through the body, leaving wounds both at the point of entrance and at the point of exit.

CONTUSED WOUNDS

A contused wound, which may be either incised or lacerated, is one in which there is bruising.

COMPLICATIONS

A wound will often be associated with damage to other structures in the vicinity, such as blood vessels, nerves or tendons; an underlying fracture may also be present. Foreign bodies may be found in the depth of a wound.

The three main dangers of wounds are haemorrhage, shock and sepsis. The healing of wounds is hindered by the presence of germs, which, being present on the skin and on most objects that cause accidental wounds, will gain access to the exposed wounded surfaces at the time of the accident. In the first instance, these germs are not very numerous and are present only on the surface of the wounds. Such a wound is called a *contaminated wound.*

Some of the germs that are present may be of a type harmful to living tissues. If they are of a virulent type, if the wound is not treated correctly, or if the natural defence mechanisms of the body are poor, these germs will invade the tissues around the wound. Such a wound is an *infected wound.* A wound that has become infected exhibits the usual signs of inflammation, becomes unhealthy in appearance and may discharge pus.

HEALING OF WOUNDS

Wounds usually heal by one of two natural methods, *first intention* or *granulation.*

In first intention healing, the edges of the wound are held together temporarily by blood clots, while new cells grow to replace those damaged by the injury. Provided there is no sepsis, which will interfere with the healing process, healing will take place in 5–10 days. First intention healing can only take place in incised wounds, the edges of which can be brought together, and kept in position, by stitching or bandaging, while healing takes place.

Granulation is a slower process that occurs in lacerated wounds and those which have become infected. Clusters of cells, called granulations, grow in the depths of the wound, increase in size and gradually grow towards the surface of the wound. On reaching the surface, new cells grow across from the skin edges to complete the healing process.

TREATMENT OF OPEN WOUNDS

The objects of treatment are to arrest haemorrhage, to treat shock and to prevent sepsis. The first two are the most important, and it is sometimes preferable to delay the preventive treatment for infection until the general condition of the patient has improved.

(a) Remove the cause of the wound, where this is possible, particularly if it is likely to cause further damage. For instance, traps, penetrating instruments or fish-hooks may be removed.

(b) Immediate steps must be taken to control any severe haemorrhage. Blood that has been clotted in a lacerated wound should not be removed by the person applying first aid.

(c) Treatment for shock should be instituted promptly.

(d) The wound should be exposed by removing any dressings that might have been applied by the owner. All instruments used in treating the wound should be sterilized if possible, and the operator must ensure personal cleanliness to prevent any further contamination of the wound.

(e) Foreign bodies in the depths of the wound, provided they are not deeply imbedded, may be removed.

(f) The hair around the wound should be clipped, and the wound cleansed thoroughly with a suitable antiseptic solution. Such substances destroy or hinder the growth of micro-organisms, but must be used in the exact strength recommended by the manufacturers. The cleansing of the wound should be gentle but thorough, making sure that the antiseptic penetrates into the depths of the wound, but taking care that the wound is not further contaminated with dirt derived from the skin. The chief value of bathing is mechanical, to wash away dirt and germs. Many proprietary antiseptics such as "Dettol" or "Cetavlon" are suitable.

(g) A suitable dressing should now be applied, preferably of sterile gauze, covered with cotton wool and bandaged. If the wound is heavily contaminated, an antiseptic cream may be used, particularly in those cases where the application of a dressing is not possible.

CLOSED WOUNDS

Closed wounds are those which do not penetrate the whole thickness of the skin.

Contusion

A contusion or bruise is produced by a blow with a blunt object, causing rupture of small blood vessels below the skin surface and varying amounts of damage to the soft tissues.

Heat, pain and swelling will be exhibited, and, in animals with a white skin, discoloration, at first red and later purple, fading to yellow at a later stage, will be present.

Treatment consists of cold compresses and firm bandaging to limit swelling. If the swelling has already developed, hot compresses will relieve pain.

Haematoma

When, following a blow, blood is lost under the skin in greater quantities than in a contusion, a rounded swelling called a haematoma is formed. Unlike an abscess, such a swelling is at first soft, and later develops a hard edge. Haematomata are commonly seen affecting the ears of dogs and cats. Treatment will be as for contusions, but surgical interference will often be required (see p. 351).

Abrasion

An abrasion is a superficial wound, in which there is some loss of the upper layers of the skin only. Such a wound will be produced by glancing blows or by being dragged along the ground in street accidents.

Although the visible wound might be slight, such injuries are often painful, and likely to become contaminated with dirt, and to become subsequently infected.

Healing of an abrasion takes place under the scab formed by the coagulation and drying of the serum which exudes from the injured surface, after the initial bleeding has stopped. Any abrasion should be thoroughly cleansed when still fresh, to prevent a contaminated wound becoming an infected one, and thus delaying healing.

Snake Bite

Although not common in Great Britain, cases will be presented of dogs and cats bitten by the adder. Massive swelling around the injured part may be exhibited, and in some cases the patient will show signs of great distress and even collapse. If the bite is in a limb, the circulation may be arrested temporarily by the use of a tourniquet. If the wound is visible, a few crystals of permanganate should be rubbed into the area. The assistance of a veterinary surgeon should be obtained as soon as possible.

Wasp and Bee Stings

Stings by these insects are common in the dog, usually in the mouth or around the lips, but occasionally on the feet. Stings in the mouth may cause considerable swelling and excessive salivation.

If visible, bee stings should be removed with forceps; wasps do not leave their stings behind. Stings outside the mouth should be freely swabbed with methylated spirit. Stings inside the mouth should be washed with a solution of bicarbonate of soda (one dessertspoonful to a pint of water). A swab soaked in a solution of one tablespoonful of household ammonia to half a pint of water, or a blue-bag, may be held over the part. In the event of marked swelling within the mouth, the assistance of a veterinary surgeon should be obtained.

Burns and Scalds

A *burn* is an injury caused to the body by dry heat, such as a fire or a piece of hot material. A *scald* is the injury caused by the effect of moist heat, such as boiling water, tar or fat. Special varieties of burns are produced by certain chemicals, excessive cold or electric currents. The distinction between burns and scalds is not of practical interest, for the signs and principles of treatment are the same in each case.

CLASSIFICATION

Burns vary greatly in both surface extent as well as in depth. According to their surface extent burns are often referred to as major or minor burns. It has been usual to describe burns according to their depth, but it must be understood that a burn is usually a combination of different degrees. Although, in the past, it has been usual to classify burns as 1st, 2nd, 3rd, 4th, 5th or 6th degree, according to their depth, it is now more usual to describe them as *superficial* (1st and 2nd degree) and *deep* (the remainder). A superficial burn is one which extends no deeper than the thickness of the skin. A deep burn is one which extends through the skin and may involve the fat below the skin, the muscles, or even the bones.

CLINICAL SIGNS

Although a small, deep burn may penetrate into the muscles, and yet cause little general upset, a large surface burn may produce severe general effects.

The appearance of a burn will, of course, vary greatly according to its depth and extent. The effect of heat on animals covered with hair can be easily recognized, as the hair is singed or destroyed. In the case of scalds, however, the effects may not be noticeable for several hours or even days.

Excessive heat applied to the skin kills the surface cells, and, except in mild cases, injures the deeper cells. The small blood vessels in the skin dilate, and fluid escapes from them and accumulates in the surrounding tissues. Some of this fluid escapes to the surface, and, where the hair has been lost, the surface is seen to be red and moist. In scalds, the fluid matts the hair together, and surface evaporation leads to the formation of thick crusts over the damaged part. Blisters are rarely seen in animals.

COMPLICATIONS

The degree of shock is very severe in cases of extensive burning, and may prove fatal. Established shock, occurring later, is equally serious and is produced by exposure, pain and the absorption of toxic substances formed in the burnt tissues.

Septic absorption, the absorption of these toxic substances into the blood, or the poisons generated by various micro-organisms infecting the damaged areas, may lead to a toxaemia or septicaemia. Death may result from the effects of shock, toxaemia or infection.

Local complications may include sepsis of the injured parts, and contractures due to the shrinking of skin associated with scar formation.

TREATMENT

Burns and scalds are extremely painful, and animals may resent interference. All cases of extensive burns or scalds should be treated by a veterinary surgeon at the earliest possible opportunity. In many cases, a suitable narcotic or general anaesthetic will be given before local treatment is commenced.

Immediate treatment to prevent and limit shock should be undertaken. Warmth, rest and the relief of pain are essential, and fluids should be offered.

The process of burning itself destroys germs present on the skin, and a burn will remain sterile for some time after the accident. It is, therefore, most important not to contaminate the burn in any way. The area should be covered with a dry, absorbent, sterile dressing and bandaged if possible. Support should be given where possible, and, if the burn involves a limb, and is extensive, a splint should be applied. Thorough cleansing of the burn should only be undertaken later, under strict aseptic conditions.

Slight burns should be treated by cleansing the affected area and applying a suitable dressing. Any loose charred remnants should be removed by swabbing with warm normal saline, and soap and water may be used to remove gross dirt or grease around the area. A suitable dressing is "tulle gras", sterile and packed ready for immediate use. Alternatively, in very mild cases, tannic acid jelly may be used, applied directly to the wound, and covered with sterile gauze and bandaged.

The long hair of animals sometimes remains attached to the injured areas, making it difficult to determine the extent of the injury. To permit the cleansing and dressing of the burn, this will have to be clipped away; such a procedure may not be possible until professional help is available.

CHEMICAL BURNS

Many chemicals produce severe burns. Among those that may be mentioned are the corrosive acids, and alkalis such as quicklime and caustic soda.

If the burn is caused by an acid, the part should be bathed in an alkaline solution such as bicarbonate of soda or washing soda. If the burn is caused by a corrosive alkali, the part should be bathed with an acid solution, made by mixing equal parts of vinegar and water. After the burn has been treated by such neutralization, a suitable local dressing should be applied.

Fractures

A fracture is said to have occurred when a bone is broken. The nature of the injury may vary from a crack to a complete break, but, however slight the injury, the condition is still, technically, a fracture.

CAUSES OF FRACTURE

Most fractures are caused by violence, applied to some part of the body.

Direct violence. When a bone fractures at the place to which violence is applied, the fracture is termed direct. This is the commonest cause of fractures, as seen in severe blows, street accidents and gunshot wounds.

Indirect violence. When a bone breaks at some distance from the area where force is applied, the fracture is termed indirect. Jumping on to the feet, and breaking one of the bones of the leg, is an example.

Muscular action. Sometimes mere force of muscular contraction is sufficient to break a bone. This will be seen particularly in the racing greyhound.

Spontaneous fracture. Occasionally, a bone will be broken without the application of violence. This is a spontaneous or pathological fracture and is due to some existing bone disease.

FRAGMENTS

The pieces of bone that are formed as the result of a fracture are called fragments. They are often sharp and jagged, and thus likely to cause further damage to the adjacent tissues. These fragments may be displaced due to muscular spasm.

VARIETIES OF FRACTURE

(a) *Simple fracture.* This is one in which the bone is broken, but there is no communicating wound between the site of fracture and the broken skin or mucous membrane. There is, of course, always slight damage to the adjacent tissues.

Simple fractures may be further classified as *transverse,* in which the bones are broken almost straight across; *spiral,* in which the bone is broken obliquely; and *fissured,* in which the bone is cracked, but not completely broken.

The term simple fracture is misleading, for the condition may be far from a simple injury.

(b) *Compound fracture.* This is one in which the bone is broken and the skin or mucous membrane punctured or torn, so that air can gain access to the fragments. Such access may be obtained either through a skin wound leading down the fracture, as in gunshot wounds; by the sharp, jagged edges of the fragments protruding through the skin; in the case of a fractured jaw, by tearing of the gum; or, in the case of fractured ribs, injuring the underlying lung.

A compound fracture allows air to gain access to the fragments, thus increasing the risks of sepsis.

(c) *Complicated fracture.* This is any fracture, simple or compound, which is complicated by damage to blood vessels, nerves, joint or vital organ, such as lung, spinal cord or brain. A simple fracture may be converted into either a compound or a complicated fracture by careless handling, or by movements on the part of the patient.

(d) *Depressed fracture.* This is a fracture in which one of the fragments is depressed below its normal level. It will occur in the skull, and may cause damage to the brain.

(e) *Comminuted fracture.* One in which the bone is broken into more than two segments.

(f) *Greenstick fracture.* A fracture, usually in young animals, owing to the softer state of the bony tissues, in which the bone is cracked and bent, but not broken across completely.

(g) *Impacted fracture.* One in which the broken ends are driven into one another.

(h) *Multiple fracture.* This term is applied when the bone is fractured in two or more places, with an appreciable distance between the sites of fracture.

GENERAL SIGNS OF FRACTURE

(a) *Pain* at or near the seat of fracture. This is not constant. Pain increases shock and every effort should be made to avoid increased pain by gentle handling.

(b) *Loss of function*, which may be partial or complete. There is always some limitation of use.

(c) *Unnatural mobility.* Movement may be noticed at the site of fracture.

(d) *Deformity.* A fractured part often appears deformed, but this sign may not be present. Comparison with the opposite side may help in detection.

(e) *Shortening.* The contracting muscles may cause the broken ends of the bone to override, thereby producing shortening of the limb.

(f) *Irregularity.* This may be noticed on the surface of the bone, in the form of a sharp edge or a bump. Swelling of the soft tissues may prevent detection of this sign.

(g) *Swelling* makes its appearance soon after the accident, due to rupture of small blood vessels and diffusion of blood around the fracture site. The swelling usually increases later, and may make it difficult to detect the other signs of fracture.

(h) *Crepitus.* A grating sound may be felt or heard when the broken ends move against one another. This and unnatural mobility should not be sought by persons giving first aid, but if noticed accidently during the course of examination give positive evidence of the presence of a fracture. These two signs will not be detected in greenstick or impacted fractures.

It must not be expected that all the above signs will be found in every case. Severe pain alone, after an accident to a limb, is in itself suspicious. Any suspicion of fracture warrants the appropriate treatment until professional assistance is available.

THE UNION OF FRACTURES (see pages 364 and 365)

PRINCIPLES OF TREATMENT

The object of first-aid treatment of fractures is twofold—to prevent further injury or aggravation, especially to prevent a simple fracture becoming compound or complicated; and to reduce the amount of pain suffered by the patient. In the case of compound fractures there are the added objects of arresting haemorrhage and preventing sepsis.

Whenever a fracture is known to exist, or is suspected, the limb or other broken bone should be handled as little as possible. The animal should be made as comfortable as possible, kept warm and its movement restricted. No attempt should be made to reduce the fracture and reset it in its correct position, but, where possible, the part should be immobilized by use of a temporary splint.

FIRST-AID TREATMENT OF FRACTURES

(a) *Bandaging.* This method, of bandaging the affected part securely to a firm part of the body, is applicable to the scapula, which may be fixed to the side of the chest, and to the bones of the lower parts of the limbs, which may thus be held firmly together.

(b) *Splinting.* Splints provide a satisfactory and permanent support for many fractures, and may be used as a temporary measure if professional assistance is not available.

(c) *Compound fractures.* The injured limb should be supported in the usual way. Bleeding should be controlled and the wound covered with a dressing. It is not advisable to cleanse the wound at this stage for fear of introducing further infection to the fracture site. A splint should be applied when possible, taking care that pressure is avoided over the fracture site, and, if possible, bandaging only above and below and not over the injured area.

Splints

A splint is an appliance which restricts the movement of an injured part. In first aid, the purpose of a splint is to prevent a fracture becoming compound or complicated pending professional attendance. At the same time, the splint provides rest to the injured part, and hence relieves pain and promotes healing. They are of particular value when there is likely to be delay before professional services are available, or when the animal has to be transported. In the dog and cat, splints can be applied to only a few areas.

Types Available

(a) *Wooden.* Straight pieces of wood, of varying length and width, may be employed, or Gooch's splinting may be cut to any desired size.

(b) *Metal.* Preformed splints, made of tin or aluminium, are available. The Mason meta splint, used primarily in fractures of the metacarpals or metatarsals, is of moulded aluminium, shaped to conform with the shape of the limb, and with provision for alteration in length. Malleable aluminium sheeting backed with sponge rubber will be found useful.

(c) *Wire.* Kramer's wire splinting, made of a framework of metal, strengthened by cross-struts, may be cut to any length, and may be easily moulded to the shape of the limb to be supported.

(d) *Plaster.* Roller bandages made of coarse material, and impregnated with plaster of Paris, are commonly used in fracture treatment. The use of such bandages to encase a limb is not within the scope of first aid. It is possible, however, to fashion excellent splints from these bandages. For this purpose, a bandage is soaked in warm water, unrolled on a smooth surface, and folded several times upon itself to form a slab of the desired length. This is then moulded upon the affected limb and secured in position by an ordinary roller bandage, used wet. The plaster will set hard and form a good splint.

Application

A splint must be firm and long enough to keep the joints immediately above and below the fractured bone immobilized. The splint should be covered with cotton-wool secured to it by adhesive plaster to prevent discomfort or damage to the skin by pressure of the hard material. When a choice of splints is available, one should be used which can be suitably moulded to the contours of the limb involved.

The limb should first be bandaged and wrapped in a layer of cotton-wool. The padded splint is then applied to the limb and bandaged firmly in position down to the limb. Care must be taken that the bandage is not applied too tightly, or the circulation may be impeded. Should any swelling occur in the limb, below the lower end of the fracture, the splint must be readjusted. Where possible, the bandage should not be allowed to encircle the limb at the actual site of fracture, for fear of causing complications.

COMMON SITES OF FRACTURE

Fracture of the Skull

A fracture of the upper part is usually due to direct violence, such as a blow on the head. A fracture of the base is usually due to indirect violence, such as a blow on the jaw or a fall on the head.

Signs. If the upper part is fractured there is frequently loss of consciousness, either immediate or gradual, together with swelling and irregularity. Fractures of the base may produce immediate unconsciousness, but there may be no swelling or other sign of injury. There may be haemorrhage from either ear or nose, or blood may pass to the stomach and be subsequently vomited. The fracture may involve the orbit, causing damage to, or prolapse of, the eyeball.

Fractures of the facial bones, except in the case of flat-nosed breeds, are not likely to cause brain injury, but may involve the facial sinuses.

Fracture of the Lower Jaw

The common sites of fracture are:

(a) At the junction of the right and left halves of the mandible, in the region of the lower incisor teeth. Such an injury may be transverse, with the detached piece of bone carrying the incisor teeth supported only by the gums, or the fractured bone may be completely detached. If the fracture is longitudinal, between the two central lower incisors, it may not be a true fracture but a forced separation of the joint between the two halves of the mandible.

(b) Just below the joint which is at the side of the face near the base of the ear.

(c) In the middle of the horizontal ramus, in the area of the premolar teeth.

The most noticeable signs of fracture of the lower jaw are deformity, irregularity of teeth and loss of power to move the jaw freely. Crepitus and bleeding from the gums are often present.

Treatment. Wounds and haemorrhage must be dealt with in the normal manner. Some support may be given by applying a wide tape muzzle, as used in restraint, but this must not be applied too tightly. Fractures at the junction of the two halves of the jawbone may sometimes be supported temporarily by tying a flat bandage round the lower jaw, over the gums, just behind the incisor teeth.

Fracture of the Scapula

Although uncommon, fracture of this bone, usually as the result of direct force, may be overlooked—particularly if other bones of the limb are fractured at the same time.

Fractures of the scapula, which are usually simple, rarely cause displacement, and there is little evidence of swelling or haemorrhage. Lameness will be exhibited and there may be some dropping of the shoulder. Pain is variable, but not usually marked, and crepitus is not a prominent sign.

Support may be given by applying a spica, binding the scapula to the side of the chest.

Fracture of the Humerus

The humerus may be fractured anywhere in its shaft, most commonly in the lower third or at the lower extremity. Fractures of the upper extremity, most likely to occur in young animals from indirect force, are uncommon; such cases will exhibit intense pain on palpation and the leg will be carried with the lower parts flexed and the shoulder extended.

Fractures in the middle of the humerus are common, and may be transverse, oblique, spiral or comminuted. Direct force is the usual cause, and haemorrhage and swelling are always present. The limb will be carried with the elbow dropped and the carpus partially flexed; the toes will be pointed outwards and the limb will appear shortened. Pain and crepitus will be exhibited.

Fractures of the lower extremity, involving the joint, are most likely to be seen when there has been impact with a moving object, such as a car, or when the animal has jumped from a high place, landing on the extended forelimb. Such fractures are usually simple, but may be associated with dislocation of the joint. The limb will be carried with the carpus flexed and the elbow extended. Pain and crepitus will usually be present, but lameness will be variable depending on the actual site of the fracture.

It is not possible to splint the upper part of the forelimb. Confinement in a small area should be enforced to prevent movement as far as possible.

Fracture of the Radius and Ulna

Most fractures of the radius involve the ulna also, but cases will be seen where the ulna only is affected. Most fractures of these bones occur in the lower segment, and are usually simple and either transverse or oblique. Comminuted fractures may be seen in older dogs. Greenstick fractures are not uncommon in young dogs. Fracture of the olecranon process of the ulna will occasionally be seen.

Fractures of these bones are usually the result of direct force. Animals with fracture of the shaft will carry the limb with a slight flexion, and the foot will be rotated outwards, producing a curvature of the limb. Swelling is variable but pain and crepitus will be present.

Treatment. The limb may be immobilized with a splint, and the animal kept in a confined space.

Fracture of the Pelvis

Fractures of the pelvis may involve any of the three pelvic bones or the acetabulum; those involving the ilium are common, but often more than one bone is involved. Separation of the pelvic symphysis may occur in young animals, and a separation of the sacro-iliac junction may be associated with other fractures or may occur by itself in dogs of all ages.

Multiple fractures are often seen but are seldom compound. The amount of displacement will be variable, but there will often be considerable damage to the soft tissues.

Animals exhibiting fracture of the ilium will usually be able to stand, and even walk with difficulty; the limb will often be rotated inwards and the injured side appears dropped below the level of the other side. Cases exhibiting fracture of the symphysis or bilateral sacro-iliac separation will usually be unable to rise or to take weight on the hindquarters. Fractures involving the acetabulum will cause varying lameness depending on their severity.

Treatment. General nursing care and confinement in a small place are the only first aid measures that can be adopted.

Fracture of the Femur

Fractures of the femur occur more commonly than fractures of any other bone. The head and neck, or any part of the shaft, may be involved.

Fractures of the head and neck, which occur mostly in young animals, are the result of indirect force. The limb will be carried in a flexed position, usually rotated outwards. There may be some swelling present, and severe pain on manipulation.

Fractures of the shaft usually occur as a result of direct violence. Those in the upper part of the shaft are the least common, and, in this position, although comminuted fractures are common, compound injuries are not often seen. Animals with fracture of the upper segment will stand with the leg shortened and hanging limp; pain is not usually marked.

Fractures in the middle of the shaft are most common, and may be transverse, oblique or comminuted, and occasionally compound. Swelling, pain and crepitus will usually be exhibited, and, if the animal attempts to walk, the leg will swing freely.

Fractures of the lower segment, often involving the joint, are seen more commonly in young animals, and may be caused by both direct and indirect violence. Compound fractures in this area are sometimes seen. Swelling is not usually marked, and the limb is usually held in a flexed position with the tarsus over-extended.

Treatment. Limitation of movement is essential to prevent further damage to soft tissues. No immobilization is possible in fractures of the upper part of the bone, but splinting is possible if the lower segment only is involved.

Fracture of the Tibia and Fibula

The common fractures seen in these bones are separations of the upper epiphysis and transverse fractures of the shaft, usually involving both bones. Epiphyseal fractures usually result from either indirect force or muscular action; fractures of the shaft result from direct violence. Such fractures are usually simple, and rarely compound.

The leg is carried flexed but may not show much distortion. Pain will be exhibited on manipulation but there is seldom much swelling.

Treatment. Immobilization by means of a splint should be carried out.

Fractures of the Carpus and Tarsus

These fractures are uncommon except in the racing Greyhound. All the usual signs of fracture will be present except that the normal mobility of the joint may be restricted by muscular contraction.

Treatment. The joint should be immobilized by bandaging.

Fracture of the Metacarpals and Metatarsals

Fracture of these bones is usually due to direct violence, often crushing injuries. All the general signs will be exhibited.

Treatment. A wide splint should be applied to the back of the injured paw to support the fracture.

Fracture of the Bones of the Digits

These are usually due to direct violence. All the general signs will be present. Support may be afforded by bandaging.

Fracture of the Ribs

Fractures of the ribs and sternum are uncommon, but some may escape detection, especially when only one rib is involved. Unless a number of ribs are fractured, displacement is not usually marked. If deformity is present, this may be detected by palpation, or may be obvious. Fractured ribs may penetrate the pleura or even the lung. This may cause a swelling under the skin containing air (*subcutaneous emphysema*) or a haemorrhage into the chest (*haemothorax*). Severe damage to the lung may result in acute signs such as cyanosis, increased respiratory rate and the coughing up of bright red frothy blood.

Treatment. Where there is no internal injury, rest is all that is necessary in simple cases. In more severe cases, some support may be given by bandaging the chest fairly tightly. General principles must be applied in all cases in which there is evidence of internal damage.

Fracture of the Spine

Direct or indirect violence may cause fracture of the vertebral column, but usually, in the dog, it is the result of road accidents or heavy weights falling on the animal's back.

Fractures of the spine may occur in any part, most commonly in the posterior thoracic or lumbar vertebrae. One or more vertebrae may be fractured, and, according to the extent of the injury and the displacement of the fragments, the spinal cord may be damaged. Injury to the spinal cord will produce partial or complete paralysis. If the paralysis is complete, sensation and movement of the body, posterior to the site of the injury, will be absent, although marked pain will be exhibited at the site of the damage. Extensive injuries, particularly in the cervical region, may result in immediate death.

Animals exhibiting fractures in the cervical region will usually be unable to stand. The head muscles will be tight, and breathing may be rapid; nystagmus is usually present. Movement of the head in any direction causes severe pain.

Fractures in the thoracic or lumbar areas result in extension and rigidity of the forelimbs, whereas the hindlimbs are limp. The back is arched over the fracture site, there is an anxious expression, often an increased respiratory rate, and intense pain on palpation.

Treatment. Euthanasia will often be necessary in these cases, and the animal must be kept as comfortable as possible pending the arrival of the veterinary surgeon.

Dislocations

A *dislocation*, or *luxation*, is a displacement of one or more bones entering into the formation of a joint. Such articular separations may be incomplete (*subluxations*) or complete (*total luxations*). A luxation is a complete separation of the articular surfaces of a joint. A subluxation is a partial separation or a change in relationship with some of the articular surfaces still in contact. A luxation may be simple or compound, but most are simple. Both fracture and luxation may occur in the same injury.

CAUSES OF DISLOCATIONS

Acute dislocations occur as the result of direct or indirect violence; chronic or recurrent dislocations are the result of degeneration of the other structures of the joint such as joint capsule or ligaments. At times, dislocations are the result of congenital deformities.

GENERAL SIGNS OF DISLOCATIONS

(a) Loss of function in the limb.
(b) Pain on manipulation of the joint, or pain around the joint.
(c) Swelling around the joint.
(d) Limited movement of the joint.
(e) Deformity, the limb assuming an unnatural position.
(f) Deviation in the length of an extremity.

The signs will vary in degree and extent according to the joint involved and the extent of the injury. The altered position of the bone-ends may be noticed on palpation. Crepitus is not a common sign, but may be noticed in a lesser form than in fractures.

TREATMENT OF DISLOCATIONS

No attempt should be made to reduce dislocations, nor to apply splints or bandages. The patient should be placed at rest in a confined space. Cold compresses may be applied to reduce swelling.

COMMON SITES OF DISLOCATIONS

Dislocation of the Shoulder Joint

This is a rare condition, owing to the strong muscles around the joint, and the absence of a clavicle which would give solid support. It may be seen occasionally in cats and racing dogs, as the result of a severe blow on the side of the humerus when the leg is partially flexed.

Acute lameness will be exhibited, and the shoulder will appear swollen and painful.

Dislocation of the Elbow

All three bones of the joint may be involved or there may be dislocation of the radius and fracture of the ulna. Dislocation of this joint is caused by direct force applied to the side of the limb when the joint is acutely flexed and the weight is on the forefoot.

The patient will not use the limb, the limb will be held slightly flexed, and the elbow will be rotated outwards. Pain will be more noticeable if the ulna is fractured.

Dislocation of the Lower Limbs

Dislocations involving the carpus, tarsus, metacarpals, metatarsals and toe joints are not common; sprains are more often seen. That most often seen in this group is dislocation of the tibio-tarsal joint.

Direct or indirect force may be responsible, often the latter in racing dogs.

Dislocation of the Hip Joint

Dislocation of this joint is the one seen most commonly in the dog and cat. The joint may be dislocated anteriorly—the most common—dorsally or posteriorly.

Most cases occur as the result of an indirect force, usually in the form of a car accident, transmitted through the femur whilst the joint is turned inwards; it may also occur in jumping or falling on to the extended limb.

No weight is taken on the limb and, in the common anterior dislocation, the thigh is rotated outward and the limb turned inwards. The leg appears shorter and the point of the hip appears higher on the affected side.

Dislocation of the Patella

Dislocations of the patella are common, particularly in the smaller breeds, where congenital abnormalities may be responsible for recurrent cases. Most cases occur in an inward direction.

When force is responsible, this is usually indirect, and may occur when an animal is turning at high speed.

In congenital dislocations, and in dislocations caused by deformity of the stifle joint, the patella may be displaced without undue discomfort to the animal. Recent dislocations may be accompanied by some pain, and the limb may be held flexed with the stifle pointing inward. Palpation reveals the incorrect position of the patella. Replacement of the patella may be accomplished by gently extending the limb and manipulating the patella into its correct position.

Dislocation of the Vertebrae

This injury is rare unless accompanied by fracture of the spine. The cause is usually direct violence and, if there is pressure on the spinal cord, the signs will be identical with those shown with spinal fractures.

Dislocation of the Mandible

These occur less frequently than fractures and are usually caused by indirect force such as chewing on large, solid objects or pulling on such an object as a lead held firmly by the owner.

The mouth is usually held in an open position and there may be excessive salivation. If the condition affects only one side the bite shifts to the opposite side of the mouth; if both joints are affected the jaw protrudes. The patient may or may not be able to close the mouth, and the eyes may appear to bulge slightly.

Dislocation of the Stifle Joint

Dislocations of this joint, other than patella luxations, are not common, and will occur only when all ligaments are ruptured. When it does occur, direct force is the cause. Subluxation, due to injury to some of the ligaments, is more common.

Lameness is always severe in acute cases but may not be very noticeable in chronic cases. The limb is carried partly flexed, with the toe pointing forward.

Sprains

A sprain is said to have occurred when the ligaments and other tissues surrounding a joint are stretched or torn as a result of violence. They are usually the result of indirect violence, such as wrenching or twisting, which forces the joint too far in one particular direction. The synovial membrane of the joint may be damaged, and the muscles may be stretched or torn, producing a combination of sprain and strain.

The joints most likely to be affected in the dog and cat are the shoulder, stifle, carpus or tarsus.

SIGNS OF SPRAIN

(a) Pain, which is more severe when the joint is moved.
(b) Loss of power, not so severe as in fracture or dislocation.
(c) Swelling, which develops shortly after the injury is sustained, due to bleeding and damage to the structures around the joint.
(d) Tenderness on palpation.

DIAGNOSIS OF SPRAIN

The diagnosis of a sprain may prove difficult, and the possibility of a fracture must not be excluded; this may not be possible without X-ray examination. In first aid, the distinction depends on discovering tenderness over a ligament rather than a bone, and the fact that the pain around the joint is increased by any movement that tends to stretch the affected ligament.

Dislocations must also be considered, and the presence or absence of fixation of the joint may help to distinguish these two conditions.

All cases in which there is any uncertainty should be treated as though a fracture were present.

TREATMENT OF SPRAIN

The affected joint must be rested as far as is possible, and it may be desirable to apply a splint to achieve this. A pressure bandage will reduce or even prevent swelling, and should be applied firmly over cotton wool. Cold compresses do not relieve pain and prevent swelling to the same degree.

Strains

A strain is the stretching or tearing of a muscle, usually as the result of a sudden wrench, particularly in the racing dog.

Lameness will follow the straining of a limb muscle, there may be loss of power, tenderness and some swelling, and further exertion is difficult or impossible.

Treatment. Rest should be enforced and, if necessary and possible, a splint may be applied. Heat applications, in the form of hot compresses or electric heating pads, can be applied.

RUPTURED TENDONS

This is a form of severe strain, in which the tendon is torn as a result of sudden violence, often indirect. It is most commonly seen, in the dog and cat, affecting the Achilles tendon. In such cases, the animal will show lameness, and will be unable to extend the limb, frequently walking with the metatarsus on the ground. The Achilles tendon will appear slack, and the ruptured ends may be palpable. Any wounds should be dressed, and the limb placed on a splint and kept as still as possible to prevent the cut ends of the tendon separating further from one another.

Loss of Consciousness

GENERAL PRINCIPLES

The causes of unconsciousness may be classified as *primary* and *secondary*. Primary cases include those in which the patient becomes unconscious as the immediate result of an injury or a disease affecting the nervous system. Secondary cases are those in which the patient loses consciousness as the result of injury or disease which first affects other systems of the body before involving the nervous system.

PRIMARY CAUSES

(a) *Head injuries.* (1) Fractured skull. (2) Concussion of the brain.

(b) *Medical diseases.* (1) Apoplexy (cerebral haemorrhage—"Stroke"). (2) Fits, epileptic and hysterical.

(c) *Poisoning.* (1) Narcotics. (2) Prussic acid, etc.

SECONDARY CAUSES

(a) Asphyxia.
(b) Shock (see page 343).
(c) Diabetic coma.
(d) Uraemia.
(e) Electric shock.
(f) Eclampsia.
(g) Heatstroke and sunstroke.
(h) Heart attack.

INVESTIGATION OF UNCONSCIOUSNESS

In many cases, where the cause is obvious, and immediate treatment is essential, history-taking is not necessary. In other, obscure cases, a history is essential and inquiry should be made to ascertain possible injuries that have been afflicted, the mode of onset of the unconsciousness, the possibility of previous attacks of a similar nature and the previous medical history of the patient.

Special physical signs are liable to occur in unconscious patients and these should be noted during examination.

(a) *Respiration.* This may be shallow or deep, rapid or slow.

(b) *Pupils.* The pupils normally become smaller when exposed to light. It should be noted whether the pupils are large or small, and whether they are equal in size. Their reaction to light should be tested.

(c) *Corneal reflex.* Attempts to touch the cornea normally result in blinking. This reflex should be tested, but care must be taken not to injure the delicate cornea.

(d) *Depth of unconsciousness.* In stupor, the animal can be roused with difficulty, the pupils respond to light and the corneal reflex is present. In coma, the animal is more deeply unconscious and cannot be roused, the pupils are usually dilated and the corneal reflex is absent.

(e) *Pulse.* The rate and character should be determined.

(f) *Odour of breath.* In cases of poisoning, the odour may give a clue as to the cause, and characteristic odours may be noticed in cases of uraemia and diabetes.

(g) *Convulsions.* Violent, irregular, involuntary movements of the limbs.

(h) *Paralysis.* Loss of use of muscles.

(i) *Incontinence.* Involuntary passing of urine or faeces.

(j) *Rigidity.* Involuntary spasm of muscles, so that they appear stiff and firm and cannot be relaxed.

PRINCIPLES OF TREATMENT

Urgent conditions must be treated immediately. The animal should be laid on its side, and, where possible, the head should be extended and the tongue drawn out. Any tight collars or coats should be removed. Warmth should be supplied and an adequate supply of fresh air ensured. No attempt should be made to give fluids by mouth, and the animal should not be left unattended.

DEATH

Death should not be assumed merely because obvious signs of life are absent. The following signs should be taken into consideration.

(a) The absence of heart-beats and the cessation of breathing.

(b) Cooling of the body is not necessarily obvious at once, and it may be an hour or two before the fall in body temperature becomes obvious to touch.

(c) The eyeball loses its firmness, the eyes lose their lustre, and the pupils are usually dilated.

(d) The muscles become limp and the jaw usually drops. After several hours, rigor mortis sets in, and the muscles gradually become stiff. This will later pass off with the onset of decay.

FRACTURE OF THE SKULL

Injury to the brain, either from a depressed fracture or a clot of blood caused by a fracture, must always be regarded as very serious. It occurs usually as the result of a blow, as in a street accident or a fall.

The signs will vary according to the severity of the injury, and the part of the brain that is affected. There may be complete or partial loss of consciousness but, usually, there is severe interference with locomotion and balance, or paralysis of certain muscles. Bleeding may be seen from ears, nose or mouth and vomiting is not unusual. The pupils may vary in size and differ in their reaction to light, or *strabismus* (squint) or *nystagmus* may be present.

Treatment consists of keeping the animal warm and completely at rest.

CONCUSSION

Concussion is the form of unconsciousness that follows a blow or fall on the head. It may last from a few seconds to half an hour; if it lasts longer, some more serious head injury must be suspected.

Mild cases may result only in slight staggering and, possibly, vomiting. In more severe cases, there is complete loss of consciousness and signs of shock are exhibited. Breathing is slow and shallow, the body feels cold and the inside of the lips appears pale. The pupils are contracted and react to light except in severe cases when they may be dilated. Whether contracted or dilated, however, they will be equal in size.

Treatment consists of complete rest and warmth. No fluids should be given.

APOPLEXY

A stroke is a condition of unconsciousness due to haemorrhage into the substance of the brain (*cerebral haemorrhage*) or clotting of the blood in the cerebral blood vessels (*cerebral thrombosis*). It is more likely to occur in old animals.

The onset is usually rapid, and often accompanied by vomiting. There is usually only partial loss of consciousness, but this will vary in severity. Attempts to stand or walk are unsuccessful, and the animal is distressed. The head is held to one side, and *nystagmus* (a continous to-and-fro movement of the eyeballs) is present. No signs of external injury to the skull are present.

The animal should be kept as quiet as possible, preferably in a darkened room. No stimulants should be given, but small quantities of water may be allowed.

FITS

Epileptic or epileptiform fits may be caused by many different agents, amongst which may be mentioned true epilepsy, virus infections such as distemper, dietary deficiencies, worm infestations and teething in puppies and kittens. The fits shown in each instance will be indistinguishable from one another, and the person rendering first aid will not be concerned with the discovery of the cause. It should be borne in mind, however, that, should virus infection be a possible cause, care must be taken to limit the spread of infection should the case be admitted to kennels or hospital.

Fits will vary in their severity, but the nature of the fit is no guide to its origin.

Mild fits may last only for a few seconds or for a minute or so. The only signs shown may be a slight shaking of the head and twitching of the facial muscles, together with some salivation and champing of the jaws. The pupils will usually be dilated, but this phase quickly passes and the animal returns to normal. The interval between fits will vary greatly.

Severe fits commence in the same way as the milder variety, but this is followed by loss of consciousness, the animal falling on its side. Violent muscle twitching is present, the respiratory rate is greatly increased, and the limbs execute racing movements. There is copious salivation, the saliva being worked into a white froth by the champing of the jaws. Loss of control of bladder and bowel is frequent. This state will last for a variable time, from a few minutes to several hours. Unless there is a fatal outcome, the twitching gradually stops, the respiratory rate returns to normal, and the animal gradually regains consciousness, remaining dazed for a while. Again, the interval between fits will vary with the cause.

Treatment. Whilst the fit is in progress, the animal should be placed in a confined space, where self-damage is unlikely to take place. Some restraint may be necessary if the fit is particularly violent, to prevent damage both to the patient and to property. On recovery, the mouth should be cleaned to remove excessive saliva, and the animal placed quietly in a darkened room. A sedative may be given, pending professional attention, but all stimulants should be avoided.

Hysteria

Hysterical fits may be a manifestation of specific hysteria, or may be associated with virus infections, or may be associated with dietary disturbances. Differentiation of the cause is not possible from the signs shown.

The onset is usually sudden, and the attack commences with violent barking or howling. The animal shows a terrified look and will rush around, barking or whining, colliding with objects in its path. Attempts are made to get into dark places, or, if in the street, the animal will rush away as fast as possible. This may be followed by partial or complete loss of consciousness, and may be followed by epileptic-type convulsions. Incontinence is usually exhibited, even if the animal has not lost consciousness.

The intervals between attacks will vary, and each attack may last only a few minutes or several hours. In the intervals the animal looks about furtively, as though seeing objects not actually present, and barks in a high-pitched way. As the attack passes, the animal may show great exhaustion and occasionally some degree of paralysis.

Hysterical dogs are not vicious, but, being very frightened, may bite if handled carelessly. The animal should be restrained and soothed, and placed in a dark room as soon as possible. No attempt should be made to give anything by mouth until the attack has passed, when a sedative may be given.

ASPHYXIA

Asphyxia, or suffocation, resulting in a lack of oxygen in the blood, will arise from any failure in respiration. There are many causes, which may be classified as follows.

(a) Obstruction of the air passages from within. This may be caused by drowning; by foreign bodies, such as a ball, wedged in the back of the throat; in unconscious animals, by the tongue folding backwards; by blood, in cases of fracture of the jaw; by vomit, when vomiting occurs in semi-conscious animals; or by food.

(b) Direct pressure on the chest or neck, as might occur in some crushing accidents. Malicious hanging or strangling will also result in asphyxia by pressure in this way.

(c) The inhalation of gases that are of no value in respiration, such as coal gas, smoke from burning buildings, fumes from cars or gas from sewers. Confinement in an atmosphere where no fresh oxygen is available will also have the same result.

(d) Complications of accidents or illnesses, such as swelling of the tissues surrounding any of the air passages, or a collection of fluid in the chest cavity or lungs.

(e) Paralysis of the respiratory muscles due to certain poisons, such as strychnine, electrocution, or fractures of the spine.

(f) Open wounds of the chest, allowing air to enter the chest cavity.

Asphyxia may be *partial*, when the obstruction allows small supplies of air to reach the lungs, or *complete*, when the animal is unable to obtain sufficient oxygen to maintain life.

Partial asphyxia results in great difficulty in breathing and respirations are jerky and irregular. The tongue will change colour, becoming blue, and this is followed by unconsciousness.

Complete asphyxia results in a complete loss of consciousness, cessation of breathing and rapid onset of death.

Principles of Treatment

Where possible, the obstruction to the breathing must be removed; this is sufficient in some cases to enable normal breathing to be resumed. When breathing has ceased, artificial respiration, possibly assisted by inhalation of oxygen, must be adopted without delay.

Drowning

Most dogs can swim well, but may become exhausted. Cats, although not naturally good swimmers, can keep afloat for considerable periods.

Treatment. Foreign matter around the nose and mouth should be removed, and the animal held up by the hindlegs for a few seconds to allow water to drain from the nostrils. Artificial respiration should be applied immediately and, on the recommencement of normal breathing, the body should be well dried. The animal should be kept warm, and given warm fluids to drink.

Choking

This is most commonly seen in cases where a rubber ball has become lodged in the back of the throat, but cases may also be seen associated with bones, solid food, hair masses or stings. An attempt must be made to remove the foreign body with the fingers, but no attempt should be made to push the object further down the throat into the oesophagus.

Choking by the tongue should never be allowed to occur. All unconscious or anaesthetized animals should have the tongue pulled well forward and maintained in this position. Blood that has collected in the throat, from any cause, should be carefully and thoroughly removed by swabbing.

Poisonous Gases

The chief ingredient of both coal gas and car exhaust fumes is *carbon monoxide*. In cases of asphyxia, the animal should be removed from the gas, and given artificial respiration combined with inhalations of oxygen.

Open Pneumothorax

Punctured wounds of the chest, as might result from street accidents or severe bites, may cause collapse of the lungs and thus asphyxia. Air is sucked into the chest cavity with every breath until the pressure around the lung causes it to collapse. Wounds on one side of the chest, in the dog and cat, are likely to cause collapse of both lungs. Any wound of the chest, involving the pleural cavity, is termed an *open pneumothorax*.

Wounds of the chest, however slight, should be covered immediately with a dressing to prevent air entering the chest cavity. Several thicknesses of lint, covered with an air-tight dressing, such as oiled silk or polythene, should be placed over the wound and held firmly in position with adhesive plaster.

RESUSCITATION

All methods that may be used to revive an animal that has apparently ceased to breathe are included in resuscitation, and include artificial respiration, administration of oxygen, cardiac compression and stimulation of the circulation.

Artificial Respiration

The animal is placed on its right side, with head and neck extended and the tongue drawn forward. The hand is placed over the ribs, immediately behind the shoulder blade. A sudden downward movement of the hand causes the chest to be compressed and the air in the lungs to be expelled. The pressure is released immediately, allowing the chest to expand by its own elasticity and fill with air. This procedure is repeated regularly at intervals of about 5 seconds. Unlike artificial respiration in the human, where the movements are rhythmical, the process is carried out, in small animals, by sudden, sharp movements.

If an endotracheal tube is available, and can be properly passed into the trachea, this may be used to provide a clear airway or may be used for direct breathing from the operator to the patient. Alternatively, the Ambu Resuscitator, consisting of a self-inflating rubber bag, connected through a one-way valve to an endotracheal tube or close-fitting face mask, may be used.

Additional Oxygen

Fresh air, which contains oxygen, is essential whenever artificial respiration is being performed. If the necessary equipment is available, this air can usefully be supplemented with additional oxygen.

Cardiac Compression

The heart of an apparently dead animal may be stimulated by rhythmical compression, simultaneously on either side of the chest, over the area of the heart. Whilst this external compression is taking place, it is essential that artificial respiration is maintained, and it will prove beneficial to have two operators.

Circulatory Stimulation

Provided there are no injuries to head, chest or abdomen, and providing there is no haemorrhage, small amounts of brandy or whisky in water may be given.

DIABETIC COMA

The dog is less liable than man to develop a coma associated with diabetes, and those cases that do occur will invariably terminate fatally.

Insulin poisoning may occur where an overdose is inadvertently given, or where the animal refuses food after a dose of insulin has been given. The physical signs exhibited will include muscular tremors, inco-ordination, circling and incontinence, and, occasionally, profuse salivation. Recovery is very rapid following the administration of glucose or sugar.

URAEMIA

In certain kidney diseases, the accumulation of poisonous substances in the blood stream which would normally be removed from the body by the kidneys—*uraemia*—may be associated with recurrent convulsions, or an attack resembling apoplexy. Severe cases may result in coma.

ELECTRIC SHOCK

This is most often caused by animals biting through live wires, and occasionally by coming into contact with live cables or railway lines. The signs will vary considerably, but the general effect is paralysis of respiratory muscles—this may or may not prove fatal depending on the circumstances.

The patient may suffer from asphyxia, shock and burns, and these injuries must be treated in the order named.

ECLAMPSIA

Eclampsia occurs in nursing bitches, particularly during the early stages of lactation and, very occasionally, during the late stages of pregnancy. It is caused by a lowering of certain minerals, such as calcium, in the blood stream.

Mild cases are associated with an increased respiratory rate, and possibly muscular tremors. As the condition progresses, these signs will become more marked, and may be accompanied by severe muscular twitching, inco-ordination of movements and marked excitement. Collapse, loss of consciousness and death may result in untreated cases.

The condition can be treated only by the administration, usually intravenously, of the necessary minerals. Professional help, therefore, should be obtained at the earliest possible opportunity.

HEATSTROKE AND SUNSTROKE

These are not common conditions in the dog and cat, but cases do occur, particularly in the bulldog. The signs exhibited will include vomiting or profuse salivation, rapid pulse, weakness of the limbs, staggering gait and finally collapse. The body temperature is considerably raised, and white-skinned animals may show redness of the skin.

Animals suffering from these conditions should be quickly placed in the cool and shade. The application of cold is the most important part of the treatment, and cold water should be applied to the head, neck and shoulders by means of a cloth, or by pouring it over the animal. If available, ice should be incorporated in the water. On recovery, the animal should be dried, placed in a cool room and encouraged to drink.

HEART ATTACK

Collapse, associated with heart disease, is usually the result of excitement or will sometimes occur after exercise. Most cases result in sudden loss of consciousness. Milder cases may be preceded by a bout of coughing, after which the animal is noticed to be standing quite still and slightly swaying; recovery takes place quickly.

Those cases that collapse may, on occasion, scream. The pulse is found to be rapid, the respirations at first slow and later accelerated. The tongue will be dark, or even bluish in colour and, on recovery, is pale. The pupils are dilated.

The speed of recovery will be proportionate to the severity of the attack. When consciousness has been regained a stimulant, in the form of alcohol, may be given.

Poisons

A poison is any substance which is liable to injure health, or destroy life, if taken into the body in sufficient quantity. Entry into the body may be by the mouth, by breathing or via the skin. The introduction of harmful substances into the body may cause damage to the digestive organs, or, if absorbed into the blood, may damage vital organs such as the brain. Poisoning may be accidental or malicious.

It must be remembered that the diagnosis of poisoning is often very difficult, and that infectious diseases may sometimes be mistaken for cases of poisoning. For this reason, it would be unwise for nursing auxiliaries to express an opinion publicly where malicious poisoning is suspected. In such cases, legal proceedings may follow the death of an animal, and all evidence, such as vomit, excreta and food eaten, should be carefully preserved for examination by the veterinary surgeon.

PRINCIPLES OF TREATMENT

(a) Medical methods of treatment for poisoning are superior to those which can be used in first aid, and, for this reason, the services of a veterinary surgeon should be obtained as soon as possible.

(b) The poison must be identified if possible, so that correct antidotes may be administered. The history supplied by the owner may help in this respect.

(c) The objects of treatment are to remove, as far as is possible, the poison from the digestive system; to neutralize the poison by means of an antidote; and to counteract the effects of the poison.

(1) *Removal of Poisons*

The first step will be to administer an *emetic*, that is, a substance that will cause vomiting. This should be given as soon as possible after the intake of the poison, before absorption into the system has taken place. Suitable emetics for the dog and cat are either a strong salt solution or a piece of washing soda, the size of a large pea. Emetics should not be used in cases of corrosive poisoning, nor in partially conscious or unconscious animals. When the stomach has been completely emptied, an aperient should be given to remove any poison from the bowel.

(2) *Antidotes*

An antidote is a substance which will neutralize the poison whilst it is still in the body, either by preventing its absorption into the blood stream, or by combining with the poison chemically to form a relatively harmless substance.

(3) *Counteraction*

Shock must be counteracted if present, and respiratory depression, present in some poisonings, may necessitate artificial respiration. The effect of the poison on the digestive system may be modified by administering demulcent drinks, such as barley water, gruel, olive oil or liquid paraffin emulsions, which soothe areas that may have been burned or irritated by the poison.

CLASSIFICATION OF POISON

Poisons may be classified as corrosives, irritants, narcotics and convulsants.

Corrosive Poisons

Corrosives may be either acid or alkaline, and are those poisons which burn the parts of the body with which they came into contact. The more important corrosive acids are sulphuric acid (oil of vitriol), hydrochloric acid (spirits of salts), nitric acid and acetic acid. The common corrosive alkalis are caustic soda, caustic potash and ammonia.

Poisoning of animals with acids or alkalis will be uncommon, but occasional cases may be met where they have been accidentally administered in mistake for a therapeutic preparation.

Administration of corrosive poisons causes severe burning of the mucous membranes of the upper part of the digestive tract. This will be followed by vomiting, colic and purgation, and will result in severe shock and, often, death. Diagnosis may be based on the signs of corrosion in the mouth, and the history.

Treatment. When an acid is mixed with an alkali a salt is formed, and this is comparatively harmless. Alkali poisoning, therefore, should be treated by giving large quantities of dilute acid such as 5% acetic acid or citric acid or vinegar. Acid poisoning should be treated by giving a dilute alkali such as 2% sodium bicarbonate, lime-water or chalk. Any burns should be flooded with water and then treated with dilute acid or alkali solution. Liberal amounts of demulcents should be given subsequently. Emetics should not be given, owing to the possibility of perforation of the oesophagus or stomach.

Carbolic acid (phenol) is an ingredient of several well-known disinfectants, and poisoning from this substance is particularly common in the cat after bathing in such preparations as Lysol. The cat is particularly susceptible and phenol is readily and rapidly absorbed through the intact skin. Signs of acute poisoning by carbolic acid are muscular convulsions and coma, with death from respiratory paralysis. Concentrated solutions are corrosive in action and death from shock will follow the intake of large amounts. Treatment should be by the administration of large amounts of demulcents, and, in the case of animals that have been bathed in carbolic acid, the substance should be removed as far as possible by using soap and water.

Irritant Poisons

Irritant poisons are those which irritate and inflame the tissues with which they come in contact. Three groups may be recognized—the animal irritants, such as decaying meat, the vegetable irritants, such as poisonous plants, and the chemical irritants, such as arsenic, lead, phosphorus, etc. The signs shown will vary according to the type of poison taken and its strength.

Irritants to the stomach act as emetics and vomiting will be an early sign. The vomiting may be severe and prolonged and, if this is the case, blood may appear in the vomit. This may be followed by colic and diarrhoea, the stools becoming fluid, offensive and sometimes blood-tinged. Staining of the mucous membranes of the mouth may be present with certain poisons, and some of the stronger irritant poisons may have a corrosive action.

Treatment should follow the principles of administering an emetic, antidote, aperient and demulcents, and general treatment for shock.

Narcotic Poisons

The narcotic poisons are those which act on the nervous system, producing sleep. The most important group, concerning the dog and cat, are the barbiturates, that may be administered in excessive doses as sleeping tablets. Carbolic acid has a depressant action on the nervous system, as does turpentine, which may be used on the skin of an animal to remove paint. Some plants also act in the same way. Opium poisoning may occur from excessive doses of chlorodyne.

Emetics may fail to act in cases of narcotic poisoning, owing to the sedative action of the substance on the stomach. They may, however, be administered in early cases, provided that the animal is fully conscious. When possible, an aperient should be given, the animal should be kept warm, and, if able to swallow, stimulants such as strong coffee with glucose may be administered. Should the breathing show signs of failure, oxygen administration and artificial respiration must be commenced.

Convulsant Poisons

Many poisons may cause convulsions, but strychnine and prussic acid are the two most important members of this group. Strychnine is no longer permitted for use in vermin baits, but is still used for the destruction of moles, and cases of poisoning may be encountered in the dog.

The first signs of poisoning are restlessness, twitching of muscles and stiffness of the neck. The muscular twitching becomes more pronounced and convulsions appear. The muscles contract, the limbs are extended and the neck is curved upwards and backwards. At first, the convulsions are intermittent, with short periods of relaxation between. These periods gradually shorten, and, if the animal is stimulated during one of the periods of rest, the spasms follow immediately. The convulsions follow one another with increasing rapidity, and death results from respiratory paralysis. Although usually typical of strychnine poisoning, similar spasms may be seen in other poisoning cases, when agents such as zinc phosphide or nitrophenide are involved.

In the early stages of poisoning, before spasms have commenced, any strychnine in the stomach should be rendered harmless by giving a dilute solution of tannic acid, a heaped teaspoonful in 2 oz of water. If spasms have started, this can only be done via a stomach tube. The animal must be kept as quiet as possible, and all stimuli that might result in the onset of spasms avoided. Artificial respiration should be given if necessary. Professional help should be obtained as soon as possible, in order that an anaesthetic may be given.

Rat Poisons

Many substances are incorporated into poisonous baits for rats and other vermin, and it is possible that these will be accidentally taken by dogs and cats, or the carcasses of rats killed by these poisons may be eaten.

Treatment for suspected poisoning must follow general principles, and specific antidotes are available in some cases if the type of poison is known.

ANTU—usually results in rapid death due to respiratory failure. No specific antidote.

Arsenic—used in some slug baits and weed killers. Antidote—hyposulphite of soda, given in a dose of 5–10 gr. in water, every hour.

Metaldehyde—used in slug baits. Causes inco-ordination, increase in pulse and respiratory rate, cyanosis and unconsciousness; convulsions and death will follow. In the cat, nystagmus is said to be characteristic. There is no specific antidote.

Phosphorus—used in rat poisons. Copper sulphate, in a dose of 2–3 gr. in water, should be given every 5 minutes until vomiting occurs, followed by 1 gr. every 15 minutes. No olive oil or liquid paraffin should be given.

Red squill—used as rat poison. This is not likely to be eaten by dogs and cats because of its unpalatable nature. If eaten it would cause immediate vomiting.

Thallium—used in rat baits. Even acute cases may take several days to develop, and result in vomiting, diarrhoea, respiratory distress, colic and thirst. Less acute cases show shedding of the hair. Emetics should be given in acute cases, followed by the administration of hyposulphite of soda.

Warfarin—the most commonly used agent in rat poisons. Produces an interference with the clotting time of the blood and damage to the capillaries, followed by haemorrhages from capillaries and small blood vessels. Treatment consists mainly of the administration of vitamin K and blood transfusions, and will be carried out by a veterinary surgeon.

Zinc phosphide—used in rat poisons. There is no known antidote.

The Digestive System

FOREIGN BODIES IN THE MOUTH

In the dog, pieces of stick or bone sometimes become wedged transversely across the roof of the mouth between the molar teeth. Pieces of soft bone may become wedged on or between one of the teeth. Needles are sometimes seen imbedded in the tongue, and fish-hooks may be fixed in either lips or tongue.

Foreign bodies in the mouth usually cause profuse salivation, movements of the jaws and tongue, and frantic rubbing at the sides of the mouth with the front paws or on the ground.

An attempt should be made to remove the foreign body with fingers or forceps but, on occasion, anaesthesia will be required. No attempt should be made to pull out a fish-hook, because of its barbed end; the shaft should be pushed still further so that the barb comes out through a second puncture.

FOREIGN BODIES IN THE PHARYNX AND OESOPHAGUS

Foreign bodies, such as sewing needles or bones, may become lodged in any part of the pharynx or oesophagus. The bones usually incriminated are either fish bones or rough, irregular bones such as chop bones, the projections on which prevent them from being swallowed.

Sewing needles are frequently found imbedded in the soft tisses of the pharynx or may transfix the pharynx. In many cases, a length of cotton thread will be attached to the needle. The thread should not be removed so as to detach it from the needle, for, if the cotton remains in the needle, it serves as a valuable guide to locate the foreign body and may even be of some assistance in its removal.

A cat with a needle or fish bone in its pharynx will often sit patiently, refusing food or drink, and salivating from the mouth.

A dog with a foreign body in the oesophagus or pharynx shows distress and frequent gulping. Food will not usually be taken but, should it be so, and the obstruction is complete, the food will be returned at once.

Treatment. With the animal held firmly, the mouth should be opened as far as possible to inspect the throat. A piece of bone, or wood, or a needle may be observed and it may be possible to remove it easily with fingers or forceps. A thread should not be pulled, but should be traced to determine if it is attached to a needle. If so, and if the needle cannot be removed, then the thread should be left in position and, if possible, the two ends of the thread should be tied together to prevent unthreading. On occasion, a gentle pull will remove the needle, but sometimes it will prove necessary to cut the needle in half with wire-cutters, and extract the two halves separately, first removing the pointed half and retaining the cotton as a guide to the second portion.

FOREIGN BODIES IN THE STOMACH

Many foreign objects may be swallowed by the dog, such as bones, balls, stones, nuts and so on and, if in the stomach, may cause little trouble except occasional vomiting. If the object is sharp, abdominal pain and blood vomiting may be exhibited.

If a foreign body in the stomach is suspected, all food and water should be withheld until a veterinary surgeon is consulted.

FOREIGN BODIES IN THE INTESTINE

Foreign bodies found in the intestine are similar to those found in the stomach. Many may cause complete obstruction of the small intestine, and even small objects may cause considerable abdominal pain as they pass through the tract. If the foreign body passes into the large intestine, the acute signs of pain and vomiting and thirst will soon disappear. In the rectum no trouble is likely to be caused unless the object is sharp.

Obstruction of the intestine by a foreign body may require surgical intervention, and any suspected case should be referred to a veterinary surgeon as soon as possible.

FOREIGN BODIES IN THE ANUS

Sharp pieces of bone, or a collection of small pieces of bone impacted into a mass, may become lodged in the posterior part of the rectum and the anus. Pins, safety pins or needles may be passed through the digestive tract and lodge in the anus.

Signs shown are those of irritation, the animal persistently licking the anus, or crying out when trying to pass faeces, or constantly straining.

Treatment. Any foreign body in the anus must be removed very carefully to avoid further damage to the tissues and to prevent great pain. The area should first be well lubricated with liquid paraffin, and a bone may then be gently removed with fingers or forceps. If a thread is found protruding from the anus a search should be made for the two free ends, which should then be knotted together. Gentle pulling may then remove the needle, but no force should be applied. If the foreign body cannot easily be removed, the animal should be referred to a veterinary surgeon.

IMPACTION OF THE ANAL GLANDS

Blockage of the ducts of the anal glands, and subsequent impaction of the glands, may lead to abscess formation. Such an abscess will usually break to the outer side of the rim of the anus.

The animal will show irritation of the area, and often great pain when the area is examined. First-aid treatment should consist of cleansing, clipping away the matted hair surrounding the abscess and washing the part gently with a mild antiseptic lotion.

ACCIDENTAL INJURIES TO THE ABDOMEN

Injuries to the abdominal wall will occur in street accidents, from staking on fences and from fights. Simple wounds should be treated in the normal way but on occasion the wound will penetrate the abdominal wall, and part of the abdominal contents may protrude through the wound. This must always be regarded as extremely serious. On rare occasions, evisceration may result from a fight or accident.

In cases of protrusion of abdominal contents the animal should, if possible, be restrained on its back. The abdominal organs that are visible should be covered with hot cloths that have been soaked in saline and then wrung out to remove excess fluid. Provided no force is required, the parts may be gently returned to the abdominal cavity. Antiseptic dressings should not be used. If possible, the saline dressing should be bound in place, with a bandage passing around the animal and held in place with a wide piece of lint or a towel. The patient must be treated for shock in the usual way.

VOMITING OF BLOOD

The vomiting of blood, or *haematemesis*, may be due to injury of the stomach in an accident; to sharp foreign bodies in the stomach; to diseases such as gastro-enteritis or nephritis; or may occur in some forms of poisoning. Blood may also be vomited that has been swallowed from some bleeding point in the mouth or nose.

The blood may sometimes be mixed with food. It is usually dark red in colour and may be clotted. If the blood has remained in the stomach for any length of time it may be partially digested and will be much darker in appearance.

Treatment. The animal should be kept as quiet as possible, and warmth should be applied. Great thirst may be exhibited, but no fluids or food should be given by mouth. A piece of ice, placed on a flannel in a dish, so that the water that forms cannot be taken, may be given to the animal to lick.

PROLAPSE OF THE RECTUM

A protrusion of the rectum, through the anal opening, will sometimes involve only the mucous lining of the rectum; in other cases, the entire thickness of the wall is included in the protrusion.

The condition is more commonly seen in young puppies or kittens, often associated with conditions producing diarrhoea and tenesmus. The characteristic sign is the protrusion of a reddish mass covered with mucous membrane, which may be normal but more often is coated with thick mucus. It may become congested and may even ulcerate.

Treatment. The protrusion should be bathed with warm water, or preferably saline, after which it should be well lubricated with liquid paraffin, and an attempt should be made to gently compress it back into place. This is more likely to be accomplished satisfactorily if only the mucosa is prolapsed. Many cases will require surgical treatment, either to effect a reduction or to prevent further prolapse at a later date. An anodyne suppository may be inserted to prevent straining until further treatment can be carried out.

The Respiratory System

EPISTAXIS

Epistaxis, or bleeding from the nose, is usually venous in origin, and may occasionally be serious. Most cases will arise from severe blows, or accidents, and may be associated with fracture of the nasal bones or, in rare cases, with fracture of the skull. Other cases may be associated with tumours of the nostrils or nasal passages, or, more commonly, paroxysms of sneezing.

Treatment. The animal should be confined and made to rest as far as is possible. Applications of cold water, or ice, should be given.

FOREIGN BODIES IN THE NOSE

Grass-seeds, blades of grass and, occasionally, splinters of wood, commonly gain access into the nose of the dog and, sometimes, the cat. Such foreign bodies will give rise to violent sneezing, and rubbing of the side of the nose with the forepaws. Epistaxis may be produced by the sneezing.

Treatment. The foreign body will sometimes be visible in the nostrils and may be removed manually. On other occasions, nothing will be visible and the advice of a veterinary surgeon, and possibly anaesthesia, will be required.

INJURY TO THE LARYNX

Wounds or blows in the laryngeal region may produce rapid swelling of the tissues, which, in turn, will lead to difficulty in breathing and, in extreme cases, asphyxia. Wounds in this area may allow the escape of air, and, in such a case, any haemorrhage is likely to be frothy in nature.

Treatment. This must follow the general lines laid down for the treatment of wounds, haemorrhage and asphyxia. Care must be taken, when dressing any wound, that fluid is not allowed to enter the air passages.

INJURY TO THE TRACHEA

The trachea may be injured in street accidents or fights, or may become lacerated by barbed wire, or by the animal falling through glass. Pain and swelling may be exhibited at the site of injury, and breathing may be noisy or distressed. Any wound penetrating the trachea will allow the passage of air through the wound during respiration. Treatment will be as outlined for injuries to the larynx.

INJURY TO THE LUNG

This may be caused by street accidents, fights, kicks, gunshot wounds, or other forms of direct violence. A fractured rib may penetrate a lung. Haemorrhage may occur within the chest cavity with no external signs of bleeding.

Signs of external injury will usually be present, together with general signs of haemorrhage and shock. There may be evidence of pain in the chest and difficulty in breathing. Bleeding from the lungs, or *haemoptysis*, may be present, in which case blood, which is usually bright red in colour and frothy because it is mixed with air, is coughed up.

Treatment. Lung injuries must always be regarded as serious. Rest is essential, and the animal should be allowed to assume the position in which it appears most comfortable. Wounds, haemorrhage, shock and asphyxia must be treated in the normal way.

The Uro-genital System

INJURIES TO THE URINARY SYSTEM

These will occur most often in severe accidents. The kidneys may be affected, or the bladder or external genital organs may be involved. Any injury to the bladder may result in frequent attempts to pass urine, which may contain blood. Rupture of the bladder, which may occur in accidents if the bladder is distended at the time of the blow, will cause severe shock and collapse.

HAEMATURIA

Bleeding from any part of the urinary tract will cause blood to appear in the urine, and this is known as haematuria. It may result from injury or disease of any of the organs that comprise the uro-genital system. Common causes are injuries to the bladder, particularly when associated with fracture of the pelvis, bites and wounds involving, particularly in the male dog, the urethra or penis, and certain bladder diseases. It is important to distinguish between haematuria and the normal haemorrhage associated with oestrus.

RETENTION OF URINE

Inability to pass urine is commonly seen in the dog and cat, and is most often due to the collection of stones, either in the bladder, blocking the opening of the bladder into the urethra, or in the urethra itself. In the male cat, the urethra is commonly blocked with sand-like material.

The affected animal will make frequent but unsuccessful attempts to pass urine, or occasionally a few drops may be passed after prolonged effort. Pain and discomfort will be shown, and distention of the lower part of the abdomen may be noticed. In the cat, the condition is frequently mistaken by the owner for constipation.

Treatment. No first-aid treatment is possible, and the case must be referred to a veterinary surgeon as soon as possible.

Affections of the Eye and Ear

THE EYE

The eye is a delicate organ, and examinations of, and treatment to, the eye must be carried out gently and carefully. Examination of the eye is usually possible with a minimum of restraint, and is best carried out in a darkened room with suitable intense illumination.

The affections of the eye most likely to be presented for first-aid treatment are injuries, foreign bodies and the prolapsed eyeball. The lids are easily examined for evidence of injury, and may be opened gently, and everted slightly to allow an examination of the conjunctiva and nictitating membrane.

Injuries to the Eye

Wounds of the eyelids are common as the results of accidents or fights. Even small injuries will sometimes produce severe swelling, and may be accompanied by excessive tear production. Treatment should follow the recognized procedures.

Burns and scalds involving the eyelids are not common, but occasionally lime or disinfectants are the cause of considerable damage.

Injury to the eyeball is not common, due to its protection within the orbit, but may be seen associated with shotgun wounds, blows or kicks. The eyeball may be injured by fracture of the orbital ring. Haemorrhage under the conjunctiva may be caused by contusion. Burns and scalds involving the eyeball are occasionally seen from boiling fat or water, lime, acids and disinfectants. Acids require neutralization with sodium bicarbonate, whereas lime burns are best treated with dilute vinegar, both cases being followed by frequent applications of sterile liquid paraffin.

Non-penetrating wounds of the cornea may be due to such things as foreign bodies, thorns, grass-seeds, motor accidents or injuries received in fights or from cat scratches.

Penetrating wounds of the cornea may be simple or may be complicated by injury to the internal structures of the eye.

Simple injuries may be treated on ordinary lines; more severe injuries should be cleansed gently, using normal saline solution that has been sterilized and, if possible, the eye should be covered with a sterile pad of gauze, bandaged into position, and fastened with adhesive tape, pending professional attendance.

Foreign Bodies

Grass-seeds commonly become lodged in the conjunctiva or beneath the nictitating membrane. Other foreign matter may enter the conjunctival sac, or even be imbedded in the cornea. All will cause pain or discomfort, excessive tear production and irritation.

It will often be possible to remove grass-seeds manually, and other foreign bodies may sometimes be removed with the corner of a moistened piece of lint, or a fine paint brush. No attempt should be made to remove foreign bodies that are imbedded either in the conjunctiva or the cornea. The eye may be irrigated with saline solution or olive oil or liquid paraffin to remove grit or sand.

Prolapse of the Eyeball

This will most commonly be seen in the short-nosed breeds, due to pressure behind the eye exerted during fights or street accidents. The prolapsed eyeball quickly becomes inflamed and congested as the eyelids close behind it. The cornea becomes dry and other damage to the eyeball may occur at the same time.

Replacement of the eye must be performed as soon as possible, for the dry cornea soon becomes ulcerated and the prolapse of the eyeball may cause damage to the optic nerve. The eyeball should be well lubricated with liquid paraffin or olive oil, and an attempt should be made to gently draw the lids over the eyeball. No force should be used, and, if it is not possible to replace the eye, the cornea should be kept well moistened, and the animal prevented from causing further self-damage, until a veterinary surgeon can attend to the case.

THE EAR

Injuries to the Ear

The ears are frequently the site of injury in the dog and cat, from street accidents or, more particularly, from bites. Wounds of the ear bleed freely, and may cause shaking of the head and irritation. Scratching at the ear will increase the haemorrhage and may even enlarge the wound.

Wounds of the ear should be treated by normal methods. If the hair is removed, this may increase the bleeding, and care must be taken, if this is done, not to cut the ear itself. If necessary, the ear may be bandaged, by folding it backwards, so that it lies on top of the head, and fixing it with a bandage that encircles the head. Large wounds may require surgical treatment later.

Foreign Bodies in the Ear

Grass-seeds commonly gain access to the ear canal, and may travel down to the base of the ear. The animal will usually show intense irritation or pain, holding the head to one side, shaking the head violently and rubbing the ear with a forepaw or along the ground.

The foreign body, if visible, should be removed gently with forceps. If this is not possible, warm olive oil should be poured into the ear. No attempt should be made to probe the ear.

CHAPTER 4

Diagnostic Aids and Laboratory Tests

J. S. WILKINSON, BSc, PhD, MRCVS

Introduction

In the following chapter are explained the principles behind the satisfactory maintenance of a diagnostic service that can reasonably be carried out in practice. All the methods described are used routinely and most are relatively simple. The function of such a service is to examine accurately and quickly various materials from patients with a view to assisting the clinician to make a diagnosis, and to assess the severity of the condition and the patient's response to treatment. The tests by themselves are of limited value and the results can only be interpreted in the light of the clinical findings. However, occasionally the results may suggest the presence of a condition not previously suspected; in these circumstances, it is wise to repeat the estimation if there is sufficient material left, or to obtain a further sample.

It is impossible to include in a book of this scope all the information that may prove of value, and a list of books which give more detailed information is included at the end of the chapter.

The value of a diagnostic laboratory depends largely upon the equipment available. However, while first-class, expensive equipment will not necessarily give first-class results, good results cannot be obtained with second-rate equipment. The following items of equipment are essential if the laboratory is to fulfil its purpose adequately.

A microscope, with $\frac{1}{3}$ in., $\frac{1}{6}$ in. and $\frac{1}{12}$ in. (oil immersion) objective lenses and a $\times 10$ eyepiece lens if any microbiology or examination of blood films is contemplated.

A cover for the microscope is essential.

A centrifuge: hand centrifuges are adequate for some investigations but are time-consuming and will not suffice for haematology or bacteriology. The separation of precipitates in the chemical tests can be achieved by filtration but this is less stiasfactory than centrifugation.

A rough balance for the balancing of centrifuge tubes before spinning.

An accurate balance for the preparation of solutions is desirable but the local chemist will no doubt help if a suitable balance is not available.

A supply of water, gas and electricity.

A lamp for the microscope.

Adequate glassware:

Storage bottles (screw-capped for solids and glass-stoppered for liquid reagents).

Test-tubes ($4 \times \frac{1}{2}$ in. and $3 \times \frac{1}{2}$ in. tubes of Pyrex glass will withstand heat and centrifugation).

Measuring cylinders (50 ml, 100 ml and 250 ml).

Filter funnels ($1-1\frac{1}{2}$ in. diameter) with papers to fit. (Whatman No. 1 are satisfactory.)

Glass rod.

Slides and coverslips.

Sample bottles (screw-capped "Bijou", holding about 6 ml, large "Bijou" holding about 15 ml, and "Universal" and McCartney bottles holding about 30 ml are suitable sizes). Camlab* produce sterile, chemically clean disposable tubes for collecting blood samples. These are relatively cheap, can be spun in the standard centrifuge bucket to give maximum yield of serum and discarded after use. (Tubes containing anticoagulants suitable for the various tests are also available.)

"Vacuum" tubes containing different anticoagulants are also available, these have the advantage that they require no syringe and therefore reduce the likelihood of contamination or haemolysis as the blood is transferred to another container.

A bunsen burner or similar heater.

Adequate storage space.

A working surface that can be cleaned easily, wood with a wax polish or Formica are suitable.

Record books.

Chinagraph pencils.

While the following are not essential they are of value in the maintenance of a good service.

A refrigerator for the storage of specimens and unstable solutions and an oven for drying and sterilizing glassware.

In addition to these general items special investigations require their own equipment.

For the blood investigations described later the following are necessary:

- Wintrobe tubes.
- Haemoglobinometer.
- Haemacytometer.

For the urine analyses:

- Urinometer, the smaller the better.
- Tubes of suitable size for use with the Clinitest tablets. (The makers of the tablets, Ames Co.,‡ will supply suitable tubes and droppers in a rack.)

* Camlab (Medical Laboratories) Ltd., Milton Road, Cambridge.

† "Vacutainers" made by Becton, Dickenson & Co., obtainable through laboratory equipment and veterinary instrument suppliers.

‡ Messrs. Ames Co. Ltd., Stoke Court, Stoke Poges, Buckinghamshire.

Black tile or piece of black perspex, white tile or piece of white perspex.
Indicator papers.

For bacteriology:

Bacteriological loop.
A 37°C incubator (this is also useful for the reticulocyte count and the estimation of trypsin in faeces. A satisfactory incubator heated by a 60-watt electric light bulb can be built for a few pounds, the most expensive item is the thermostat).

For blood chemistry:

A boiling water bath (a small saucepan or beaker is adequate).
A colorimeter, either of the comparator type, or photoelectric, is necessary if more accurate results than can be obtained by unaided visual methods are desired.

For faecal investigation:

A pair of dissecting forceps.
A pair of mounted needles are useful.

Running a Laboratory

GENERAL RULES

The following rules should always be observed.

1. Keep the laboratory clean; unsatisfactory results may arise from contamination of glassware.
2. Keep it tidy, many breakages occur through untidiness.
3. Carry out all tests as soon as possible and dispose of all samples as soon as they have been fully examined.
4. Label all reagent bottles, samples and test-tubes used in tests clearly.
5. Keep all poisonous reagents under lock and key.
6. Keep clear records and keep records away from the sink and work bench where they may get splashed.

LABELLING AND RECORDING

This is probably the most important part of laboratory practice.

There is no value in taking a sample, testing it and recording the results if there is no certainty from which animal it came, and there is no point in knowing from which animal it came if the results are not correctly recorded. Zinc oxide plaster makes a most efficient label, it is smooth enough to write on easily and does not come off if wetted, as paper labels will. Pencil, ball points and permanent inks are satisfactory for writing the labels but washable inks must be avoided. Always label the lids or corks of the containers as well, this ensures that the right cork goes back in the right tube.

If one sample only is being tested it is wise, but not absolutely necessary, to label any test-tubes in use. If two or more samples are being tested it is essential, and for this a chinagraph pencil can be used. If serial dilutions of the same sample are being used each tube should be labelled. Chinagraph wax can readily be removed with a little ether.

Similar rules, of course, apply to any slides that are made. Special ink is available for labelling glassware permanently or a diamond "pencil" can be used.

Accurate recording of results is essential for the satisfactory running of any laboratory. A small duplicate booklet for each type of sample examined or sent away is satisfactory, one for urine, one for blood, one for faeces. Even if no blood examinations are carried out in the laboratory it is worth making a note of the date on which they were sent; this will serve as a check in case the laboratory reports are held up and inquiries have to be made.

Records should show:

1. The date of the sampling and how the sample was obtained.
2. The date of testing.
3. The reference, possibly the surgery number, the owner's name, the dog's age, breed and sex, and, if known, the dog's name.
4. The results of all the tests.
5. The date the results were entered in the surgery books. Entering the results in the case records will, of course, depend on the methods employed in the practice. They should be written down and put where the surgeon in charge of the case will see them before or at the same time as he next sees the case. There is little point in doing the tests if the results are not available when needed.

PREPARATION AND CARE OF GLASSWARE AND LABORATORY EQUIPMENT

New glassware should always be carefully washed before it is used.

It should be scrubbed with a good detergent (Teepol) and rinsed two or three times in really hot running water. If it is to be used for collecting blood or storing serum it should finally be rinsed in distilled water. It is advisable to dry it in an oven as this sterilizes it as well; stoppers should be put on as soon as the bottles are cool enough to handle.

Used glassware should be rinsed very well in cold water (if infected, stand in 2% Lysol for 24 hours) immediately after use; serum, urine and faeces are frequently very difficult to remove once they have dried. It should then be washed in detergent, rinsed and dried in an oven. Glassware should not be left lying about in the laboratory; as soon as it is cool it should be stored carefully in a cupboard, which should be kept tidy.

Microscope slides should be scrubbed with a nailbrush in hot soapy water, rinsed very well with hot running water and dried with a cloth which does not leave fluff. Coverslips, which are very fragile, should not be washed but cleaned with a tissue (Kleenex, Scottie or Kimwipe) immediately before use. Once clean, slides can be stored in absolute alcohol and *dried carefully immediately before use.*

Probably the most valuable piece of apparatus in a practice laboratory is the microscope. This must be treated with respect and requires to be kept as clean as any good glassware. The "stage", the part on which the slide rests, sometimes gets contaminated with material that is being examined and should be cleaned regularly. If the material is infected, it should be swabbed off with a piece of cotton wool just moistened with methylated spirit.

To function properly the lens must be clean and free from scratches. Never use a harsh cloth on microscope lenses; soft paper tissues (Kimwipes) are most satisfactory. The "oil-immersion" lens should be wiped free of oil as soon as it has been used. The mirror should be kept clean and occasionally it may be necessary to put a drop of oil on the focusing devices. The microscope should never be left uncovered. It should either be kept in its box or in a safe place under a polythene bag or glass bell-jar. Never try to take a microscope lens apart to clean the inside. This is an expert's job and, if necessary, the lens should be taken out and given to such an expert for cleaning.

All electrical apparatus should be kept clean, and for safety ensure that it is adequately earthed and that it is far enough away from the sink not to get splashed. If there is any doubt about the serviceability of any equipment it should be checked; if it is not functioning properly it will probably stop working when it is needed most.

DESPATCH OF SAMPLES TO OUTSIDE LABORATORIES

This activity is covered by quite strict postal regulations and all packages must be labelled "PATHOLOGICAL SPECIMEN". In addition, "FRAGILE WITH CARE" may help to ensure safe arrival.

The first thing to ensure is that all bottles are adequately stoppered. A waterproof screw-cap tightly screwed is the best, but corks pushed well home and secured with Sellotape are satisfactory.

The next most important precaution is sufficient packing; at least three thicknesses of corrugated cardboard should be used, or, if the container is a small one, cottonwool in a small box will suffice. As a final safety precaution, a polythene bag will prevent any leakage.

Always include with the specimen a note giving details of the case, nature of the specimen, any preservative used and a reference. All containers should be clearly labelled and the labels must be well secured. Where possible avoid having samples in the post over the week-end; if there is any doubt about their arrival by Saturday morning keep them in the refrigerator until Sunday afternoon or Monday morning and post them then.

PRESERVATION OF MATERIAL

Do not use preservatives unless it is necessary; urine and faeces, provided that they are correctly bottled, will keep in reasonable condition in a refrigerator for 4 days. Serum will keep less well, and whole blood is practically valueless for many investigations after 36 hours. Serum can be stored in the freezer compartment for several weeks with relatively little change.

If no refrigerator is available a few crystals of thymol will reduce bacterial and fungal growth in urine and will not interfere with the tests; whole blood should be sent away or examined immediately.

In warm weather, faeces should be examined immediately, particularly if egg counts are to be done.

PRESERVATION OF POST-MORTEM MATERIAL

There are three important points to remember; firstly, that it takes a lot of formalin to fix tissues; secondly, that it takes formalin a long time to penetrate tissues (even though the outside of a large piece of tissue may be well fixed, the inside will continue to decompose); and thirdly, that while fixing is going on the tissue becomes very firm and rigid. Soft tissues pushed into a narrow-necked bottle and then fixed can frequently only be removed by breaking the bottle.

Therefore, there are three rules to be observed when preserving post-mortem material:

1. Use plenty of formalin, say 20 volumes of formalin for every one of tissue.
2. Cut large organs open so that the formalin penetrates more quickly. Better still, remove a piece which is big enough to show all the abnormalities but no more (it may be necessary to cut more than one piece from an organ).
3. Fix the tissues in a bowl first, when they are well fixed transfer to a wide-necked bottle.

For a small piece of tissue, fixing will be complete in about 24 hours but larger ones may take 2 to 3 days, even longer.

Vomitus needs no preservation; its high acidity prevents bacterial action.

If there is any likelihood of the material having to go to an analyst for examination for poison and there is the possibility of a lawsuit, it is as well to keep with it a bottle of the same batch as that in which the vomitus is stored. This will answer any suggestion that the bottle was contaminated before the material was put into it. If the vomitus was collected from bedding some of this should also be saved.

The Collection of Material for Examination

Several points have to be borne in mind when dealing with samples for analysis.

The most important of these is absolute cleanliness, both from the infection and chemical aspects. There is no point in putting a sample into a dirty bottle and there is no excuse for hazarding a patient's health by using dirty techniques. It is, therefore, essential to use clean sterile bottles and sterile catheters and needles.

Samples should be tested as soon after collection as possible since delay frequently results in deterioration.

COLLECTION OF URINE

Dogs in particular, and sometimes bitches, will urinate on the floor of the waiting room or surgery; provided that the floor is clean the urine can be salvaged with a pipette or old syringe. The same applies to kennel floors or yards. If the animal is an in-patient, a sample can usually be collected when it is taken out first thing in the morning. Practically anything can be used, but for bitches a small shallow dish or saucer is best and a saucepan is most convenient for dogs. A kidney bowl can be used for both sexes.

If the patient is presented at surgery and there is space available, it can be "walked", though this method is rarely successful.

If none of these methods is satisfactory the patient can be catheterized. This method is not without drawbacks, it may result in cystitis and damage to the urethra, and in some cases it is impossible to pass even the smallest available catheter.

It is possible to make satisfactory catheters from polythene tubing provided that the sharp edges of the cut end are carefully rounded. This can be done with a nail file, with sandpaper or by very carefully heating in a small flame. It is important when boiling any catheter that it should not be bent or coiled; for this reason a long sterilizer should be used. If catheterization is considered necessary, a suitable size catheter should be boiled, allowed to cool, and all the water shaken out. Catheterization is a two-man job in most cases, and it is wise to muzzle the patient before starting. If the patient is a dog, the operator, if right-handed, should stand facing the dog's right side. The penis is held in the left hand (it is usually easier to put the left arm between the dog's hindlegs). The prepuce is retracted using the right forefinger; when the penis is extruded the prepuce is held back with the left hand. If there is much preputial fluid it can be cleaned off with a piece of damp cotton-wool. The catheter, with stylet in place, is inserted into the urethral meatus and gently but firmly pushed as far as it will go. When resistance is felt, the stylet is withdrawn an inch or so and the catheter pushed further in. Eventually the stylet can be removed entirely and the tip of the catheter pushed into the bladder.

It is wise to have two containers for the urine since the first few drops may be contaminated with preputial and prostatic fluids. This is collected into one container and saved in case there is insufficient urine in the bladder. The main portion is collected into the second bottle; it may be necessary to squeeze the bladder gently through the stomach wall in order to get sufficient urine for testing. When the sample has been taken the catheter is carefully withdrawn, washed well, resterilized, and stored in a suitable container. It should not be left lying about or be stored coiled.

The sample bottles must be carefully labelled with the owner's name, the animal's name and its age, breed and sex, or with a record number depending on the system used. Similar precautions have to be taken when catheterizing bitches.

Bitch catheters are usually metal, and of wider bore than those used on dogs. There are two methods normally used. The simplest, but not always the easiest, is to insert the left forefinger into the vagina, locate the urethral meatus on the floor usually 1–2 in. anterior to the clitoridal fossa. The catheter is then introduced below the finger and guided into the meatus.

The second and more frequently used method involves the use of a vaginal speculum and lamp. The speculum is inserted (remembering that the vagina is almost vertical for the first inch or so). The speculum is opened and the lamp arranged so that the urethral meatus can be seen and the catheter is then introduced gently. As this instrument is metal it is most important that no undue pressure is exerted at any time, since it is possible to perforate the bladder wall. The bitch must be firmly held, preferably with the hindquarters practically over the end of the table, thus reducing the likelihood of her sitting on the catheter and perforating the bladder. Bitches with vaginitis or open pyometra should only be catherized in an emergency, since the risk of infecting the bladder is very great.

A fairly close watch should be kept for 2 or 3 days on any animal that has been catheterized. The frequent passage of small quantities of urine, sometimes even blood in the urine, may indicate that there is an infection present and this should be reported.

If a bacteriological examination is required, catheterization is, of course, the only acceptable method for collection of urine.

COLLECTION OF FAECES

This normally presents little difficulty. The simplest method is to provide the owner with a suitable container and ask him to collect a sample.

If the dog is a boarder, faeces can be collected from the run, using a wooden spatula or palette knife. If it is a communal run, however, it is important that the run is clean and that the dog is watched. This will avoid the possibility of material from the wrong dog or stale faeces being collected. It may be possible to collect a sample directly from the dog as it defaecates and this should be done if the patient has severe diarrhoea.

If neither of these methods is satisfactory, it is usually possible to extract a small quantity of faeces from the rectum. Using a finger-stall lightly lubricated with liquid paraffin or vaseline, the middle finger is gently introduced into the rectum. As with catheterization, this is a two-person procedure and must be done gently to overcome constriction of the anal sphincter muscle. It may be necessary to do this two or three times to get sufficient material for analysis.

Store faeces in a wide-necked jar or plastic container.

COLLECTION OF VOMITUS

This will usually have to be collected from the bedding or floor of the kennel. A wooden spatula, or better a palette knife, or preferably two, will do this job satisfactorily. The sample is transferred to a suitable container.

Occasionally it is necessary to make a dog vomit and a variety of emetics may be used; in these circumstances the sample can usually be collected directly into the container. (See also section on Preservation of Material.)

COLLECTION OF BLOOD SAMPLES

This requires more skill and practice than the previous techniques.

The needle must be sterile and dry. Since frequent boiling soon takes the edge off a needle it is best to dry sterilize it. After washing and shaking dry, the needle is put into a small glass tube with cotton-wool at the bottom to protect the point and a small pledget of cotton-wool is put into the top of the tube. This should then be "cooked" in an oven Regulo 1 or similar setting for 3 hours.

Blood is usually taken from the radial vein, the one used for giving intravenous injections. The technique for taking blood is very similar to that for giving injections. An area over the vein is clipped and cleaned with spirit, the vein is raised by constricting the limb above the clipped site and the needle, which must be sharp, inserted. The vein should not be kept raised for long before sampling and if the flow is satisfactory a better sample of blood is obtained without keeping the vein raised. However, in small dogs the flow rate may be slow and raising the vein is then necessary.

For most dogs a 15-mm 10/10 needle is quite satisfactory; for large dogs a bigger needle should be used. It is better not to use a syringe since haemolysis frequently occurs when transferring the blood into the bottle. Disposable needles are now in common use and have the advantage of being sterile and sharp without any maintenance problems.

A most satisfactory arrangement is a short length of polythene tubing fitted into the hub of the needle. With a little practice the receiver and needle with polythene can be held in the one hand. In this way there is less spillage. If the sample needed is whole blood, the receiver must be gently shaken to mix the blood with the anticoagulant; if serum is wanted, shaking must be avoided. When sufficient blood has been collected the assistant should put his thumb over the shank of the needle, thus preventing leakage from the vein when the needle is withdrawn. The needle should never be withdrawn while the vein is still raised.

After the needle is out a small pledget of cotton-wool is placed over the site and held firmly in place with sticking plaster. This should be removed within a few hours.

If serum is required the receiver is put on one side to allow the clot to form and shrink. If there is an incubator available, 30 minutes at 37°C, followed by 30 minutes in a refrigerator will help the process. This should leave quite a large amount of serum which can be carefully poured off into another clean bottle or tube. If there are some red blood cells that are not trapped in the clot it is better to remove the serum with a narrow glass pipette. If a centrifuge is available, this can be used to get the last of the serum from the clot, or to remove any red cells that may have been decanted with the serum. Do not spin blood samples for longer than 10 minutes or at more than 2500 rev/min.

If "clotted blood" is to be sent away for analysis it is wise to allow the serum to separate and send this. A few red cells do not matter since these can easily be spun down by the laboratory. If the blood, clot included, is sent through the post considerably haemolysis frequently occurs.

COLLECTION OF MATERIAL FOR BACTERIOLOGICAL EXAMINATION

The bacteriological examination of blood is a specialized job and microscopic examination of even a thick film is unlikely to be of value, since very few organisms will be present. The organisms have to be incubated in a suitable medium to allow them to reach sufficient numbers to be readily examined. The sample should be taken into a sterile syringe and immediately transferred to a suitable medium (this will be supplied by the laboratory that has agreed to make the examination).

Direct smear. The slide can be held against some purely superficial lesions; possibly a gentle squeeze will help to express pus from a furuncular lesion.

Swab. The bacteriological swab is a small pledget of absorbent cotton-wool wrapped firmly round a stick, usually about 6 in. long. This is stored in a test-tube with a bung of, usually, non-absorbent, cotton-wool. The whole has been sterilized. It is important that the absorbent cotton-wool is firmly adherent to the stick, otherwise it may fall off while being used. For swabbing many lesions, the usual length is unneccessarily long and sticks about 3 in. long are sufficient. Swabs are used for collecting bacteria from any skin lesion, eyes, nose, ears, vagina and tonsils.

If the lesion is exposed, no preparation is necessary. The swab stick is withdrawn from the tube taking care that it does not touch the neck, which may not be sterile. The cotton-wool is then worked well over the surface to be examined until it has picked up sufficient material to be well damped. It is then returned carefully to the tube. The tube is labelled, stating the reference and the site of the lesion, and stored in the refrigerator until examined or despatched.

If the lesion is less open it may be necessary to reduce contamination by cleaning the surrounding skin. This is particularly so in the cases of furunculosis and some ear conditions. Here, any scabs or debris should be removed and the area cleaned with cotton-wool before the swab is used.

It is important that enough fluid is taken up on the swab to prevent it drying out before examination.

The bacteriological loop. This can be used to make smears directly from infected sites. It may sometimes be necessary to dilute the material with a small drop of sterile saline solution in order to make a good smear.

Aspiration (paracentesis). Certain diseases, of which tuberculosis is one of the more important, will cause the accumulation of fluid in the body cavities.

The sample must be taken with a sterile dry syringe using a wide bore, 1–2 in. needle, depending on the size of the dog. The site is clipped and cleaned with disinfectant and, if necessary, infiltrated with local anaesthetic. The needle is introduced, at least 10 ml withdrawn (the bacteria are likely to be well diluted and the larger the volume examined the higher the chance of demonstrating their presence), and transferred to a sterile container. A non-sterile dish should be available in case it is necessary to withdraw more fluid as part of the treatment of the condition. Label the bottle, again noting the source.

This method can also be used for withdrawing pus from a closed abscess. Pus is very viscid and a wider bore needle is usually necessary. In some cases the pus is so thick that the method fails.

COLLECTION OF SAMPLES FROM CASES OF SKIN DISEASE

Skin scrapings. The mites which cause some skin diseases live in the deep layers of the skin and to be of any value the material should be primarily from these layers.

Reagent. Ten per cent potassium hydroxide solution.

Equipment. A used knife blade (too sharp a knife does not scrape well).

Procedure. Always take the scraping from the edge of the lesion as it is here that the mites are likely to be commonest.

Moisten the area to be scraped with a little potassium hydroxide, anchor the skin between finger and thumb of one hand and gently scrape the lesion until pinpoints of blood develop. Transfer the material to a suitable labelled container, a small glass jar or test-tube will do.

Hair. If it is suspected that the skin condition is due to ringworm the patient should be examined under the Wood's lamp (ultraviolet light). The infected hairs will fluoresce a brilliant yellow; this must not be confused with blue and white fluorescences, which are due to a variety of compounds.

If the animal cannot be taken to the Wood's lamp the lesions should be very carefully examined, possibly under a magnifying glass. Infected hairs are frequently broken and any such hairs should be removed with forceps and put into a small tube, corked and labelled.

Blood

INTRODUCTION

Blood consists of fluid matrix in which are suspended or dissolved a large number of chemical substances and the blood cells. These cells and chemical substances do not vary a great deal in the normal dog, but in disease there is frequently a marked increase or decrease in their numbers or concentration. The degree of change frequently reflects the severity of the condition (see Table 4.1, p. 242).

The study of the cells is called haematology.

HAEMATOLOGY

Clotted blood is valueless for haematology and therefore an anticoagulant must be used. Different laboratories like different anticoagulants and if the sample is to be

TABLE 4.1

NORMAL VALUES IN HAEMATOLOGY (DOG)

Haemoglobin	(g/100 ml)	12–18
ESR	(mm/hr)	0·0–1·0
PCV	(%)	37–55
Buffy coat	(mm)	0·5–2
Total white-cell count	(thousand/mm^3)	6–18
Total red-cell count	(millions/mm^3)	5·5–8·5
Differential count		
Juveniles	(/mm^3)	0–200
Polymorphs	(thousand/mm^3)	5–10
Lymphocytes	(thousand/mm^3)	1·8–3·8
Monocytes	(/mm^3)	250–1050
Eosinophils	(/mm^3)	200–1000
Basophils		Rare
Reticulocytes		0–1·5% of red cells

sent away it is as well to find out which anticoagulant is preferred. For most purposes, sequestrene (known also as EDTA or ethylene diamine tetracetic acid or disodium versenate) is the best. This is readily soluble and little difficulty should be experienced with clotting if reasonable precautions are taken. Two mg/ml of blood is sufficient and more than this should not be used. The tube or bottle should be shaken gently to ensure mixing while the sample is being taken; if there is a mark to which the bottle should be filled do not overfill or clotting may result due to insufficiency of the anticoagulant. As soon as sufficient blood has been withdrawn, cap the bottle and mix well by rotating. Do not shake vigorously as this will cause haemolysis. *Heparin should not be used as an anticoagulant for haematology.*

Blood films should be made with absolutely fresh blood and this can really only be done satisfactorily if there are three people available, one to hold the dog, one to bleed, and the third to make the films from blood directly from the needle. If this is not practicable, smears can be made from the collected blood but this should be done immediately, particularly if anticoagulants other than sequestrene are used.

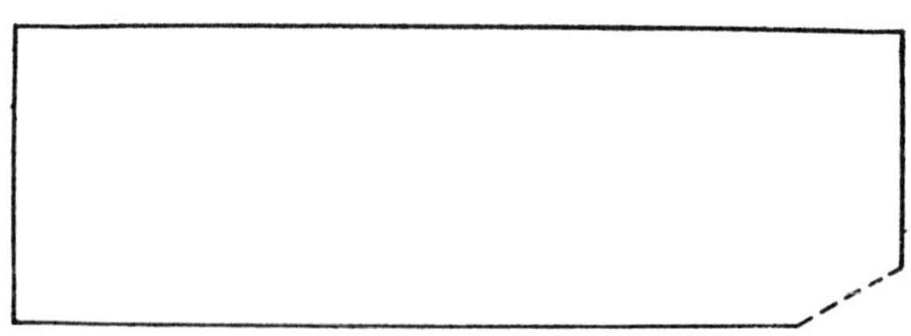

Fig 4.1. A spreader. The corner of a slide is scored with a glass file and broken off.

There are three precautions to observe when making blood films.

1. The slides must be cleaned really well; particularly they must be free of grease.
2. A suitable spreader should be used (Fig. 4.1).
3. Not too much blood should be used for a thick film is valueless for differential counts.

TECHNIQUE FOR PREPARATION OF BLOOD FILMS

Put a small drop of blood on to the slide at one end and draw the spreader into this. Allow the blood to spread along the spreader. If the drop is too large, lift the spreader up (this will take sufficient blood with it) and put it back on a clean portion of the slide. Push it gently and firmly along the slide; this should give a good even spread with possibly some tailing at the further end. It is most important that the blood be pulled along behind the spreader, not pushed along in front. Blood cells are fragile and if pushed in front of the spreader many will be destroyed.

Always prepare three or four films at a time: this allows for failure in staining, breakages and second opinions.

Wave the slides gently in the air until they are dry and then store face downward on a piece of clean blotting paper. Once again, label the whole blood and the slides clearly. Wax pencil is suitable, or the films can be labelled by writing in the centre of the film with an ordinary pencil (Fig. 4.2). This is probably the best method since there is little likelihood of the "label" coming off during staining.

In examining blood samples one is looking for changes in numbers, size and shape of the cells; these facts will give some indication of whether there is an anaemia, the type of anaemia, whether the patient is making an attempt to overcome it, whether there is an infection and, if so, whether acute or chronic.

Some of the leucocytes are controlled by the hormones of the adrenal gland and changes in the numbers of these cells may suggest changes in adrenal function.

Of rather less importance because the conditions are rarer, are diseases of the organs responsible for forming the different types of cells.

Always remember to mix the blood sample well before any is withdrawn for testing.

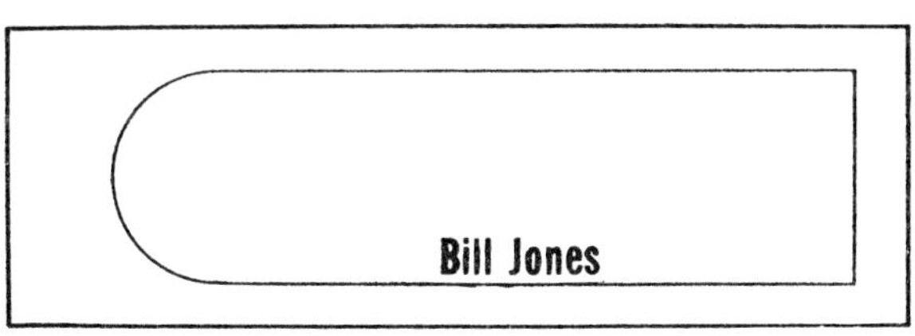

Fig. 4.2. Method of labelling blood film with a lead pencil.

HAEMOGLOBIN

This is the one chemical test that is routinely performed as a part of a haematological investigation. There are a number of tests of varying accuracy which can be used.

Probably the most commonly used method in the smaller laboratory is the Haldane haemoglobinometer. This consists of a small box with a ground glass back; in this are two tubes, one containing a standard solution of carboxyhaemoglobin and one graduated. Into this second tube is placed about 0·5 ml of distilled water and 20 μl (mm^3) of blood. These are mixed well and then coal gas is blown gently over the mixture, converting all the haemoglobin to carboxyhaemoglobin. Water is added to the unknown until it matches the standard and the percentage of the "unknown" haemoglobin is read directly from the graduations on the tube.

The Sahli haemoglobinometer works on the same principle but uses acid haematin instead of carboxyhaemoglobin.

The physical characteristics of blood that are of interest are:

The ESR (erythrocyte sedimentation rate). If a sample of unclotted blood is allowed to stand the cells will, due to gravity, sink through the plasma. Certain diseases may accelerate this fall and the rate at which it occurs can often give some indication of the severity of the animal's condition. This test is done in a special tube (Wintrobe tube) which must be carefully filled by means of a long thin pipette and then fixed upright in a piece of plasticine. The tube is graduated in millimetres and the distance that the erythrocytes have fallen in 30, 60 and 90 minutes is recorded.

The packed cell volume (PCV or haematocrit). For this test an electric centrifuge is necessary.

The Wintrobe tube, after the ESR has been measured, is spun at 3000 rev/min for 30 minutes and the level again recorded. This is the PCV.

It is usually possible to see three distinct layers after spinning. The largest is the erythrocytes, and is deep red, the next is paler and is due to platelets (thrombocytes) and on top of this is the buffy coat which consists of the different types of white cells. (The size of this layer is a rough guide to the number of white cells in the blood.)

The haematocrit, with the total erythrocyte count, gives a measure of the size of the cells or, with examination of the films to give some idea of the size, an indication of the number of cells present. Low haematocrit values will be found in anaemia and high values when there is much loss of water (haemo-concentration) as is seen in severe diabetes and severe nephritis.

TOTAL CELL COUNTS

Special pipettes are usually supplied with the equipment, but these are not absolutely essential since the dilutions can be done with ordinary laboratory pipettes. It is essential to have a counting chamber; this is a thick glass slide with a central platform which is, usually, $\frac{1}{10}$ mm lower than the rest of the slide. There is a channel on each side of this area which prevents seepage of the blood mixture.

On this platform are very accurately engraved a series of squares whose pattern and size vary according to the type of chamber. The best is the improved Neubauer. The chamber and coverslip must be completely free of grease and, in view of the delicate nature of the apparatus, only the softest material should be used for cleaning.

White cell count. The pipette is carefully filled to the 0·5 mark with well-shaken, or fresh, blood and then to the 11 mark with a special fluid (2% acetic acid with 0·01% gentian violet); this gives a dilution of 1 in 20. This fluid destroys the red cells and stains the nuclei of the white cells so that they are more easily seen. The blood and the fluid are carefully and thoroughly mixed in the bulb by rotating the pipette. There is a small white bead in the bulb which helps the mixing. (So that no mistake is made the bead in the pipette used for erythrocyte counts is red.) The pipette should be put on one side for about 5 minutes to make sure that all the red cells are destroyed. After this period the pipette is rotated well again to make sure that the leucocytes are equally distributed throughout the fluid. The first three drops, i.e. the fluid in the capillary stem which contains no cells, is discarded and then the tip of the pipette is placed on the counting chamber and a little of the mixture allowed to flow under the coverslip. This requires care and the troughs should not be allowed to fill. The chamber is put on to the microscope stage and the lighting and focusing carried out. Counting should be delayed for a few minutes to allow the cells to sink; they will then all be in focus. There should be no movement of the cells; this will occur if there is too much fluid present. Also if the light source is too hot and too close to the chamber this will cause evaporation.

When all the movement has ceased the count can be made using the low-power lens. Start at the top left-hand small square and proceed along to the right, drop down a row and move back along this row and so on until one big (1 mm) square is completed. Make a note of the number of cells counted at the end of each line of small squares. Count at least four large squares; on some chambers this can be done with one filling, but with others it has to be done by removing the coverslip, cleaning and drying this and the chamber, and refilling. Remember to mix the cells well again before each refill and discard two or three drops from the stem each time.

Cells on, or touching, a line should be included in the square to the right or below. In this way they will be counted once only. It is necessary to count more than one large (1 mm) square since there is a considerable variation in the cells per square, from the same mixture; this is due partly to faults in mixing and partly to chance; counting 4 overcomes this variation. The improved Neubauer has an area of 9 mm^2 engraved; this is subdivided into nine large squares (1 mm area). The four corner squares are further divided into sixteen squares and the centre square is divided into twenty-five squares which themselves are divided into sixteen small squares (1/400 mm^2). The four corner squares should be counted for white cells.

It is important to remember here that the pipette must be absolutely clean and dry before use and must be cleaned immediately after use. Wash well in cold water until all the blood is removed, rinse in hot water and shake dry, rinse in methylated spirit and finally acetone, allow to drain. If needed in a hurry the pipette can be warmed on the microscope lamp but if dried in this way it must be allowed to cool before further use.

The calculation of the total white-cell count from the actual count. Let x be the number of cells counted in 4 large (1 mm) squares, then

$$\frac{x}{4} = \text{the number of cells in one square.}$$

The depth of the chamber is 0·1 mm, therefore the volume for each square is 0·1 mm³.

Therefore, there are $x/4 \times 10$ cells per mm³, but the blood was diluted $\times$ 20. Therefore,

$$\text{No. of cells per mm}^3 \text{ of blood} = \frac{x \times 10 \times 20}{4}$$

$$\text{or } x \times 50.$$

This calculation obviously only applies to counts with chambers of 0·1 mm depth and with large squares of 1 mm area. Usually, sufficient information upon which to base calculations is etched on the chamber.

A very simple diluting technique (Unopette*) is available. This consists of a length of capillary tube of known volume which fits a small plastic bottle containing a fixed volume of diluent. The capillary tube is filled with blood which is then transferred into the plastic bottle. The mixture is allowed to stand, then resuspended and transferred to the counting chamber. The capillary and bottle are then discarded.

Red-cell count. This investigation is even more time-consuming than the white-cell count and until considerable experience has been gained the results are very unreliable. More accurate information can be gained from the PCV and estimation of the size of the cells from examining the film.

EXAMINATION OF BLOOD FILMS

In order to examine the cellular element of blood it is necessary to stain the cells. Special stains are used to show the differences in the cells; these stains are the Romanowsky stains and are a mixture of dyes which stain different portions of the cells different colours. There are a large variety but the simplest stain to use is Leishman's and this gives very satisfactory results.

Procedure. The dried film is flooded with Leishman's stain for 2 minutes; this fixes the film. After this time, double the volume of buffered distilled water† is added and the slide rocked gently to mix the stain. It is left 5–7 minutes to stain and then washed in buffered distilled water until the film has a pinkish tinge. This should take no longer than 2–3 minutes.

* Unopette—Becton, Dickenson, U.S.A. In the U.K. Unopette is obtainable from Becton, Dickenson U.K. Limited, York House, Empire Way, Wembley, Middlesex.

† pH 7·0. Proprietary tablets are available for the preparation of this solution.

The back of the slide can be wiped dry and most of the moisture shaken off the front. The slide can then be stood on its side to drain or it can be carefully blotted with filter paper or blotting paper.

The film should be examined with the low-power lens to get an overall picture of distribution of the cells and the quality of staining. If the film is a reasonable one and staining is satisfactory a more detailed examination can be made with the high-power lens. This lens can be used for differential counts and for an appreciation of changes in red cell shape and size. The oil immersion lens should only be used to examine unusual cells. If the film shows a lot of small black granules the stain needs filtering.

The differential white cell count. This is the most important examination carried out on a blood film since the relative percentages of the different types of white cells are a valuable diagnostic acid. The leucocytes are not evenly distributed throughout the film; lymphocytes are commoner in the body than elsewhere and polymorphs accumulate in the tail. All forms are commoner at the edge of the film than in the middle. This has led to the development of three methods for doing counts. Of these three the "battlement method" is the most satisfactory (Fig. 4.3). Each "step" is two fields long; in this way a reasonable area is covered and the sites chosen for the count counteract the variations in distribution of the different types of cell.

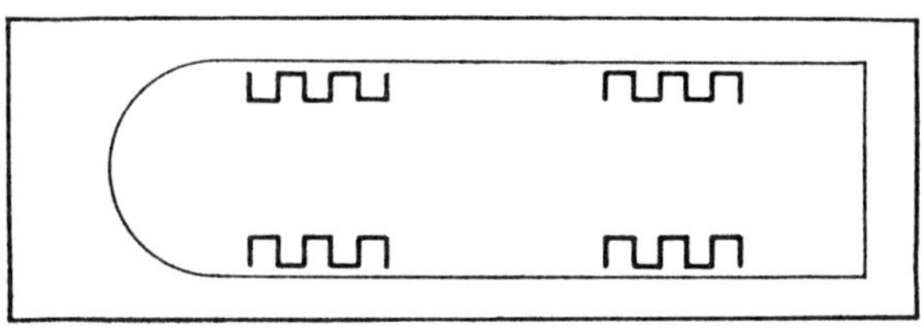

Fig. 4.3. "Battlement" method of counting, each "step" represents two fields.

When doing a differential count the more cells counted the more accurately will the count reflect the true picture. Count 100 cells for each 10,000 cells in the total white cell count.

The simplest method of keeping count is using squared paper; mark off blocks ten squares by ten squares. For each cell counted put a letter in each small square, N for neutrophil, L for lymphocyte, M for monocyte and E for eosinophil. When two blocks are filled 200 cells have been counted. Count the number of each type of cell noted and express them as numbers/mm^3.

The commonest white cell is the neutrophilic polymorphonuclear leucocyte commonly known as the neutrophil or polymorph. This cell has relatively little colouring matter in the cytoplasm (minute red granules may be seen occasionally), and a nucleus which varies from a horse-shoe shape in the young forms through two, three and four lobes up to twelve to sixteen lobes in very old cells. High number of these cells (neutrophilia) is seen as a response to bacterial infection, either general or local. A reduction in number (neutropenia) is sometimes seen in virus diseases.

Fairly closely related to the neutrophil is the eosinophil which has large red granules in the cytoplasm. This cell is relatively uncommon and an increase (eosinophilia) is seen in allergy, worm infestation and in insufficiency of the adrenal glands. A decrease (eosinopenia) is rare and may be seen in hyperactivity of the adrenal glands or in severe distemper.

The basophil, with blue-staining granules in the cytoplasm, is extremely rare in the dog.

Myeloid leukaemia is rarely seen in the dog; in this condition cells which are the early stages in the development of these leucocytes and are normally confined to the bone marrow, occur in the blood.

Agranulocytosis or granulopenia, that is a reduction in all these forms of leucocytes, may occur in the dog, as it does in man, as a result of treatment with a drug which depresses the bone marrow activity.

After the neutrophil, the commonest cell is the lymphocyte; sometimes these are subdivided into large and small lymphocytes, but for routine purposes this is not necessary. These cells have relatively little cytoplasm, the large form having more than the small. The significance of changes in numbers of these cells is not always certain but an increase (lymphocytosis) is frequently associated with a chronic infection and with some virus diseases. Lymphatic leukaemia is occasionally seen, in which cells normally confined to the lymphoid tissues appear in the blood. A lymphopenia sometimes occurs in hormonal diseases, particularly where there is excessive production of adrenal hormones, in distemper and in chronic interstitial nephritis.

The monocyte is an even more enigmatic cell than the lymphocyte. It is found in increased numbers in chronic disease.

The film will also show some very small blue "cells" with red granules; these are platelets. There appears to be very little indication for doing platelet counts in veterinary work but with experience it is possible to say whether they are present in excess or in numbers below normal.

RETICULOCYTE COUNT

In cases where there is anaemia, it is worth knowing whether the bone marrow is active or whether the anaemia is due to a failure of the marrow to produce new cells. This can be done with a technique known as supravital staining.

Newly produced red cells contain the remnants of the nuclear material as a network of basophil, i.e. blue-staining material. This material cannot be demonstrated by the usual staining techniques but if a drop of fresh, and therefore living, blood is mixed with stain the network, or reticulum, takes up the stain.

THE CHEMISTRY OF BLOOD

Introduction

It is wise, when bleeding a dog for chemical tests, to avoid sampling within 8 hours of a meal. This ensures that all the constituents are at the "baseline" or "fasting" level for that patient.

For most tests the presence of the blood cells is undesirable and they are eliminated either by spinning "whole blood", i.e. blood which has been taken into an anti-coagulant, and recovering the clear plasma, or by allowing blood to clot and removing the serum. These two fluids differ in that plasma contains the clotting protein fibrinogen, but serum contains none. The first method has the advantage that the plasma can be separated from the cells within 15 minutes of sampling, but there are some tests which can only be carried out on serum and as most of the others can be done on serum as well as plasma the former is the most frequently used.

Anticoagulants

The clotting process is a complicated one which depends on a number of enzymes and, at one step in the process, the presence of calcium.

Anticoagulants fall into two groups:

1. Those which "block" calcium: EDTA, oxalates, citrates and fluorides.
2. Those which interfere with an enzyme system: heparin and fluorides. For most purposes *heparin* is the best anticoagulant to use (2 mg/ml blood) but for glucose estimations fluoride is used.

For the following tests serum is usually used:

Enzyme tests (transaminases, alkaline phosphatase).

Sodium and potassium. (In man plasma is used for potassium estimations; this is unnecessary in the dog since the concentration of potassium in the cell is low whereas in man it is high and rapidly leaks out of the cells.)

Protein tests (including tests for specific antibodies).

Calcium and magnesium.

In these tests plasma may be used:

Glucose (but see later).

Inorganic phosphate (though, provided that no undue delay occurs, serum or whole blood can be used).

Cholesterol.

For glucose it is customary to use whole blood; erythrocytes are living cells and will continue to use glucose after blood has been withdrawn. It is therefore necessary to prevent this glycolysis if accurate results are wanted. For this reason a fluoride anticoagulant (sodium fluoride 10 parts, thymol 1 part; 10 mg/ml blood) is used. The fluoride destroys the enzyme systems concerned and the thymol prevents any bacterial growth. Plasma can be used, but the concentration of glucose is higher in plasma than in the cells and therefore higher results will be obtained.

Urea also may be estimated, depending on the technique used, on whole blood, serum or plasma, but as with glucose, plasma and serum values will be slightly higher than whole blood values.

Constituents of Blood

Normal dog serum is usually quite clear or only slightly opaque and practically colourless. A pink or red colour shows that the sampling technique is faulty or that the equipment is dirty or wet and that haemolysis has occurred. Some samples, particularly if taken too soon after a meal, are cloudy, sometimes as dense as milk; this is due to fat and is called lipaemia. The serum may be yellow and this suggests jaundice, though very occasionally the colour may be due to a pigment related to vitamin A. The urine test for bilirubin will differentiate between them.

The compounds existing in the highest concentrations in the blood are the proteins. These are placed into two main groups:

1. Albumin; this is a single compound whose properties and functions are very similar in all species but whose chemical composition varies slightly from one species to the next.
2. The globulins; a very complex group in which at least twenty-eight different proteins have been identified. Fibrinogen is present also.

Albumin acts mainly as a means of maintaining the fluid content of blood at the normal level through its osmotic pressure. It can also act as a transport mechanism for fats, calcium and bilirubin.

The globulins act as transfer systems for fats, copper and iron and the γ globulins include the antibodies to infectious agents.

Among these proteins are the enzymes, proteins which assist some vital reactions to take place; a large number of enzymes are present in blood and only a few are of known clinical significance.

Possibly next in importance to the proteins is glucose. Glucose is the prime source of energy for all tissues, and, in fact, if the level in the blood drops too low there is an interference with brain function and fits will result. Insulin is a hormone produced in the pancreas and is necessary for the use of glucose, and where insulin is in short supply, as in diabetes mellitus, the level in the blood rises. On the other hand, if the pancreas is producing too much insulin, glucose is used too quickly and the level in the blood falls below the normal level.

The estimation of blood glucose is therefore valuable in both these conditions. Diabetes can be diagnosed on urine tests alone, but estimating blood glucose will help to assess how severe the condition is and how it is responding to treatment. The excess of insulin can frequently only be differentiated from brain disease by showing that the blood sugar level is very low.

Probably the most important constituent of blood from the practical aspect is urea. The body is unable to store protein in excess of its needs and therefore any digested protein that cannot be used immediately is excreted. It is converted to urea by the liver, transported in the blood to the kidney and there passed out with the urine. In kidney disease, and one or two other conditions, there is an inability to remove the urea from the blood and the level rises. The degree of increase is a reasonable measure of the severity of the condition and routine testing for urea is a very good guide to the progress being made by the patient. Frequently related to the failure of kidney function is the level of inorganic phosphate in the blood. Phosphates are very important substances in the body, not only as a part of bone but also as an important compound in the chemical changes occurring in the cell. Excess phosphate is excreted by the kidneys and when the kidneys begin to fail the phosphate level begins to rise.

The rise in phosphate and urea is paralleled by a rise in the serum creatinine level; creatinine is a breakdown product of protein metabolism.

It must be emphasized here that the mechanism of illness in uraemia is not fully understood. Urea itself is not very poisonous in dogs, as they can tolerate large doses of urea given intravenously. It is thought that the illness is due to the failure of the kidneys to excrete substances like the phenols, sulphates, and phosphates. Urea is, however, easier to measure than these and for this reason it is used as an indicator of kidney disease.

The urea level can rise above normal in some conditions that are not primarily due to kidney disease. Poor heart function, with insufficient blood reaching the kidneys, will put the urea level up and excessive water loss will have the same effect.

The electrolytes (sodium, potassium, calcium, magnesium, copper, cobalt and iron) are important in a variety of ways and, with the exception of calcium and magnesium, complicated to estimate.

Changes in sodium and potassium occur in certain hormonal disease; calcium is affected by a number of factors such as bone breakdown and milk production; a low calcium level is the cause of milk fever in cattle (though here changes in magnesium and phosphate frequently occur also) and in eclampsia in bitches; magnesium disturbances seem to be rare in dogs. Iron is, of course, necessary for the production of haemoglobin and cobalt and copper also play a part here. Cholesterol, from which bile salts, the adrenal steroid and the sex hormones are produced, varies quite considerably. It is low in severe debilitating conditions and high in deficiency of thyroid function and in uncontrolled diabetes. Chloride is lost in cases where there is severe vomiting.

The changes of bicarbonate and carbon dioxide and of the pH of blood have not been fully investigated in the dog.

Chemical Methods

Introduction. The methods of estimating these compounds are varied but the majority are colorimetric and depend on reacting the substance under test with another substance. The amount of colour produced is proportional to the amount of test substance and is compared with:

1. The amount of colour produced by treating solutions of test substance of known strength (standard solutions) in exactly the same way.
2. A solution of a different substance having the same colour and amount of colour as the standard solutions.

3. With tinted glass, having the same amount of colour as the standard solutions.

This comparison may be done (1) by eye, (a) diluting the stronger to match the weaker and calculating the concentration of the unknown from the amount of water added, (b) in a comparator block, or (c) in a visual colorimeter, or (2) with a photo-electric colorimeter.

Turbidometric methods, in which a turbidity or cloudiness is produced, are sometimes used; in these, the comparison can be made by eye or in a colorimeter.

The titrimetric method is sometimes used in which small amounts of a reagent are added to the test substance until the reaction is complete. The end is usually marked by a colour change in the solutions and the amount of unknown is proportional to the amount of reagent added.

The simplest methods for assaying urea are "stick" methods, but they sacrifice some degree of accuracy for simplicity and speed. Azostix (Ames Co. Ltd.) and Urastrat (W. Warner & Co.) are both satisfactory. More accurate colorimetric methods are available and very satisfactory enzymatic test kits are available. These require a water bath and colorimeter but give more accurate results. Both the "stick" tests and the enzyme test kits should be used according to the makers' instructions.

Glucose can also be assayed by simple though less accurate stick methods and enzymatic test kits. Destrostix (Ames Co. Ltd.) will help to demonstrate whether the blood glucose level is high or low, which is all that is needed for initial diagnosis. The more accurate methods (as, for example, Boehringer glucose assay) should be used if day-to-day checks are required.

The Tintometer Co., Salisbury, have produced a handbook describing colorimetric methods for practically every blood and urine investigation using a comparator box with tinted glass standards. If further analyses are considered this reference should be consulted. Commercial kits* are now produced for a wide variety of tests which make them suitable side-room techniques. A range of serum enzymes can now be easily estimated and these are useful for checking for liver and pancreatic diseases. Chemical supply houses should be consulted as to what is available.

Urine

INTRODUCTION

The composition of urine varies considerably according to the animal's diet and needs, and also varies during the course of the day. To obtain the maximum amount of accurate information from urine examination these tests should be carried out on a 24-hour sample, that is, all the urine passed during a 24-hour period. This, however, is not possible in practice and provided that the limitations of the method are appreciated, the "grab" sample technique is satisfactory. Care must be taken in interpreting some tests, and some should be repeated on a second sample before using the result to establish a diagnosis. As with examination of blood, tests on urine are either physical or chemical.

* Firms include Boehringer, Sigma and Warner.

EXAMINATION OF URINE

Physical Properties

Colour. This may range in the normal animal from pale yellow or almost colourless to dark brown. The natural colour in the urine is due largely to urochrome, a pigment of endogenous origin. The variations in colour of the urine in a normal animal depend on many factors, including species, concentration, diet and exercise.

Abnormal colours are due to bile pigments, haemoglobin, blood, myoglobin—this is seen during azoturia and imparts a coffee-brown colour to the urine—and drugs, e.g. phenothiazine gives a red colour, methylene blue a blue colour, dinitrocresol and other similar compounds give a bright chrome-yellow colour. Greenish fluorescence is occasionally seen in dog urine and this may be associated with colouring matter in the food.

Turbidity. Carnivore urine is usually clear, but becomes cloudy on standing; this is often accompanied by an increase in pH due to the presence of micro-organisms that can decompose urea into ammonia, and the alkalinity then causes the precipitation of phosphates. Abnormal turbidity may be due to the presence of pus, mucus, bacteria, inflammatory cells, prostatic or vaginal secretions.

Odour. This varies with species and condition; the odour is sourish in dog and cat. Acetone and acetoacetic acid impart a sweetish small, and drugs such as camphor, phenols, cresol, turpentine and garlic impart their own odour.

Consistency. This varies according to species, condition, diet and fluid intake. Inflammatory changes in the urinary tract may give rise to urinary mucoproteins, which may make the urine viscid.

Reaction (acid or alkaline). When fresh, normal carnivore urine is acid (pH 5–7), changes of pH may occur in abnormal metabolic conditions. A lowered pH may result from increased acid secretion in diabetes mellitus and other conditions involving increased fat metabolism. An increase in pH results from the activity of urease positive organisms (that is those which can turn urea into ammonia) (see above); a high pH in a fresh sample of dog urine indicates cystitis, but, if not fresh, may indicate bacterial contamination. It is rare to find acid urines with pH values below pH 5.

Tests for pH may be made with wide and narrow range indicator papers.

Specific gravity. This varies widely with time of taking sample, health, fluid intake, degree of exercise and sweating. It is inadvisable to draw conclusions from an observation of the specific gravity of a single urine sample; more than one sample should be examined. The normal range in the dog is 1·012–1·060 and in the cat 1·020–1·040.

Values are low in polyuria, as found, for example, in chronic interstitial nephritis in the dog, and in diabetes insipidus (1·001–1·005); high values (but not outside the normal range) may be found in acute nephritis in the dog in various fevers, and often in diabetes mellitus. A so-called "fixed-level" value of about 1·008-1·010 may be found in severe cases of renal insufficiency when this value remains constant irrespective of diet and fluid intake. This corresponds to the sp.gr. of protein-free plasma filtrates. Specific gravity is measured with a urinometer.

Chemical Tests

Note. Before testing, all urine samples should be made clear by filtering, centrifuging, or by standing to allow any deposit to settle.

Proteins. Recent developments in analytical technique have revealed that many normal urines contain traces of protein although these are in quantities that are too small to be identified by normal chemical techniques. Small quantities of protein are known to pass the normal glomeruli and there is good evidence for reabsorption of albumin and globulin in the proximal tubule.

Protein is pre-renal (haemoglobin, myoglobin), renal (acute fevers, nephritis), or post-renal (lower urinary or genital tract) origin. Spermatozoa are frequently found in dog urine and this indicates that there is a leak of seminal fluid into the urinary tract. This fluid is protein rich and will give positive results with protein tests. Severe cystitis will cause an exudation of serum into the bladder and this will also give positive results. In cases of nephritis, where there is little glomerular damage and, therefore, little protein loss, the urine will be free from protein as shown by the usual tests. It is obvious, therefore, that one must be careful in assessing the significance of proteinuria, and it is worth examining the urinary sediment microscopically for spermatozoa and for bacteria which may be causing cystitis.

Sulphosalicylic acid test. In a small test-tube or on a piece of black perspex place one drop of 20% sulphosalicylic acid. This is followed by one drop of urine. Protein is indicated by a faint turbidity (0·01%) to a descrete heavy precipitate (possibly as high as 1%); compare with normal urine. Report as + to ++++.

Albustix. These are strips of stiff paper, one end of which is impregnated with tetrabromphenol blue buffered to approximately pH 3·0 with a citrate buffer. Urine containing protein gives a colour change—yellow through green to blue—depending on the concentration of protein. This test is not satisfactory with urines of high (alkaline) pH.

Reducing substances. Most normal urines when boiled with an alkaline solution of a copper salt cause no change; a few, however, reduce the copper to the metallic form causing, depending on the amount reduced, a colour change from pale green to bright yellow or brick red. (It is very unusual for a normal urine to contain sufficient reducing substances to produce the complete reaction.) Glucose will produce this colour change and so will lactose or milk sugar. Glucose is found in the urine in dabetes mellitus and in very small quantities in occasional cases of kidney disease; lactose is sometimes found in the urine of lactating and suckling animals. Lactose is not used by the animal; if, therefore, any be absorbed, as occurs if the mammary gland becomes distended, or if the alimentary mucosa is disrupted, then it is excreted unchanged.

Several substances other than glucose and lactose reduce these reagents and may be responsible for false positives. These substances include creatinine, uric acid, glucuronic acid and glucuronides. Pentoses and fructose also reduce copper but as yet they have not been positively identified in animal urines. The use of certain drugs increase the normal output of glucuronides and may result in a definite "positive".

Clinitest tablets. Using the "standard" dropper provided, put five drops of urine and ten of water into a tube, add one tablet and allow to react, watching all the time. Fifteen seconds after the reaction has ceased shake the tube and compare with colour chart provided. When the concentration is high, the final colour may be brown rather than yellow, but a yellow colour will have occurred during the reaction and for this reason the test must be watched throughout.

Demonstration of glucose in urine. It is important to show whether or not the reducing substances in the urine is glucose. For this purpose the test papers containing the enzyme glucose oxidase (Clinistix) are used. These are dipped into the urine. If glucose is present the enzyme reacts with it, liberating oxygen in an active form which turns an indicator in the strip purple within 1 minute. This test is given by glucose only but if the strip is allowed to stand for a long time after dipping, the atmospheric oxygen may turn it purple. It is not sufficient to rely only on Clinistix, both this *and* Clinitest should be used.

Ketones. The most satisfactory test for ketones in urine is that of Rothera and its developments. The ketone bodies usually encountered are acetone, acetoacetic acid, and beta-hydroxybutyric acid. Transient false positives may result from the presence of organic sulphides (mercaptans) and excessive pyruvate will give a very blue reaction. These are as yet of no known clinical significance in small animals. Ketone bodies occur in urine as the result of carbohydrate starvation, e.g. in diabetes mellitus.

Acetest tablets. These are a modification of Rothera's mixture. Place one drop of urine on a tablet, allow to stand for 30 seconds and compare with colour chart provided. Report as trace (+), moderate (++) or strong (+++).

Blood and blood pigments. There are several tests for the presence of blood in urine. The three most important are (a) the identification of red cells microscopically, (b) spectroscopic examination, (c) the benzidine or *o*-tolidine tests. There are several modifications of the last. Blood may be present either as haemoglobinuria or as haematuria. Haematuria may become haemoglobinuria as the result of degeneration of the red cells. Haemoglobinuria or myoglobinuria (which also gives a positive reaction with benzidine or tolidine) are pre-renal conditions (that is, they are present in the blood before it reaches the kidney). Haemoglobinuria or haematuria can be differentiated by microscopic examination of the sediment. Absence of debris or cells indicates pure haemoglobinuria, erythrocytes or debris indicates haematuria. A previously red sample which becomes clear on spinning, with a red deposit, is normally haematuria. Haematuria indicates haemorrhage at some point in the urinary tract, e.g. bruising of the kidneys, inflammation or tumour of the bladder and wounds of the urethra (usually the result of catheterization).

Test for blood. If all urines are examined microscopically there is no need to test for blood chemically. The reagents used are carcinogenic, a good reason for avoiding this test.

Occultest. Put two drops of urine on the filter pad, put a tablet on top and flood the tablet with two drops of water. Watch for speed of development and intensity of the blue colour. Report + to ++++. Haemoglobin may be distinguished from myoglobin by spectroscopic examination.

Bile salts and bile pigments. Bile pigments appear in the urine of animals suffering from various disorders affecting the pigment (haemoglobin) metabolism of the body. It has long been held that the presence of bilirubin in the urine is a good indication of obstructive liver disease, but it is becoming increasingly obvious that this is not the case in the dog. Bilirubin, which is insoluble in water, is transported from the reticulo-endothelial system to the liver as a complex with serum albumin. In the liver this complex is broken down and bilirubin converted to the water-soluble glucuronide. In man this is apparently the only site of production of a water-soluble bilirubin compound. In haemolytic jaundice there is an increased production of the glucuronide excreted in the bile, but there is no regurgitation into the vascular system. In obstructive jaundice, conjugation occurs normally but owing to the obstruction the bile cannot reach the intestine and bilirubin, glucuronide and bile salts are regurgitated into the vascular system and are excreted by the kidney. Testing for bilirubin is therefore a useful procedure in the diagnosis of these two conditions. However, in the dog this happy stage of affairs does not exist, serum bilirubin being a much lower concentration than it is in man, which suggests a more efficient excretory mechanism. The enzyme necessary for conjugating bilirubin has been shown to exist in the kidney and up to 20% of dogs which show no impairment of their liver function by other tests excrete detectable quantities of bilirubin in their urine. Presumably conjugation is occurring in the kidney. In addition, there are a number of cases in which liver function, as estimated by serum changes, is severely impaired but in which no bilirubinuria occurs. It has also been shown that 5% of normal cats excrete bilirubin.

It may or may not be justifiable, but it is assumed that trace and even mildly positive reactions are without clinical significance in the dog. However, strongly positive reactions may indicate an obstructive condition, either intrahepatic or in the extrahepatic duct system or an increase in haemolysis. Hayes test (for bile salts) should be positive only in obstructive conditions but positive results occur in normal dogs.

In the absence of information to the contrary it is assumed that species other than the cat and dog simulate man in their metabolism of bilirubin.

Ictotest tablets. Put five drops of urine on the special mat provided, put a tablet on the mat and flood it with two drops of water. Note the intensity of the purple colour developed within 30 seconds.

Tests for pH, protein, ketones, glucose and blood are now available on one dipstick (Labstix*) and this has proved a most valuable side-room technique.

* Ames Co.

Microscopic Examination of Urine

Considerable information can be gained about the state of the urinary tract by examination of the sediment in urine. For satisfactory results this must be done on fresh urine.

Put 10 ml of urine in a centrifuge tube and spin at 2500 rev/min for 5 minutes. Discard most of the supernatant fluid (or use for the chemical tests) and mix the sediment gently but well with two or three drops of Sedistain.*

There may be no deposit, but usually some bladder epithelium cells will be present and crystals are common. "Casts" occur also; these are cylinders of material, protein, fat or cells, which have been washed down from the kidney tubules where they are formed (Fig. 4.4).

Urinary Deposits

These may be divided as follows:

Deposits

Cellular	Inorganic/Organic	
Excess of these nearly always associated with disease	Rarely pathological, normal result of metabolism. May increase, e.g. alkaline phosphate in infected urine (see above).	
	Acid	Alkaline
	Urates	Phosphates
	Cystine	

Cellular Deposits

Epithelial cells. These are present normally in small numbers, some from the vaginal epithelium in females. Transitional epithelial cells may be seen in cystitis, cells from the kidney tubules may be seen in nephritis.

Leucocytes. Rounded, granular. If the urine is also rich in protein and casts, the pus is likely to have come from the kidney. Pyuria is also seen in prostatitis, metritis and vaginitis. In haemorrhage, red and white cells are present in the proportion in which they are found in the blood.

* In the United Kingdom obtainable from Arnold R. Horwell Ltd., 2 Grangeway, Kilburn High Road, London, NW6.

Red blood cells. Nearly always pathological (but remember that oestrus in the bitch will give haematuria). If from the kidney the cells will form cylinders.

Spermatozoa. In dog urine.

Parasites. Capillaria spp. in foxes and foxhounds.

Bacteria. Cocci, coliforms, proteus. Urine sometimes contains contaminants, bacteria are present but there is no other evidence of inflammation in tract.

Tumour cells. For example, from papilloma of bladder.

Casts. These are structures moulded into the renal tubules; look for parallel sides. Hyaline casts are simple protein and are most frequently globulin. This precipitates more readily as the concentration and acidity increase, therefore the more severe the disease, the more casts. Epithelial casts retain their cellular structure and form granular casts as they degenerate; lipoid casts also occur. All these forms may be stained with bilirubin. Blood casts are indicative of glomerular bleeding and on degeneration form copper-coloured haem casts.

Inorganic/Organic Deposits

Crystals

Uric acid. Usually tinged brown. Rhomboid plates, rosettes of spindle-shaped crystals, clusters of parallel crystals.

Amorphous urates. In strongly acid urine. Resemble red, yellow or brown sand in miniature (dissolve on warming). There is a predisposition to these in dalmatians.

Calcium oxalate. A small amount in all urines. The crystals are four-sided or dumb-bell shaped. They are soluble in hydrochloric acid, but not in acetic acid.

Cystine. Flat regular hexagons. Increased cystine in urine appears as a sex-linked condition occurring only in the male.

Triple phosphate. Magnesium ammonium phosphate. Prismatic crystals with oblique ends (knife rests, coffin lid) or feathery or leaf-shaped, often agglomerated into star-shaped bodies. If found in fresh urine, they indicate retention, or alkaline fermentation (pyelitis, cystitis). They will deposit if the urine is allowed to stand.

Amorphous phosphates. Granular sand-like precipitations, grossly resembling sedimented white cells.

Calcium carbonate. Crystals dissolve in acid, giving bubbles of carbon dioxide (as with normal cattle urine). They are usually yellowish spheres with radial striation but these crystals are rare, particularly in small animals.

Sulphonamide crystals. These are sometimes seen in patients that are being treated with sulphonamides. The shapes vary very much according to which drug is being used.

Many other crystals not readily identifiable may be seen in urine but can be ignored as their significance is uncertain.

Urinary calculi

The factors involved in the development of urinary calculi are not fully understood, but a knowledge of the composition of the stones is sometimes of value in treatment.

Phosphate stones. These are the commonest stones: they are found particularly in bitches and in certain breeds which have a tendency to develop them.

They may be large or small, rough or smooth, single or multiple. Usually the single stones are rough, two or more are smooth. They are not infrequently associated with an alkaline urine.

Test for phosphate. Scrape a little of the stone into a tube and add a drop of concentrated nitric acid, follow this with a drop of 10% ammonium molybdate and warm gently. A yellow precipitate indicates phosphate.

Cystine stones. There seems to be little connection between the amount of cystine in the urine and the development of cystine stones. These are usually small, round, and smooth, and yellowish in colour and cause obstruction of the urethra. Occasionally larger stones confined to the bladder are seen.

Test for cystine. Scrape a little of the stone into a test-tube, add a drop of 10% sodium cyanide and a drop of 20% ammonia solution. Allow to stand for 5 minutes and then add a very small crystal of sodium nitroprusside. The development of a magenta colour indicates the presence of cystine.

Urate stones. The Dalmatian has a high excretion of urates and has a tendency to develop stones of this type. Again they may be small or large, are usually smooth and are pale green or brown. The larger stones are frequently markedly laminated.

Tests for urate stones. A little of the stone is treated with concentrated nitric acid, warmed gently until the residue is dry and allowed to cool. A drop of 20% ammonia solution is added and if urates are present a purple colour develops.

Oxalate stones. These stones are readily distinguishable by their very crystalline structure and considerable hardness. They are perhaps the least common stone.

Test for oxalate stones. Crush a little of the stone into a tube, add a drop of concentrated sulphuric acid and a few grains of resorcinol. Allow to stand for up to 30 minutes when a greenish-blue colour develops if oxalates are present.

It is not infrequently found that calculi are not composed entirely of one substance. For example many cystine stones contain some phosphate and for this reason tests for all the common constituents should be carried out on each stone.

These compounds described are not the only ones which cause urinary calculi. If further tests are necessary the calculus may be sent away or other textbooks consulted for methods.

Faeces

The examination of faeces can be of value in the differential diagnosis of wasting diseases.

As with urine, it is important to examine the sample as fresh as possible.

EXAMINATION OF FAECES

Take note of the colour, consistency and smell, and look for blood or mucus and adult worms (Figs. 4.5 and 4.6). Drugs will affect the colour; iron treatment will cause very black faeces, much fat or the absence of bile will cause pale faeces. Fatty faeces are usually very bulky and often smell of rancid butter.

Physical Examination: Microscopic

Direct smear. Mix a small amount of faeces on a slide with a drop of Lugol's iodine, using the bacteriological loop. Carefully lower a coverslip over the suspension, avoiding air bubbles as far as possible. Examine under low power and look for:

Muscle fibres. The degree of digestion can be assessed by the structure. If digestion has failed, the muscle fibres stain brown and will be clear cut and the striations may be visible, and the nuclei well preserved. "Blurring" of the nuclei, striations and edges of the fibre indicate that some digestion is occurring (Figs. 4.7).

Starch granules. Stain vivid blue or black with iodine and this colour change can sometimes be seen with the naked eye (Fig. 4.8).

Fat globules. These are present in normal faeces and it is only safe to say that they are in excess in extreme cases (Fig. 4.8). If preferred, Sudan red can be used instead of iodine; this stains the globules red.

Worm eggs may be seen at this stage but if they are not, further concentration methods have to be used before saying that they are absent.

Chemical Tests

It is sometimes worth testing faeces for the presence of digestive enzymes and of these the easiest to measure is the protein digesting trypsin.

Mix well 1 g of faeces with 10 ml of a 1% solution of sodium carbonate, transfer one drop to a piece of X-ray film (either undeveloped or the dark portion of a developed film). Make sure that the drop is applied to the emulsion side of the film. Place in a small dish and cover with a piece of moistened filter paper or blotting paper. Do not allow this to touch the film. Incubate at 37°C for 30 minutes and then rinse gently in cold running water. If trypsin is present the emulsion will have been digested and washed away in the rinse, leaving a clear area. If none was present the emulsion will have remained intact though swollen due to the action of the fluid.

Trypsin is present in the normal dog to a dilution of at least 1 in 10 (frequently as high as 1 in 2000); values lower than this are strongly suggestive of reduced digestive function.

Microbiology

INTRODUCTION

It is sometimes possible to diagnose a specific condition by demonstrating the presence of the causal organism, whether bacterial, viral, protozoan, fungal or parasitic.

In practice, simple techniques can be usefully employed in showing the presence of significant bacteria or viruses. Examination can be either of the living or of the dead stained organism; this latter method is used particularly in bacteriology.

EXAMINATION OF MATERIAL FOR BACTERIA

The techniques used for the demonstration of bacteria are very similar, regardless of the material examined. It is particularly important to observe cleanliness in all techniques. Some of the organisms involved are transmissible to man and care must be taken to avoid this. It is important to examine all material as fresh as possible.

A wide-necked jar of 2% Lysol should be available for the disinfection of used slides and pipettes and a second bottle for disinfection of the bench in case of accidents.

Preparation of Material for Staining

Swab and loop. If the swab is very moist a direct smear is satisfactory; if the material does not spread well or the swab is rather dry a drop of sterile saline may help.

Dry the smear at room temperature and fix by passing through a flame two or three times. Fixing is complete when the slide, when held against the back of the hand, is just too hot for comfort. It should never be overheated. The smear is now ready for staining.

Fluids. In these the bacteria should be concentrated by centrifugation at 1500 rpm for 15 minutes. This applies to urine and pleural and ascitic fluids. After centrifugation the supernatant is discarded either by pouring or with a pipette; a few drops should be left. The sediment is resuspended in this fluid and a loopful transferred to a slide and a smear made. If tuberculosis is suspected some of the material should be saved in case animal inoculation experiments are necessary.

Methods of Staining

Some information of the type of organisms present can be gained by noting their shape and arrangement in the material and this can be done with a very simple single stain technique. Further identification can be made with a differential stain which depends on the chemical characteristics of the bacterial cytoplasm.

Certain bacteria, including the *Mycobacterium tuberculosis*, have a high concentration of waxy substances which makes them resistant to staining. However, they can be stained using heat and a strong stain, and the stain is then very difficult to wash out. This property is used in looking for these organisms which are called acid-fast organisms. The stains mentioned can be obtained ready prepared from a number of sources.

Methylene Blue

Reagent. One per cent methylene blue. This is the simplest stain to use.

Procedure. To save stain and fingers, with the wax pencil draw a circle round the smear, which holds the stain. Stain for 3 minutes and then wash with tap water. Shake excess water off the slide, wipe the back clean and blot the front with filter paper or fluffless blotting paper. This procedure requires care, since it is very easy to wipe the material off the slide. Alternatively, the slide may be stood on end to drain or warmed very gently over the Bunsen burner. Discard paper used for blotting. When the stain is dry it is ready to examine.

A development of this stain—polychrome methylene blue—is used for examining tissues for anthrax bacilli. Polychrome methylene blue is methylene blue made up in very dilute (1:10,000) caustic potash and allowed to "ripen", that is, to react with oxygen in the air for about 12 months. It is used primarily in large animal work, to demonstrate anthrax in the blood of cattle which have died suddenly. The bacteria stain dark blue but the disintegrated capsules stain a purplish colour. Anthrax does occasionally occur in the dog.

Differential Staining Technique

Gram's method. This method depends on the fact that certain bacteria which are treated with methyl violet and then iodine and finally with acetone or alcohol retain the dye, while others do not. Those that do retain it are called Gram-positive and those that do not are Gram-negative. The Gram-negative organisms are stained with a red stain so that they can be readily differentiated.

The technique requires considerable practice but will give useful results.

Reagents: (1) methyl violet—0·5%; filter before use,
(2) iodine solution (Lugol's iodine),
(3) acetone,
(4) 0·05% basic fuchsin.

Procedure. Stain in (1) for 20–30 seconds and pour off excess stain. Hold slide at an angle and wash off rest of stain with (2), allow iodine to act for 30–60 seconds. Wash off iodine with water and treat with acetone for 1 second. Wash with water. Stain with basic fuchsin (3) 2–4 minutes; wash with water and dry. The slide is now ready for examination.

The Gram-positive organisms stain deep blue-purple while the Gram-negative organisms are red.

Staining for "Acid-fast" Organisms

Ziehl–Neelsen method: Reagents: (1) strong carbol fuchsin,
(2) 3% hydrochloric acid in 95% ethanol,
(3) 1% methylene blue.

Procedure. Flood the slide with stain (1) and warm until steam rises and stain for 5 minutes warming occasionally. It is important that the stain does not evaporate and it may be necessary to "top up". Wash with tap water. Destain with alcohol (2) until only a faint pink colour remains (2–3 minutes). Wash with water. Counterstain with methylene blue (3) for 20 seconds. "Acid-fast" bacilli stain bright red, the background material and other bacteria are blue. This test is most usually done on faeces from cattle.

Examination of Smears

Examine as for blood films, using the low-power first, then the high-power and finally the oil immersion lens.

When a suitable field has been found turn the objective lens turret so that no lens is in the way and put a drop of oil over the field. Slide the oil immersion lens into position and rack the lens down very carefully into the oil using the fine adjustment focus. Watch this procedure, not through the microscope, but from the side. When the lens is in the oil, focus very carefully making sure that the lens does not press on to the slide. After putting the lens into position rack it up; if it is too low this prevents damaging the lens.

Examination of Material for the Presence of Virus

Sometimes in the course of virus disease, there develop within the cell accumulations of material called inclusion bodies.

They may occur in the cytoplasm (cytoplasmic) or within the nucleus (intranuclear) and they cause marked changes in the disposition of the cell or nuclear contents.

In virus hepatitis these inclusion bodies sometimes develop in the nuclei of some of the liver cells and in distemper in the cells of the bladder mucous membrane and elsewhere. Unfortunately, their absence does not rule out the possibility of either of these diseases and occasionally inclusion bodies have been seen in the bladder of dogs not known to be suffering from distemper. These bodies can unfortunately only be demonstrated in post-mortem material.

Reagent. Leishman's stain.

Procedure. For liver disease, a small portion of liver (1 cm^2) is cut out and dabbed on to a slide several times. This is called an impression smear. For distemper, the lining of the bladder is scraped with a not too sharp scalpel, the material is then transferred to a slide and mixed with a drop of saline and spread.

When dry, the smears are stained with Leishman's stain as for blood films. The nuclei of the cells in the liver are examined for the quite marked changes which accompany the inclusion body. Normally, the coloured material (chromatin) is fairly evenly spread throughout the nucleus, and the nucleolus is centrally placed, but with the development of the inclusion body this chromatin is concentrated round the outside of the nucleus and stains very intensely, and the nucleolus is pushed to the edge. This leaves the centre of the nucleus clear and within this clear area can be seen the inclusion body (Fig. 4.9).

In distemper, the development of the darkly staining inclusion body within the cytoplasm will push the nucleus to one side and may distort the cell wall.

Demonstration of Worm Ova and Coccidia

Concentration method. Reagent. Strong sugar solution (133 g sucrose in 100 ml water with 1 ml liquid phenol BP).

Procedure. Put 1–3 g of faeces in a screw-capped bottle containing a few glass beads and add about 30 ml of water. Shake well until the faeces are completely dispersed and then filter through some coarse muslin. This will hold back the larger debris but allow the eggs through. Centrifuge the fluid for 5 minutes at 1000 rev/min; discard the supernatant fluid. Replace with sugar solution and mix deposit and sugar solution well. Centrifuge again for 2 minutes at 1500 rev/min; this will bring the worm eggs to the surface.

Just touch the surface film with a flat-ended glass rod. (This will pick up a drop of fluid containing the ova) and transfer to a slide. Apply coverslip and examine under the low power for worm eggs and high power for coccidia. Note presence of eggs or coccidia and relative proportion of each type (Figs. 4.10 and 4.11).

Demonstration of Mites and Fungi in Material from Cases of Skin Disease

Direct examination. In some cases of demodectic mange, where there is a secondary bacterial infection, it is worth examining the pus without staining. The lesion is raised between finger and thumb and some of the pus transferred either directly or with a loop or pipette to a slide. A coverslip is applied and the material examined for the presence of long-bodied (demodex) mites.

If there is a particularly heavy infestation of round-bodied (sarcoptes) mites the direct examination may be of value. (As a general rule one of the concentration techniques should be used.)

Reagent. Ten per cent potassium hydroxide solution.

Procedure. Place the material on a slide with a drop or two of potassium hydroxide solution and mix well; apply coverslip. Warm gently (the material must not be boiled); this dissolves much of the debris and clears the remainder. Allow to cool and examine under the low-power lens. Look for the presence of round-bodied or long-bodied mites (Figs. 4.12 and 4.13), and the presence of ringworm (fungal) spores in the broken hairs.

Concentration techniques. These techniques are used for mange mites only.

Procedure. To the material in a centrifuge tube add about 10 ml of potassium hydroxide and heat in a boiling water bath for 5 minutes. Centrifuge for 2 minutes at 1000 rev/min and discard the supernatant fluid. Transfer some of the sediment to a slide, apply coverslip and examine under the low power.

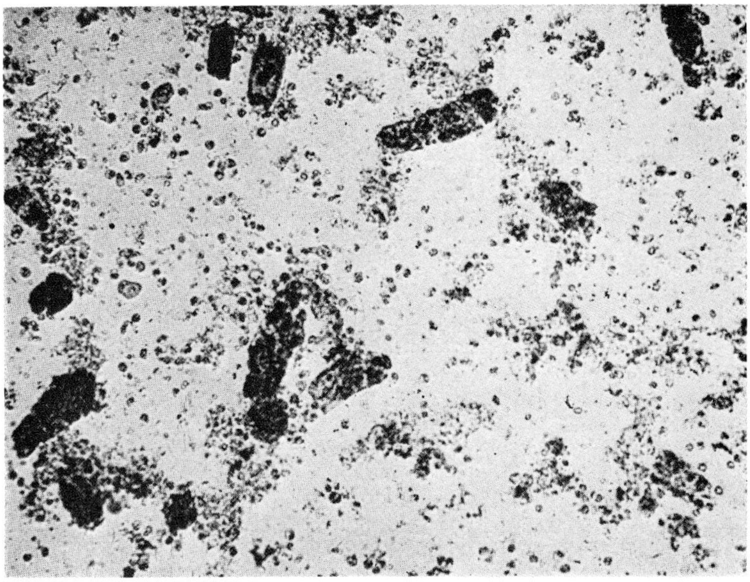

Fig. 4.4. Urinary sediment showing casts and cells, mostly polymorphs.

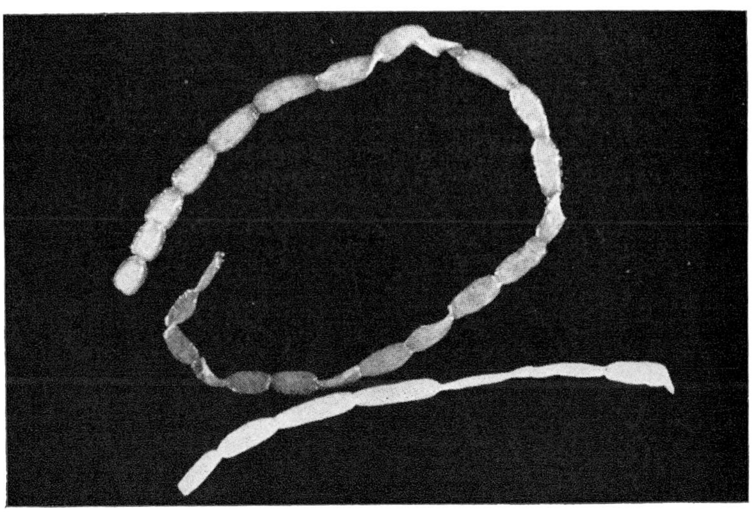

Fig. 4.5. Tapeworm.

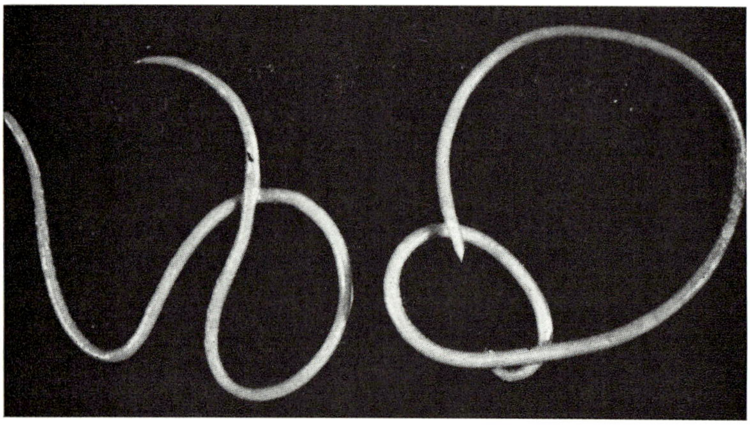

Fig. 4.6. Roundworm.

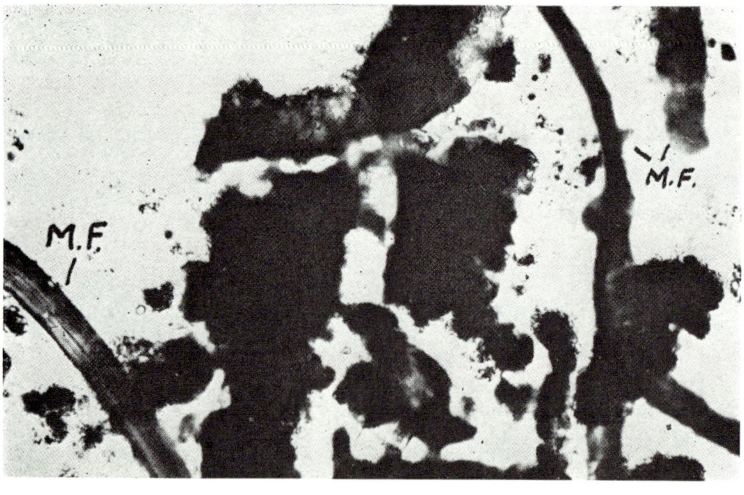

Fig. 4.7. Suspension of faeces with iodine showing muscle fibres (MF)—note striations in the fibre in the bottom left corner.

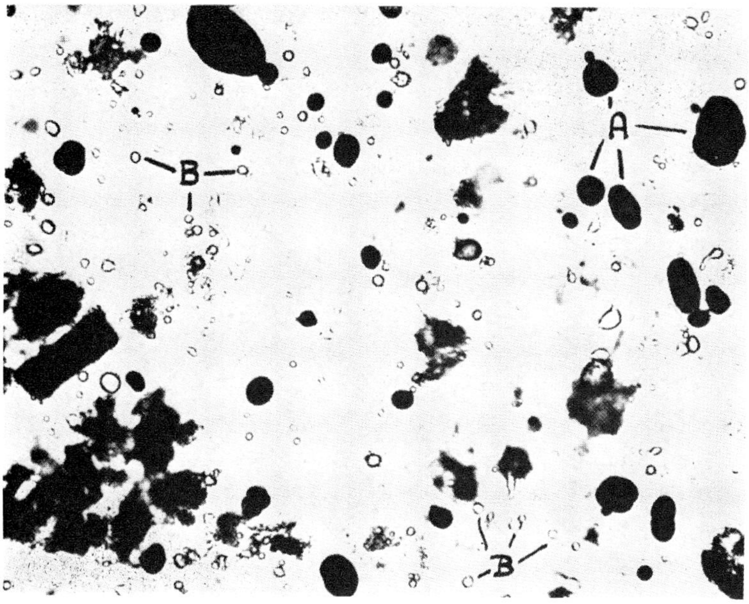

Fig. 4.8. Suspension of faeces with iodine showing black or dark blue starch grains (A) and clear fat droplets (B).

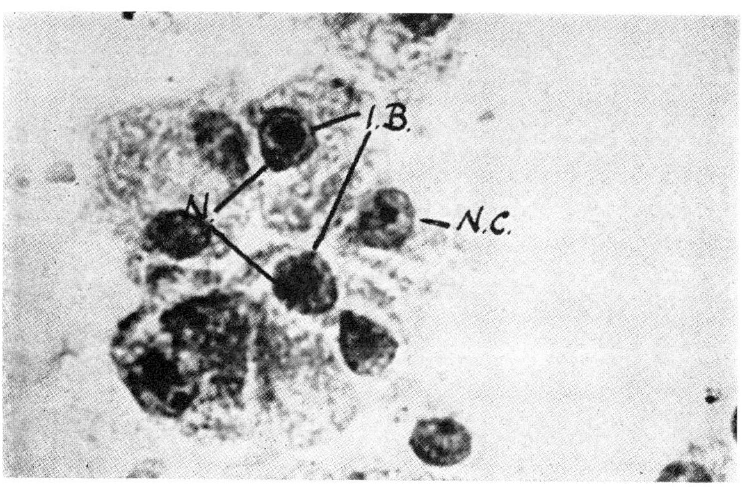

Fig. 4.9. Impression preparation of liver showing normal cell nucleus with central nucleolus (NC) and two nuclei with inclusion bodies (IB) and nucleolus displaced to edge of nucleus (N).

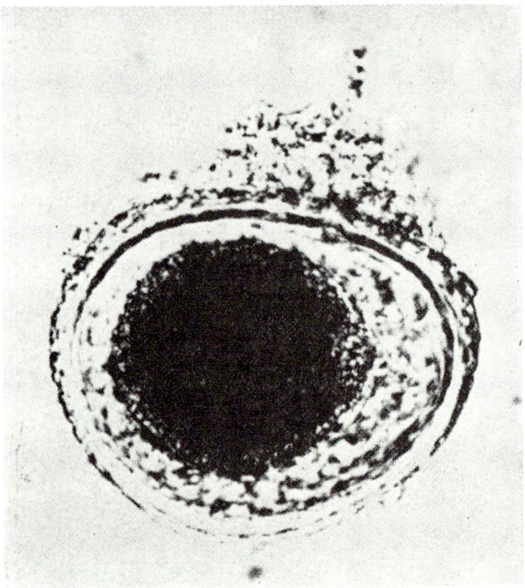

Fig. 4.10. Roundworm ovum.

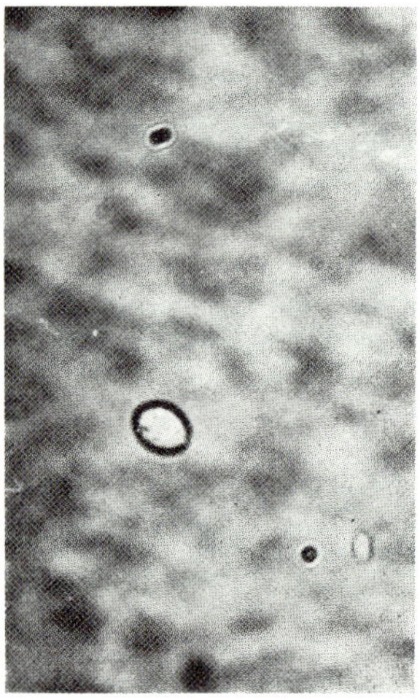

Fig. 4.11. Coccidial occyst.

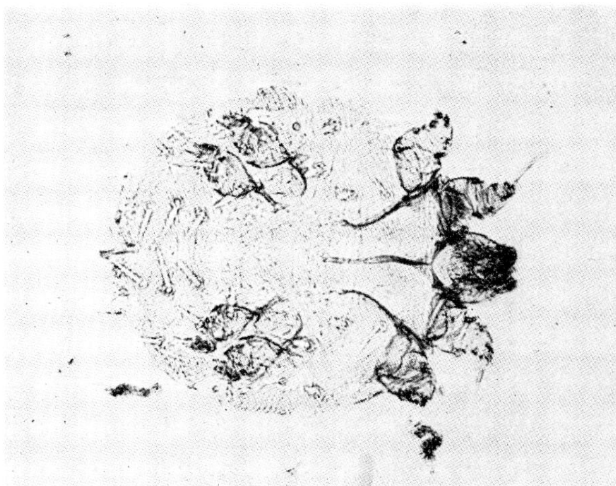

Fig. 4.12. Round-bodied mite.

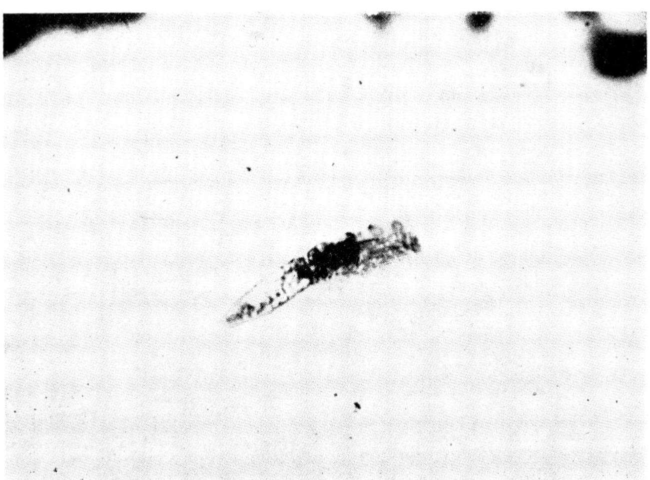

Fig. 4.13. Long-bodied mite.

Further concentration can be achieved by discarding only 5 ml of the supernatant and replacing this by the concentrated sugar solution used for demonstrating faecal parasites. Mix well and centrifuge again for 2 minutes at 1500 rev/min; transfer the surface film with a flat-ended glass rod to a slide and examine under a coverslip.

For ringworm-infected hairs. If a Wood's lamp is available for examining the hairs this is the most satisfactory method of demonstrating the presence of the ringworm fungus.

The lamp should be allowed to run for about 5 minutes to "warm up"; the hairs should be placed in a small metal dish. Some glass fluoresces in ultraviolet light and some is impervious to it, so the material should not be examined in the tube. A metal dish will give a very black background and any fluorescence will be easily seen.

Further Reading

BAKER, F. J., SILVERTON, R. G. and LUCKCOCK, E. D. (1966), *An Introduction to Medical Laboratory Technology*, 4th edition, Butterworths.

Colorimetric Chemical Analytical Method, 7th edition, The Tintometer, Ltd., Salisbury, 1970.

Laboratory Aids to Diagnosis, 2nd edition, British Veterinary Association, 1964.

MEDWAY, W., PRIER, J. and WILKINSON, J. (1969), *Textbook of Veterinary Clinical Pathology*, Williams & Wilkins, Baltimore.

SCHALM, O. W. (1965), *Veterinary Haematology*, Bailliere, Tindall & Cox.

CHAPTER 5

Theory and Practice of Nursing

(a) THE ETHICAL ASPECTS

D. G. EARNSHAW, MA, BSc, MRCVS

ETHICS may be defined as a set of rules which regulate one's conduct and behaviour in regard to professional duties. Generally one might say, in a practical sense, that ethics is superimposed on good manners and correct behaviour towards one's fellow creatures. Accordingly the animal nursing auxiliary will require some knowledge of the correct behaviour towards her employer and the other people with whom she may come into professional contact in the course of her daily work. Such people will include her colleagues of similar rank, clients and owners of animal patients who may require veterinary service, relatives of clients or other persons acting for clients, breeders of small animals, owners of kennels or catteries, pet-shop personnel, animal welfare workers, RSPCA inspectors, representatives of firms selling veterinary drugs, medicines, surgical equipment, appliances, etc., veterinary students attending the practice to gain experience, the police, or representatives of the Press, radio or television.

The outstanding personal virtues required by the RANA are discretion and a sense of responsibility, sympathy, tact, cool-headedness, cheerfulness, firmness, the ability to inspire confidence and to take a personal interest in patients and their owners. One must also possess some sense of reserve on occasion and weigh one's remarks carefully.

Most veterinary practices have some policy in regard to the large number of routine problems encountered daily. The RANA must get to know the practice policy and be able to follow it intelligently. These routine problems will to a large extent be concerned with inquiries from clients on such matters as surgery hours, vaccination, costs of veterinary services, location of kennels, catteries, etc., as well as actual "calls" or requests for specific veterinary attention.

The RANA will often be the recipient of information, much of which, if not actually confidential, should not form the subject of gossip outside the practice. She should endeavour to treat information obtained or overheard during consultations, etc., with reserve and discretion. Clients expect their confidences to be respected and the RANA must be extremely discreet in her responses to such confidences. A sympathetic yet tactful attitude is desirable. Some occasions will call for firmness but it should not be forgotten that the relationship which clients have with the veterinary surgeon is often rather delicate. Professional considerations aim at serving the public at large, if necessary, at the cost of one's own comfort.

In her attitude to other people working in the practice she should appreciate that there is usually some sort of protocol based on position, seniority, age, etc. Rarely, however, is this obvious, and people who work together for a period soon adjust themselves to the situation. If one is a newcomer, one is in the position of learning and should be willing to do so from senior and more experienced people at all times. If roles are reversed then one should be as helpful as possible to the newcomer.

The RANA may be asked embarrassing questions relating to her employer or the practice. These must be received impartially and the questioner referred to her employer for the answer.

Many questions will be too difficult or unanswerable as far as the RANA is concerned. If so, she can show her competence by finding out the answer or putting the questioner in the position of discovering the answer for him or herself.

One important aspect of the RANA's behaviour is that she should shoulder her responsibilities and even if she commits some heinous sin she must be open about it. It is often possible to reduce the consequences of a foolish or negligent action if the information is known in time. Therefore, the RANA should not be afraid of letting her employer or more senior colleague know of any mistakes as soon as possible when there is some chance to minimize their effects.

The legal liability of the RANA is that of a servant or employee. She will have certain rights in law in respect of her terms of service, wages, free-time, absence through illness, safe and suitable working place and conditions, etc. She also has certain responsibilities towards her employer; to safeguard and further his interest, to treat his property, etc., with care, to behave carefully towards clients, remembering that her employer will have some liability for whatever actions she may perform during the course of her employment. In the average practice where lay staff are employed, little or no obvious attention is paid to these legal considerations and everybody works together without restriction and with a spirit of cheerful comradeship.

(b) HYPODERMIC INJECTIONS

D. G. Earnshaw, MA, BSc, MRCVS

Where drugs, or nutrient fluids are to be given to an animal, other than by mouth or per rectum or via another natural orifice, and where it is desired that they should be absorbed into the system, they are administered parenterally. This implies that the drug, etc., must be dissolved in a liquid (usually sterile water) and injected beneath the skin into the subcutaneous space by means of a syringe and a hollow needle.

All injections made through the thickness of the skin may be referred to as hypodermic injections. Many of them will be subcutaneous, as described above, but some are made into muscle tissue (intramuscular) and some directly into veins (intravenous).

Less commonly injections are made into the peritoneal cavity (intraperitoneal), into the chest (intrathoracic), or into the heart (intracardiac). Intraspinal injections are also used for special purposes such as regional anaesthesia.

Some substances require to be given by a specific route, others may be given by any route. For example, atropine, given as pre-medication, may be given subcutaneously half an hour or so before its effect is required; if given intravenously, its effect occurs within a few minutes. Chlorpromazine often produces a local reaction if given subcutaneously, and it is, therefore, usual to give it by deep intramuscular injection or by intravenous injection. By the former route it takes about 45 minutes to act, whereas after intravenous injection its effect is evident within a few minutes. Sodium thiopentone (a short acting anaesthetic) is irritant to subcutaneous tissues and should always be given intravenously.

Nutrient fluids may be given intraperitoneally, intravenously, or subcutaneously.

Drugs are usually labelled in respect of the routes of administration, or, if they are not, this information is available on the leaflet enclosed in the package, or from the *British Veterinary Codex*.

The absorption of drugs into the circulation and the manifestation of their effect is quickest by the intravenous route, taking up to a minute or two in most cases, usually of the order of 20–30 minutes by the intramuscular route—and perhaps slightly longer, say 30–40 minutes, if injected subcutaneously.

The addition of hyaluronidase to large volumes of infusions given subcutaneously increases the rapidity of their dispersion and absorption.

THE TECHNIQUE OF MAKING AN INJECTION

Injections are usually prepared in sterile liquid form in rubber-capped vials containing a large volume of the preparation or in small glass ampoules containing a single dose. Less commonly used preparations are cartridges for use in dental-type syringes and hypodermic solvellae or tablets which are dissolved in a little water to make up the solution which is then sucked into the syringe. The hypodermic tablet may, alternatively, be crushed in the dry syringe, then a small volume of water aspirated to dissolve it.

To extract a quantity of liquid from the rubber-capped vial the procedure is as follows. Firstly, clean off the rubber cap by swabbing it over with alcohol and allow evaporation. Check the contents carefully and compute the dose you require. For example, if a vial holds 10 ml of a drug with a concentration of 5 mg/ml and you wish to administer a dose of 15 mg, the volume of the preparation to be withdrawn into the syringe would be 3 ml. Affix a needle of appropriate size on to the syringe, withdraw the plunger to the 3 ml mark and plunge the needle through the rubber cap, invert the vial, and inject 3 ml of air into the solution, immediately withdrawing the plunger again to the 3 ml mark. If there are great differences of pressure between the inside of the vial and the outside, the contents of the vial may bubble out or air may be sucked in. Care and practice will ensure that this procedure is carried out efficiently without waste.

The site of injection is selected, the patient restrained as necessary, and the needle quickly inserted. When the RANA is satisfied that the needle is correctly sited, the plunger is pressed home steadily, but not too quickly, so that the contents of the syringe are expelled into the tissues. It is good technique to hold up a fold of skin when inserting the needle and to press down on the skin on either side of the needle when it is being withdrawn. After an injection has been made, the site should be briskly massaged. Immediately after use, the needle and syringe are rinsed out with clean, cold, sterile, distilled water; they can then be resterilized.

Clipping and disinfecting of the site of needle entry is not normally necessary in small animals when giving ordinary subcutaneous or intramuscular injections. It is helpful to clip the hair and swab the skin over the site of intravenous injections with spirit or ether.

The main sites for subcutaneous injections are the sides and back of the neck, the wall of the chest behind the shoulder and elbow, and the inguinal region. Intramuscular injections can be made into the muscles, behind and in front of the femur (thigh), in the gluteal region on either side of the midline or into the muscles of the upper arm behind the line of the shoulder blade and humerus. The sites for intravenous injection are the radial veins in the forelimbs of dog and cat, the small saphenous veins in the hindlegs of the dog and the jugular and sublingual veins of both species.

Intraperitoneal injections are usually made in the midline, an inch or two behind the umbilicus. In this case a short fillet needle is used and the insertion through the skin and the abdominal wall made separately and in an oblique direction. Therefore, there is less danger of penetration of a viscus, and the hole through which the needle is inserted tends to be closed after its removal by the pressure above. It is, of course, preferable that the bladder and colon should be empty, though this is not always possible.

Syringes are made of plastic, glass, glass and metal, nylon, nylon and metal, or metal alone. The nozzle, on which the needle is mounted, is situated at one end of a graduated barrel, either centrally or at the side (eccentric). A plunger or piston fits into the barrel from the opposite end, and the plunger is usually prevented from falling out by a cap over the barrel.

Syringes are often designated according to the capacity of the barrel, viz. 1 ml, 2 ml, 5 ml, 10 ml, 20 ml. There are syringes of larger capacity, but they are not in common use.

Syringe nozzles may be of different types. The commonest at present in use in veterinary practice is the Record. In future, it is probably that Luer nozzles will come into wider use. Luer nozzles are now commonly used in practice.

Needles have a point, which may be of long or short fillet, a hollow shank, of which there are different bores, and a hub or mount which fits over the nozzle of the syringe. A needle should be mounted by a screwing motion and it will then remain firm.

It is preferable to use as small a bore needle as will allow the solution to flow through it, since small needles do less damage to the tissues and are less painful. Short needles are, of course, relatively stronger than long ones of the same bore.

Most veterinarians have their own preferences with regard to suitable size needles. Needles should be sharp and points can be touched up on an Arkansas stone.

Nowadays, many syringes can be sterilized in one piece, and plunged straight into boiling water; however, since there are still a number of less robust type, it is wise to find out what sort of syringes are in use in the practice in which you are employed.

Sterile, disposable syringes are now in common use and many practices use these exclusively. They are cheap to buy, require no sterilizing and aie in all respects convenient.

(c) CARE OF PATIENTS

Caroline J. Franklin, RANA

Introduction

For the most part, treatments to patients carried out by the RANA will be those ordered by the veterinary surgeon. For example, she will be specifically told what drugs to give, when and by what route to give them. By careful observation and a sympathetic approach, she will, however, learn to make the minor adjustments that speed recovery and may even save life. This is possible because she spends a great proportion of her time in the hospital, unlike the veterinary surgeon, who is normally obliged to visit it for relatively short periods each day. In order to know when certain measures must be taken, the RANA must first observe the patient and draw inferences from her observation; but before an assessment may be made of an abnormal animal, it is essential to be familiar with the normal state. For this reason, many trainees are strongly advised to work in boarding or breeding kennels before taking up ANA work.

APPEARANCE OF THE NORMAL DOG

In normal health, the dog is bright eyed and elert. He reacts to stimuli, such as the noise of a chain leash or the clatter of bowls when his meal is prepared. He sleeps lightly when he is not playing or being exercised. His coat lies in the position normal for his breed (e.g. if he is a Labrador the hairs point backwards) and the skin is supple enough to slip back into position if pinched into a fold. He has a keen appetite, produces a firm motion without undue effort at least every 24 hours, and urinates without discomfort. His temperature is between 38·3° and 38·7°C (100·9–101·7°F), and he pants only after exercise or if hot.

SOME POSSIBLE SIGNS OF ILL HEALTH

By contrast, a diseased dog may be dull eyed and unresponsive to stimuli. He may sleep much more than usual, or be abnormally restless; his coat takes on a "staring" appearance, and the skin loses its elasticity. The appetite may diminish, constipation, diarrhoea or tenesmus (non-productive straining) may occur, and urinary incontinence or retention may set in. The temperature may be above or below the normal range (raised or subnormal respectively) and heavy, shallow or panting respirations take the place of normal breathing.

Admission of Patients into the Hospital

Patients are not normally admitted into the hospital without the veterinary surgeon's sanction. If the veterinary surgeon is absent, however, and an emergency case—e.g. a road accident victim, or an animal having fits or collapsed with heat-stroke—is brought to the hospital, it would be reasonable for the RANA to admit it.

NAME OF HOSPITAL NAME OF VET. SURGEON

NAME OF OWNER:

ADDRESS:

TEL. No. (HOME & OFFICE):

NAME OF PATIENT:

BREED:

AGE OR DATE OF BIRTH:

SEX:

REASON FOR ADMISSION:

DATE(& TIME) OF ADMISSION:

ITEMS BROUGHT WITH PATIENT:

DATE	Urine	Motion	Appetite	Fluid intake	Temp.	Pulse	Respiration	Treatment

Fig. 5.1.

Should clients put pressure on the lay staff to take in patients for their own convenience, this should be resisted. Cases of mange, feline influenza and other infectious conditions can be unintentionally admitted to the hospital in this way.

It is important to obtain a detailed case history before the owner leaves. This may involve questions concerning the recent past, or the dog's whole life. For example, if the patient is admitted for abdominal surgery, the RANA should inquire if it has had normal bowel action and appetite recently; if the patient is about to whelp, she should ask if it has done so before, at what age, when it was mated, what its recent behaviour has been, and if any obstetrical complications have occurred in the past.

When admitting the pet of a new client, the RANA should obtain full details of the owner. This will obviate the need to make later inquiries which may well prove irksome. A client who receives a bill correctly addressed and who is asked for his office telephone number as well as his residential one, will be impressed by the efficiency of the practice. A suggested admission form which can also be used as a clinical record is shown here (Fig. 5.1).

The RANA should always ascertain that patients admitted for procedures involving general anaesthesia have been starved in accordance with instructions. In some cases, the veterinary surgeon may have asked the client to administer some premedicant drug, or withhold a drug that is normally given regularly, and this should also be checked.

Should the patient be highly nervous, the RANA may be required to administer a sedative and ask the client to wait until it takes effect.

Many clients require reassurance when leaving an animal for surgery, and a brief, simple explanation of what is to happen to their pet can do much to allay their fears. Questions such as: "He isn't likely to die, is he?" are best dealt with by a non-committal reply, for example: "There is always some risk involved in general anaesthesia, but the veterinary surgeon would not consider anaesthetizing your dog unless the benefits of the operation outweighed that risk. Naturally we shall take every care of him."

An indemnity form has to be signed by clients leaving animals in many veterinary hospitals, and the RANA should ensure that all signatures are legally valid. If necessary, juvenile pet-owners should be asked to obtain their parent's authority for veterinary procedures to be undertaken.

Clean kennels should be held in readiness so that admitted patients can be made comfortable on arrival.

Routine Care of In-patients

GROOMING

The in-patients should be groomed daily and just before discharge as a matter of routine, unless this is contra indicated by their condition. Discharges should be wiped from the eyes with cotton-wool dipped in boiled water or saline; the external ears can be gently cleaned with cotton-wool dipped in warm olive oil; and the anal area and urinary orifices should likewise be kept clean, clipping away soiled hair if necessary. Any ectoparasites, such as fleas, lice, ear mites, or skin lesions, should be reported to the veterinary surgeon in charge of the case, who will give instructions for treatment. The patient's bedding and toys should be carefully de-infested by immersion in disinfectant and application of an insecticide, or by burning if the owner allows. If the RANA is not familiar with the grooming techniques required for each breed of dog, she would do well to consult a book on the subject. The hospital should have a good basic grooming kit, and brushes, etc., should be disinfected if necessary after use. Autoclaving may be a useful means of sterilizing them, although some nylon brushes are warped by this process.

BEDDING

The following materials are used for bedding material for dogs in veterinary hospitals: barley-straw, wood-shavings, wood-wool, palliases, blankets, foam plastic, newspapers. Wood-wool and newspapers seem to have found most favour. Plastic foam is particularly suitable for paraplegic patients. Newspaper has the advantage of being cheap, easily available, hygienic, a good reflector of light, easily disposable, absorbent, a good insulator and providing a light background against which discharges, vomit, afterbirths and so on are easily observed. Blankets used for hospital kennels must fulfil certain requirements; they need to be warm, light, non-toxic, easily cleaned and cheap. Recently several veterinary surgeons have waxed enthusiastic over the use of nylon fur fabric for this purpose. Nylon fur fabric is warm, light, non-toxic, comfortable, easily cleaned and sterilized; it repels dog hairs, is virtually fireproof and is reasonably cheap. Contact dermatosis is not normally a serious hazard of nylon fabrics, especially if undyed. Animals appear to find it very comfortable. The fabric is obtainable at most departmental stores and costs about £2 per yard of 48-in. width. One yard of 48-in. fabric is sufficient to provide a mat for the average dog cage or fibreglass compartment.

Animals should always have their bedding changed as soon as possible after it is soiled, and care must be taken to ensure that it is clean, dry and free from infection. Bedding can carry organisms from a dog that may be resistant to them to another patient whose resistance has been lowered by disease. Substances such as blood, pus and hair on bedding material may cause infection or irritation of an operation site, if bedding is taken from one kennel to another, or if a patient is placed in a kennel that has not been cleaned since the last occupant. Dirty bedding material should be washed or disposed of as soon as possible, since excreta and discharges on it will serve as a breeding ground for bacteria, and may be a source of parasites, as well as attracting vermin.

Beds will require to be removed from a kennel or cage while an animal is recovering from anaesthesia, or if an unconscious patient is admitted.

Beds require to be cleaned between occupants with as much care as the kennels. Individual patients must be assessed in order to decide whether they will use their beds for sleeping in or merely chew them up. Fibreglass beds are probably the most durable and hygienic.

FEEDING

Routine daily feeding of in-patients is best carried out at the same time each day, the time in many hospitals being late morning. If possible, the RANA should find out from the owner what time an animal is accustomed to having his feed so that this time can be adjusted a few days before admission to the hospital. For example, a dog used to being fed at 10.0 p.m. might suffer a digestive disturbance if suddenly switched to a 10.0 a.m. regime.

Hygiene in the hospital kitchen is, of course, all-important. All rejected food should be discarded, and the contents of partially used cans placed in dishes and refrigerated. Feeding bowls are best boiled after each use, but, failing this, should be scrubbed with detergent, immersed in disinfectant solution for a time and finally rinsed. Disposable bowls, made either of aluminium foil, expanded polystyrene or papier maché, are currently finding favour in many establishments.

Special feeds may be required for certain patients at intervals during the day. For example, an animal which has had a panhysterectomy to correct toxic pyometra will require foods rich in glucose to counteract the toxaemia and foods rich in easily digested protein to aid the healing process. Glucose solution is usually supplied *ad lib* to such patients, and light, nourishing foods, such as Complan, Farex, and chicken broth of the type prepared for infant feeding, are offered three or four times a day. These feeds should be administered punctually, and the animal coaxed to eat if necessary.

Patients with respiratory conditions that impair their sense of smell, or with painful mouth lesions or persistent anorexia (loss of appetite) may need to be force-fed. This procedure requires a great deal of patience and understanding of the animal—a very reluctant patient may vomit voluntarily after force-feeding, thus undoing all the good work. Force-feeding should be done at intervals of 2 to 3 hours. Suitable foods are: beaten egg, protein hydrolysate, meat soup and lactols; water and glucose solution may also need to be given by this method. Equipment used may be an ordinary teaspoon, a specially modified spoon with a "hood" and spout, a long-necked bottle, an invalid feeding cup, or an old hypodermic syringe (without a needle attached). The liquid is introduced into the side of the mouth without forcing the teeth apart, the animal's chin is tilted upwards, and, if necessary, gentle pressure is applied to the larynx to encourage swallowing. Small quantities only are given at a time to prevent choking. At the end of the feeding session, the patient almost always has a certain amount of spilled food on its chest, and should be wiped clean. Force-feeding equipment requires thorough cleaning, a bottle-brush being ideal for the modified spoon and invalid feeding-cup.

THE COLLECTION OF SAMPLES FROM PATIENTS

Urine

If it is required for physical and chemical tests, which are usually carried out in the practice laboratory, urine may be collected in a clean, dry vessel, such as a kidney dish or an old cup, when the patient is exercised. The simplest technique is to carry the vessel behind one's back, lead the dog and wait until it has actually started to pass water before slipping the vessel under it to catch the stream of urine. Even the most suspicious animal has difficulty in witholding urine once the bladder has started to contract. When taking samples from male dogs, make sure that foreign material, e.g. bark from a tree against which they urinate, does not contaminate the samples. Should a client be asked to collect a sample, make sure he knows receptacles such as meat-paste jars or jam-jars are unsuitable—these could be a source of protein or sugar which would confuse laboratory findings. The urine should be examined as soon as possible, or it may be refrigerated, or a few crystals of thymol added to preserve it.

It is almost impossible to obtain a urine sample from a cat by the method described above. Cats that are in the habit of using a dirt tray, however, will often continue to use it even if the litter is removed. The urine can be withdrawn from the tray with an old syringe. Cats and small dogs can often be made to pass urine by applying gentle manual pressure to the bladder through the abdominal wall. Failing other methods, urine samples can be salvaged from the floor or ground, provided these are known to be chemically inert and free from contaminants.

In order to take a urine sample for bacteriological examination, it is essential to introduce a sterile catheter into the urinary bladder and collect the urine in a sterile container. This is because urine passing through the penis or vulva can easily pick up bacteria from the skin and hair. The bacteriologist needs to identify organisms present in the urinary tract, not those on the body surface.

Faeces

Faeces samples can be taken from the ground on which they are passed, if required for parasitological examination. It is important to be sure that they are fresh, and were passed by the right patient. Alternatively, a faeces sample may be obtained by the introduction of a finger, protected by a lubricated finger cot, into the rectum. As much material as possible should always be presented for examination; this is because tests may have to be repeated several times in the case of a negative diagnosis. The middle part of the motion should be taken, since this part is least likely to be contaminated.

To obtain a faeces sample for bacteriological examination, sterile swabs of cotton-wool on wooden sticks or metal wires are used. After cleaning the perineal area, the swab is inserted into the rectum with a gentle twisting action. One end of the stick or rod is inserted into a cork, so that the swab end can be placed in a test-tube, whose mouth is stoppered by the cork. Since there is a tendency for cotton-wool swabs to become dry (thus slowing down tests at the laboratory), the test-tube should be carefully stoppered and sealed to prevent loss of moisture from the sample. It is then labelled clearly to prevent accidental re-use, and dispatched quickly.

Vomit

If a patient is suspected of having eaten poison or a foreign body, any vomitus it produces should be kept for the veterinary surgeon to examine. Vomitus for dispatch to an outside laboratory should be collected in a clean stainless-steel or enamel kidney dish or gallipot, and placed in a stoppered container. No preservative is required, since vomit contains hydrochloric acid produced in the stomach.

Sputum

This can be obtained by inserting a sterile swab of the type previously described into the mouth.

EXERCISING

Whether the patients go into an exercise-run or are taken out individually on a lead, this provides an excellent opportunity for the RANA to observe them. She should note if they are keen to go outside, if their gait is normal or appears to be hampered, either by muscular weakness or by an abdominal operation wound. Orthopaedic patients can be checked to see if they are placing weight on the affected limb; ophthalmic patients to assess their reaction to daylight and obstacles. The patient should be observed while it passes urine and faeces, and the latter can be examined later for signs of intestinal worms. Even partially paralysed patients will benefit from being assisted outside for a few minutes in the fresh air.

The Care of Weakly and Paraplegic Patients

Very weak and debilitated patients require extra attention because they cannot do things for themselves; for example, they may be unable to move towards their water bowls or change their position in the kennel. An animal that is paralysed or one which takes 2 or 3 days to recover from anaesthesia will require turning every 2 hours or so. This is because fluid can collect in the lower lung of an animal lying on one side, causing hypostatic pneumonia. Similarly, an animal that cannot move away from the spot where it has passed a motion may get its coat soiled and will require constant changes of bedding. When cleaning the coat, a mild shampoo or antiseptic solution should be used, and then rinsed off thoroughly. The area should be patted dry with a towel, and baby talc applied liberally. A mild antiseptic cream such as Savlon may be used on the anus if this becomes sore. It is best to hold the feeding and drinking bowls for such patients, rather than placing them close to the animal and leaving them with him. Patients which are weak but not paralysed may need support when they are exercised, and should be fed a laxative diet if their condition does not contra-indicate this. They will probably need to be provided with blankets, although care must be taken to ensure they do not become entangled in these. In order to recover their strength, weakly patients will require a nutritious diet and plenty of sleep. Weakly cats may be unable to groom themselves adequately, and will benefit from having this done for them.

The Care of Premature Puppies and Kittens

Premature mammals are born with less hair than full-term ones, and as a result their skins require special care. A bedding material should be selected that will not cause irritation. The environmental temperature requires careful control, since dogs and cats, unlike some other species, have a non-functional temperature-regulation mechanism at birth. There is thus as much danger of burning very young puppies and kittens, by the use of hot-water bottles and infra-red lamps, as there is of chilling them by failing to provide sources of heat. Hot-water bottles should be filled with hot, not boiling water, and should be wrapped in a blanket or towel. The "ribbed" variety are more satisfactory than smooth ones. A thermometer in the pen is invaluable when infra-red equipment is in use.

Since the under-developed skin of premature animals absorbs nutrients more readily than that of full-term ones, some authorities advocate the rubbing of cod-liver oil onto the skin. Oral feeding, however, is more widely practised. The proprietary dog lactols and human milk substitutes are satisfactory sources of nourishment until the young are strong enough to suck from the dam. For giving the milk food, an eye-dropper, small hypodermic syringe, pen-filler, or premature-baby feeding bottle, are suitable. A small amount of the feed should be given to each animal at blood-temperature every 2 hours during the day and every 3 hours during the night. The abdomen should be firm to the touch after feeding, and the young animal should appear full when supported by the shoulders. It should be stimulated to defaecate and urinate by gently touching the genitals with a piece of cotton-wool. This substitutes for the vigorous licking by the dam. Gentle rubbing of the stomach will assist in preventing indigestion.

The Preparation and Administration of Enemata

An enema is a fluid preparation for injection through the anal sphincter into the rectum and lower colon. There are four main types of enema:

1. *The evacuant enema.* This is used to empty the rectum, for example prior to certain abdominal operations, to relieve constipation or to remove foreign bodies from the rectum.
2. *The enema which acts as a vehicle for drugs.* Some drugs are effective when given by the rectal route, and are then incorporated into an enema. An example is chloral hydrate.
3. *The enema as a diagnostic aid.* Barium sulphate enemata may be given prior to radiography. The shape of the rectum is thus shown, and abnormalities such as rectal diverticula may be clearly observed. A gas-producing enema may also be used before radiographs are made of the rectum. Gases show up as dark areas on the plate, thus providing a contrast between the rectum and adjacent tissues.
4. *The nutritive enema.* If nourishment cannot be given by mouth or by using a stomach tube, foodstuffs are sometimes given into the rectum, following the use of an evacuant enema. Enemata can also be used as a means of replacing fluids lost if the patient is dehydrated, for example normal saline might be given per rectum to replace chloride ions lost from the stomach after excessive vomiting. Nutrients are absorbed through the rectal wall to a certain extent, although

this method is generally a last resort. Suitable fluids are glucose-saline solution, Brand's essence of chicken or beef, and protein hydrolysate (Protogest, Ovigest).

The enemata commonly used in practice may be made up of mild soap and water (never use carbolic), made by adding soap until no more will dissolve, or glycerine and water in equal parts. Alternatively midwife's enemata, containing sodium salts in weak solution, are available in polythene disposable packs with a nozzle. These are very suitable for use in small animal practice. Enemata are given at blood temperature.

Several different types of equipment are used for the administration of enemata. A simple filter funnel with a length of soft rubber tubing attached may be used, the enema flowing down the tube by gravity when the funnel is filled and raised above the level of the patient. One type of enema syringe resembles a hypodermic syringe, but is much larger and has a blunt nozzle in place of the needle. It is usually made of stainless steel or glass. The disadvantages of this are that great force is required to press home the plunger, although finger-grips are provided to facilitate this, and there is some danger of puncturing the bowel if extreme caution is not exercised. The third alternative is Higginson's syringe. This is a length of soft rubber tubing into which a bulb is incorporated. At one end is a nozzle and at the other a valve and suction cup. Both ends of this apparatus are immersed in order to fill it, the suction-cap adhering to the base of the vessel containing the enema. Squeezing the bulb has the effect of expelling air from the tube, so the enema then enters it. During administration the valved end is held well above the patient while the bulb is again squeezed.

The patient should be prepared for the administration of an enema by applying Vaseline to the anal ring and clipping hair away from the area if necessary. The nozzle of the syringe or tube is likewise lubricated with Vaseline, and is then pushed through the sphincter. Rubber nozzles require to be held in place. The patient's hindquarters may be raised slightly to facilitate the flow of the enema. The operator is well advised to stand to one side of the patient rather than directly behind him so as to avoid being splashed by an unexpected expulsive effort by the patient. In order for the enema to have maximum effect, it is advisable to exercise the animal for a time before allowing him to evacuate the contents of the rectum.

Approximate quantities for administration are:

cats, Chihuahuas, etc.	$\frac{1}{4}$ pint (0·14 litres),
Spaniels, Terriers	up to 2 pints (1·14 litres),
very large breeds	up to 3 pints (1·70 litres).

An alternative to the evacuant enema which is rapidly becoming popular is the suppository. Paediatric suppositories, usually of glycerine, are commonly used, and suppositories containing local analgesic may provide relief from painful conditions of the rectum. The manufacturers' instructions should be carefully followed, as suppositories often have a protective wrapper which requires to be removed, and some suppositories need to be moistened before use.

Very young animals may sometimes be induced to defaecate by introducing a suitably lubricated and protected finger through the anal ring with a gentle twisting action. A thermometer may also be used for this purpose.

Great care should be exercised when giving enemata to cats, particularly if repeated administration is required. This species tends to become shocked when given enemata, and, moreover, those requiring evacuants are frequently constipated, and therefore dehydrated and debilitated, beforehand.

Temperature, Pulse and Respiration

The temperature of an animal and its pulse and respiration rates are affected by its metabolic rate. This is generally speaking higher in carnivores than in herbivores and, within a species, higher in smaller animals than in larger ones. Thus the metabolic rate of a puppy is higher than that of an adult and that of a Chihuahua higher than that of a Labrador. An increase in the metabolic rate of an individual animal may be caused by exercise or fever. It also occurs in heat-stroke, to which puppies are particularly susceptible; in this condition, the body heat regulation mechanism ceases to function, and the temperature rises rapidly. Excitement, resulting in adrenaline release, can also raise the metabolic rate.

THE THERMOMETER: TAKING THE TEMPERATURE

The clinical thermometer consists of a bulb containing a reservoir of mercury; an evacuated capillary tube, having a kink or constriction near its junction with the bulb; a thick glass jacket, enclosing the two former items which optically magnifies the capillary tube. Veterinary thermometers differ from those used for humans in that they have a short spherical, rather than an elongated, bulb. The principle on which the thermometer works is that mercury expands when warmed, thus travelling along the capillary tube. Its linear expansion is proportional to the change in temperature when it is warmed.

When taking the temperature of a patient, the thermometer is first shaken to cause the mercury in the tube to fall down to a point near the kink. The patient's rectum should be empty. The patient is restrained and the thermometer, which may be lubricated with Vaseline or mild soap, is introduced into the rectum with a gentle twisting action. Difficulty in introducing a thermometer into a cat's rectum may sometimes be encountered, because this species has an internal anal sphincter. Gentle pressure on the anus with the thermometer for a short time will usually be followed by relaxation of the muscle. It is then held, with about half its length in the rectum, for at least the time stated on the thermometer, but preferably for 3 minutes. It may then be removed, and the bulb wiped with a piece of cotton-wool (thermometers should never be rinsed under a hot tap, as this can cause the mercury to expand so much that it bursts the tube). The thermometer is then held horizontally and rotated until the magnified scale can be clearly seen, and the temperature can be read off. Because of the kink in the tube, the mercury does not contract and return to the reservoir bulb immediately on withdrawal of the thermometer. The RANA should however, avoid touching the bulb with her hand. Finally, the thermometer is placed in a jar of antiseptic solution, such as benzalkonium chloride.

Possible causes of a rise in temperature are mentioned above. A drop in temperature may be caused by impending parturition; toxaemia (the presence of toxins in the blood system); impending shock; and impending death, frequently associated with haemorrhagic or dehydrating conditions.

It is important to bear in mind that in many febrile (feverish) diseases, an alternating rise and fall in temperature may occur. Thus, if the patient's temperature is taken only once every 24 hours, a normal reading may be obtained. In order to get a true picture of the disease-pattern when fluctuations in temperature occur, the temperature should be checked every 4 hours.

TABLE 5.1

NORMAL TEMPERATURES

Dog	Cat
38·3–38·7°C	38·0–38·5°C
(100·9–101·7°F)	(100·4–101·6°F)

Guinea pig	39–40°C (102.2–104°F)
Rabbit	38.5–40°C (101.5–104.2°F)
Rat	37.5°C (99.9°F)
Hamster	36–38°C (98–101°F)

Like humans, some individual animals have a high or subnormal "normal" temperature, and this may have to be taken into account.

PULSE

The significance of taking the patient's pulse lies in the fact that the nature of the pulse reflects the state of the heart, and hence that of the blood-pressure. Sphygmomanometers, used for measuring blood-pressure, are rare in veterinary practice, and other apparatus used to measure blood-pressure quantitatively is complex, and requires the insertion of a fine catheter into the carotid artery. The pulse can be felt in any artery conveniently near the surface. The veins are not suitable, since pulsations in blood draining from the capillary bed are negligible. The pulse most usually felt is in the femoral artery where it crosses the medial aspect of the thigh, above the stifle. With a little practice, this can be done at the same time as the temperature is taken. Alternative sites for taking the pulse are the volar aspect of the carpus and under the root of the tail. The normal pulse rate range for a dog is 62–130 per minute, according to size, and for a cat 110–130 per minute. The dog has a characteristic rhythmic irregularity in its heartbeat which, if detected in the pulse, may be discounted. There is a variety of terms used to describe the character of the pulse: if the rate is elevated, the pulse is termed "frequent", the opposite condition being "infrequent". If an abnormally large volume of blood passes under the fingers with each pulsation, the pulse is "large", the opposite being a "small" pulse. If each pulsation takes a short time, the pulse is "quick", and if each pulsation takes a comparatively long time, it is "slow". The pulse may also be described as "hard" or "soft", "wiry", "intermittent", "strong", "weak", and "running down". Any apparent idiosyncrasies in the pulse should be reported to the veterinary surgeon, who may then check the findings and possibly carry out auscultation. In the moribund animal it is sometimes impossible to detect a pulse, but it is best to continue to attempt to save the animal's life until more conclusive evidence of death is available.

RESPIRATION

The respiration rate is best taken when the patient is either unaware of the RANA's presence (e.g. while dozing in its cage), or when it has been in her company for some while and is therefore completely relaxed. Animals placed on the examination-table or recently taken from their kennels are likely to be mildly excited, and their respiration rate will consequently alter. The respiration rate should not, of course, be taken while the animal is panting, since this is a form of accelerated respiration employed to regulate the body-temperature. A respiration is regarded as comprising inspiration and expiration (between which a short pause occurs), so that it is necessary to count either inspirations only or expirations only, but not both. The normal values for dogs range from 15–30 respirations per minute, and for cats from 20–30 respirations per minute. As well as being asked to check the respiration rates of hospital in-patients, the RANA may well be asked to measure that of an anaesthetized patient. If the respiration rate and the tidal volume (that volume of gas expired by the patient in a single expiration) are known, then the minute volume is the product of these two factors, i.e. the total volume of gas expired per minute. Hence, in "positive-feed" methods of inhalation anaesthesia, the correct flow-rate of gases can be selected. If an animal ceases to breathe, or is short of oxygen, the build up of carbon-dioxide in the tissues has the effect of stimulating a special respiratory centre located in the medulla oblongata, and nervous impulses are produced to recommence respiratory movements.

The following abnormal types of respiration occur:

(a) *Hypernoea*: the number of respirations per minute increases. This occurs if the animal is short of oxygen, or shocked.

(b) *Dyspnoea*: difficult breathing. This occurs when there is obstruction of the respiratory passages, for example by mucus or as a result of contraction of the bronchioles. Breathing is frequently stertorous, i.e. grating, and the abdomen moves more than normal in order to supplement the movement of the intercostal muscles and diaphragm. Dyspnoea occurring during anaesthesia may be an indication that the endotracheal tube is kinked, or has been inadvertently passed into one of the bronchii.

(c) *Deep respiration*: a greater volume of air than normal is inspired. This occurs when there is a need for extra oxygen, for example at high altitudes.

(d) *Shallow respiration*: a smaller volume of air than normal is inspired. This may be caused by extreme weakness, or because respiratory movements are inhibited by pain, as for example if ribs are fractured or in cases of pleurisy.

(e) *Cheyne–Stokes respiration*: a period of normal respiration is followed by one of apnoea, which is suddenly succeeded by a deep breath. The cycle then recommences. Cheyne–Stokes respiration may occur during anaesthesia and if the patient loses consciousness. Cheyne–Stokes respiration in a collapsed patient may be an indication of imminent respiratory failure.

(f) *Apnoea*: the cessation of breathing. This often occurs during the induction of thiopentone anaesthesia, and is not a cause for alarm. It can also occur if surplus oxygen is supplied during maintenance of anaesthesia. In other cases, however, the onset of apnoea is an indication for artificial respiration.

The Administration of Medicines

With present-day equipment, it is possible to administer drugs by many different routes. In some cases, the choice of route is made largely for its convenience. In others, various factors have to be considered:

1. The speed of effect of the drug: parenteral administration enables the drug to be rapidly absorbed.
2. Compatibility of the drug and the route: some drugs cannot be given by certain routes, for example thiopentone sodium given subcutaneously causes sloughing of the skin, and insulin is destroyed by the digestive juices if given orally.
3. Compatibility of the route and the disease: for example, it is inadvisable to give liquid medicine to a patient with a respiratory infection.
4. The patient's temperament: a fractious animal may defy attempts to administer drugs orally, topically or intravenously.
5. The convenience of clients and veterinary staff: it is impractical to present an animal four times daily at the veterinary hospital for injections if the drug may be given satisfactorily by the oral route at home.

Routes for the administration of drugs may be summarized as follows:

A. Systemic routes:

Intravenous
Intra-muscular
Subcutaneous
Intraperitoneal
Intracardiac
Intrathoracic
} parenteral, i.e. by injection.

Oral (inc. inhalations)
Rectal

B. External routes:

Application to	mouth and nose
	eyes
	ears
	mucous membranes
	skin

The main advantage of the oral route is that there is no penetration of mucosa or epithelium, and the risk of introducing infection is thus minimized. Moreover, most clients are able to give drugs orally, while only a minority are prepared to give them by injection. The disadvantages of the oral route are the dangers of choking and aspiration pneumonia already mentioned; the variability in the speed of absorption of the drug; the fact that some patients spit the drugs out, which means it is difficult to give accurately measured doses; and the fact that the method cannot be used for animals like hamsters, which retain foodstuffs in their cheek pouches. Drugs given orally include: fluids, semi-solids (electuaries), pills, tablets, capsules and powders.

The procedure for administering tablets, pills or capsules to a tractable dog is as follows: open the mouth gently, throw the tablet onto the back of the tongue, close the mouth, and, if necessary, restrain the head and stroke the larynx to induce swallowing (Figs. 5.2–5.5). If the dog is vicious, it is more practical to give the tablet in a tit-bit such as meat, butter or chocolate, or to grind it thoroughly and mix it with his meal. To administer a tablet to a cat, the head should be firmly grasped with the fingers spread apart, as a bowler grips a cricket ball. As the head is bent backwards, the mouth falls open, and the procedure is then the same as for a dog. If the cat resists such treatment, it may be necessary to hold the "scruff" rather than the head, and to have an assistant to hold the forelegs and prevent the cat moving backwards. A blunt object may be used to poke very gently the tablet over the back of the tongue into the throat.

The giving of fluids is slightly simpler. The required dose is first put into a bottle, spoon or hypodermic syringe. The operator stands beside the dog and administers the drug into the cheek pouch, simultaneously holding the head tipped back. There is no need to prise open the jaws. The head is then restrained until swallowing occurs (Figs. 5.6–5.8) and again the larynx may be stroked if necessary. When giving fluids to the cat, the jaws require to be opened, as this species does not have such generous jowls as the dog. It is generally found that the use of a syringe, which can be inserted between the carnassial teeth, greatly facilitates this procedure.

Powders may be given in the form of an electuary (usually made up with honey or treacle) or mixed with water, or they may be merely tipped on to the tongue.

Local Applications

Drugs and other agents, such as heat or cold, may be applied to specific areas of the body in order to remedy localized conditions.

HOT APPLICATIONS

These are applied in order to dilate the blood vessels of the area, which has the effect of increasing the number of white blood cells, thus speeding the healing process. Oedema (swelling), such as occurs in sprains and strains, may also be reduced as fluid is carried away from the area by the dilated vessels.

Poultices are one of the most effective means of applying heat. Kaolin is the commonest material in use, but bread, bran or mustard, or any similar substance which retains heat, may be used. The kaolin is usually heated in the tin in which it is supplied, with the lid removed. It may be placed in a saucepan of boiling water or in the boiling sterilizer. It is then spread on a piece of gauze or gamgee tissue, which is covered with another piece of gauze to prevent kaolin adhering to the animal. If the kaolin can be borne on the back of the hand, the patient will tolerate it, and the poultice may now be applied. A thick, insulating layer of cotton-wool is placed on top of the poultice, and the whole is bandaged in position. This procedure needs to be repeated about four times daily.

Fomentations of hot liquids are frequently used to bathe developing abscesses; water and saline are the liquids of choice. Epsom salts may be used to harden the area of a wound where protection is impractical; for example, when a shallow cut on the pad occurs. Fomentations should be applied with swabs of cotton-wool, at as high a temperature as the patient will tolerate; they are best carried out at least three times a day.

Rubefacients are drugs which, when massaged vigorously into an area, cause inflammation which speeds the resolution of sprains and strains. The heat generated at the time of their application is a source of comfort to the patient. Embrocations of the type used by athletes come into this category; soap liniments are widely used in veterinary practice, being particularly favoured in equine work.

COLD APPLICATIONS

These cause vasoconstriction, thus reducing haemorrhage and swelling caused by loss of fluids from dilated blood vessels (extravasation). Intense cold has a local analgesic effect. Cold applications are also used to lower the body temperature in cases of heat-stroke. Refrigerated water and saline may be used for cold compresses, and swabs dipped in these solutions may be bandaged over cuts to reduce haemorrhage until the veterinary surgeon can attend. For heat-stroke cases, crushed ice is wrapped in a cloth which is placed collar-wise around the neck, and ice may be placed in the orifices and round the feet. Volatile substances, such as ethylchloride, may be sprayed on to the skin. In evaporating, they absorb heat from the body surface, thus causing a temporary local analgesia. The disadvantage of this method is that a risk of frost-bite exists. Similarly, carbon dioxide "snow" or liquid nitrogen are sometimes used as topical local analgesics.

ELECTRICAL APPLICATIONS

Ultraviolet lamps are beneficial in that the radiation produced stimulates conversion of ergostearol in the skin to vitamin D and so they are sometimes used in cases of rickets. It is important to protect the patient's eyes when using them.

Infra-red radiation helps to relieve rheumatism and fibrositis. Care should be taken to ensure that the patient is not too close to the lamp, and is turned at intervals to prevent uneven heating of the area.

Diathermy may also be employed to relieve fibrositis and rheumatism. Heat rays are produced by high-frequency electricity. The operation of the diathermy machine requires considerable skill, since minute adjustments require to be made according to the patient's response.

Low-voltage electric currents are sometimes applied to the paralysed limbs of animals suffering from paraplegia. The source of electricity is held a short distance away from the end of the limb, and the current switched on for brief periods. This stimulates the muscles to contract in the same way as a nervous impulse would, and so helps prevent disuse atrophy—a wasting away of muscular tissue. In the event of the patient recovering use of his nervous tissue, the limbs are in a much better state than they would otherwise be.

Bandaging

Bandaging materials used in small animal work include: white cotton open wove, white crepe, tubular stockinette (Tubegauze), elastic adhesive, non-elastic adhesive. The white-open-wove type of bandage is also available impregnated with plaster-of-paris for the support of fractured limbs. Choice of bandaging material is governed by the purpose for which the bandage is being applied. The commonest shape of bandage is the "roller", a ribbon-shaped strip wound into a cylinder. This is available in widths of $\frac{1}{2}$ in. 1 in., 2 in., 3 in. and 4 in. for small animal work. Alternatively, the tubular bandage may be used, particularly on the extremities or head. The triangular bandage, used extensively in human first aid, is practically unheard of in veterinary work, although the "many-tailed" bandage is ideal for use on the abdomen and chest.

The functions of bandages are as follows:

1. To provide support for the tissues, for example support of the abdominal musculature (herniation). Oedematous tissues also require support, and a tight bandage is sometimes used in an attempt to reduce oedema.
2. To support fractured or dislocated bones until long-term therapy is carried out.
3. To retain dressings, for example poultices and impregnated tulle, in position.
4. To prevent self-mutilation of wounds, or lesions such as eczema; foot bandages may be applied to prevent the ears being damaged by the claws.
5. To arrest haemorrhage: the effect in this case is twofold; the rough surface of the

dressing, usually gauze, and the pressure exerted on the tissues both encourage clotting.

6. To correct deformity. This application is used most in developing animals, where a support bandage will sometimes prevent a bone from growing crooked.

GENERAL RULES TO OBSERVE IN THE APPLICATION OF BANDAGES:

1. Ensure that the bandage is tightly and evenly rolled before application; a loosely wound bandage is most unsatisfactory in use. If the bandage is accidentally dropped during application, it should be carefully rewound.

2. Unroll a short length at a time; as far as possible, keep the roll of bandage almost in contact with the patient.

3. Hold the roll of bandage in such a way that the "outside" surface of the roll lies against the body of the patient. This makes for better control. It is permissible, however, to twist the bandage when dressing awkward sites, in order to obtain greater purchase, particularly if a non-elastic material is being used.

4. Each revolution of the bandage should overlap the preceding one by two-thirds. This prevents unsightly edges from showing and helps to ensure even pressure distribution.

5. Avoid applying bandages so tightly that the circulation is impaired. When bandages are applied to the lower limb, it is advisable to include the foot, as it may otherwise swell.

6. The bandage should be secured by tying and/or with adhesive tape. Safety pins, which may be removed by the patient and swallowed, are not suitable.

Bandaging Techniques

The simple spiral

This is suitable for the lower limbs and the tail. The bandage is applied obliquely round the circumference of the appendage, and is thus more secure than if merely wound horizontally.

The figure-of-eight

The bandage is passed obliquely round the limb, alternately upwards and downwards. This is particularly useful for the elbow and hock joints, and could also be used for bandaging the top of the head, using the ears to anchor the dressing.

The spica

A series of parallel turns are made in one direction around the area to be bandaged, and then another series around another adjacent structure, to provide stability. This technique is used for bandaging the shoulder, several turns being placed first round the elbow.

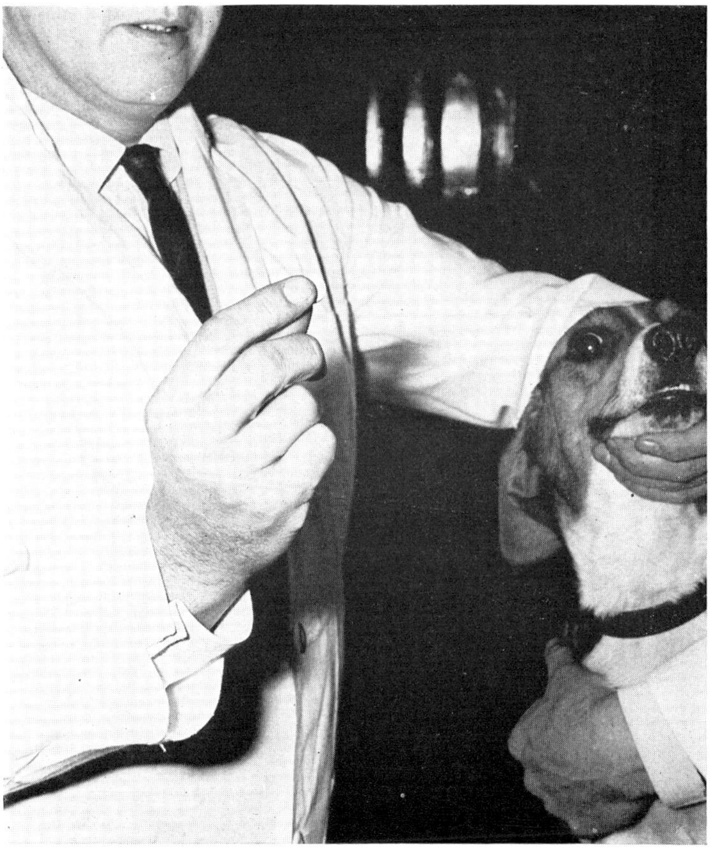

Fig. 5.2. Dosing dog with tablet. (Photographs by courtesy of Burroughs Wellcome & Co.)

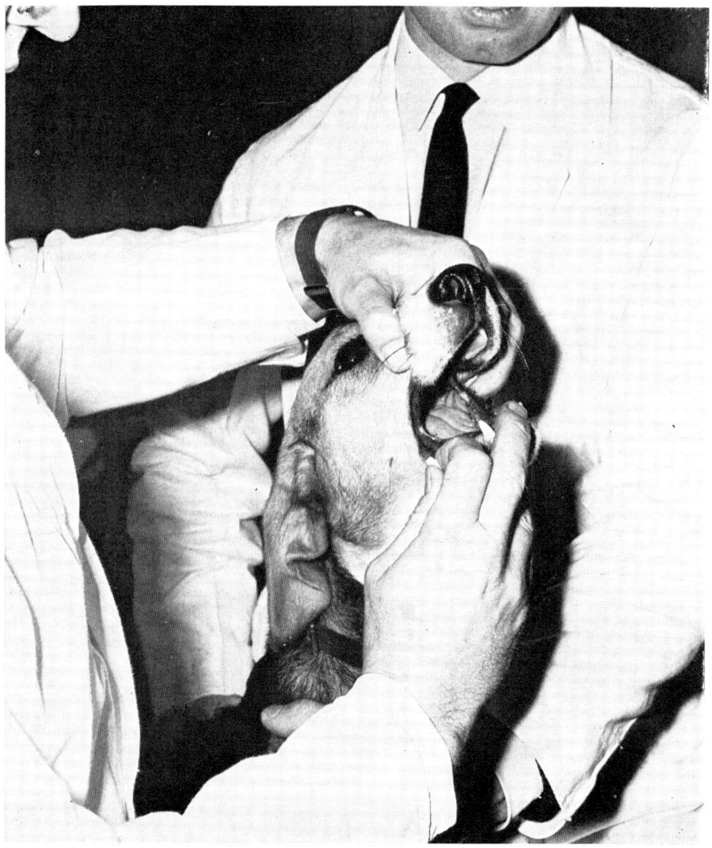

Fig. 5.3. Dosing dog with tablet. (Photograph by courtesy of Burroughs Wellcome & Co.)

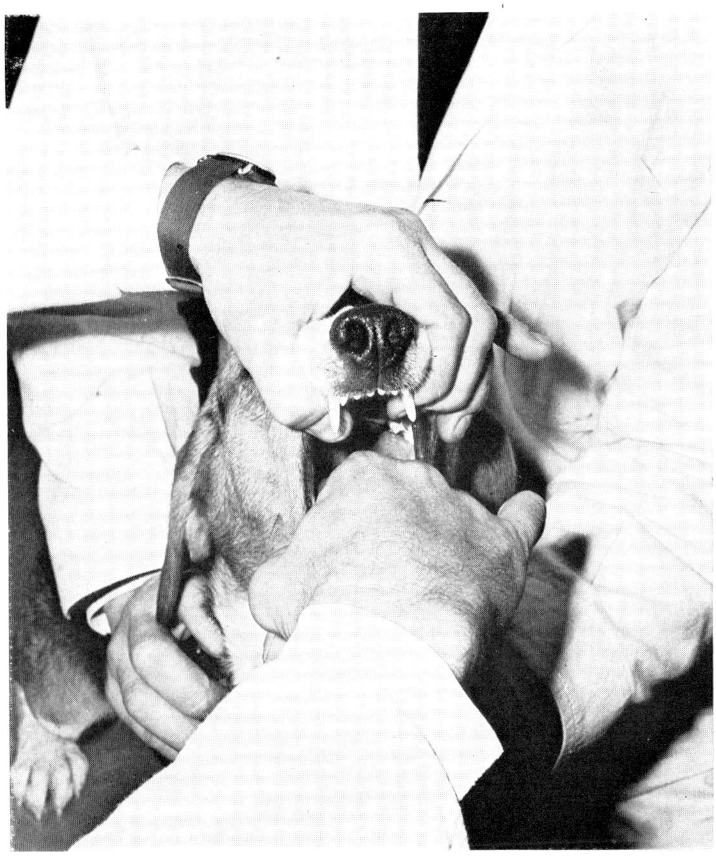

Fig. 5.4. Dosing dog with tablet. (Photograph by courtesy of Burroughs Wellcome & Co.)

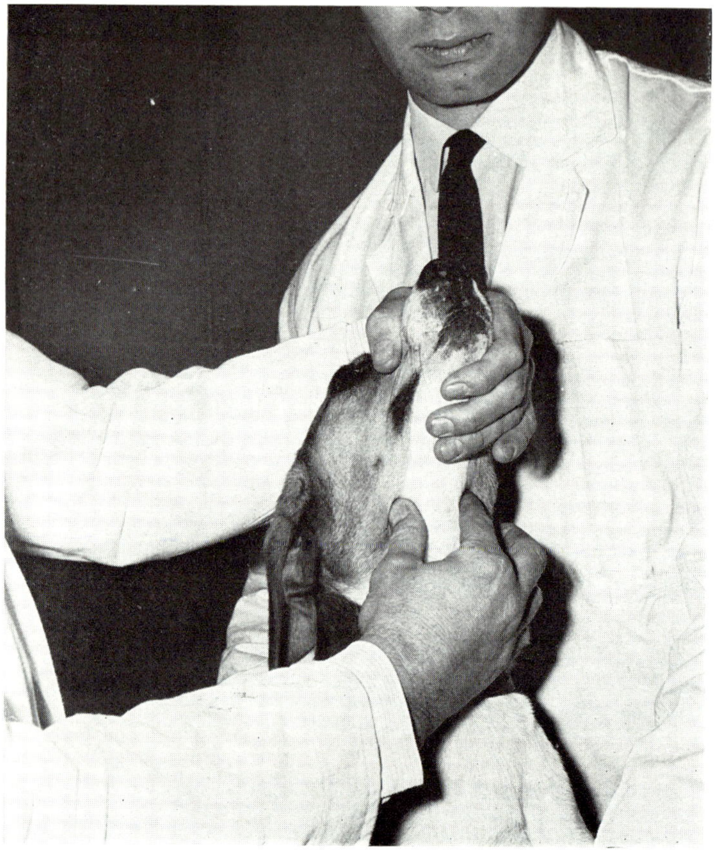

Fig. 5.5. Dosing dog with tablet. (Photograph by courtesy of Burroughs Wellcome & Co.)

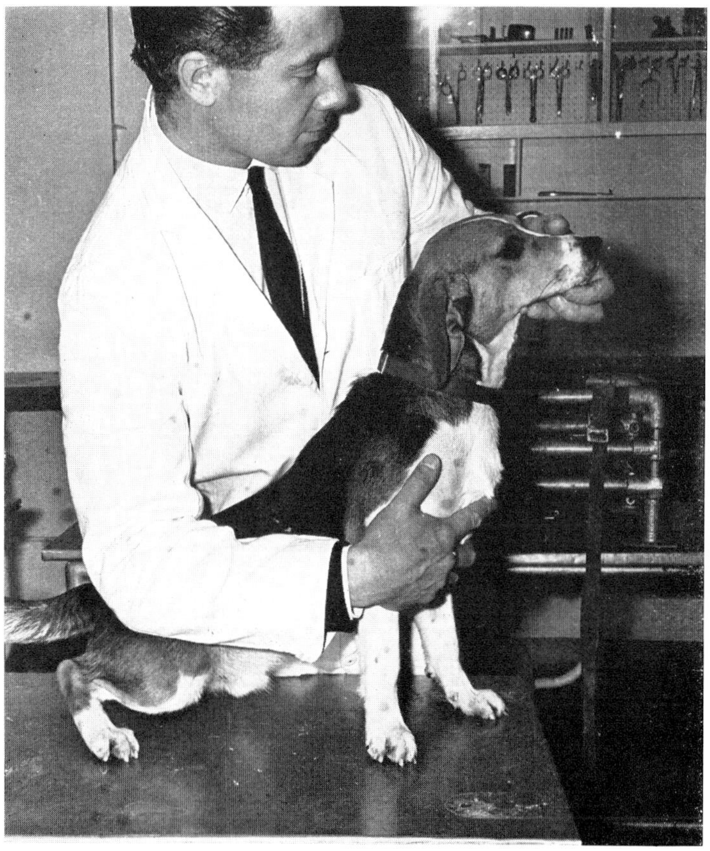

Fig. 5.6. Dosing dog with fluid. (Photograph by courtesy of Burroughs Wellcome & Co.)

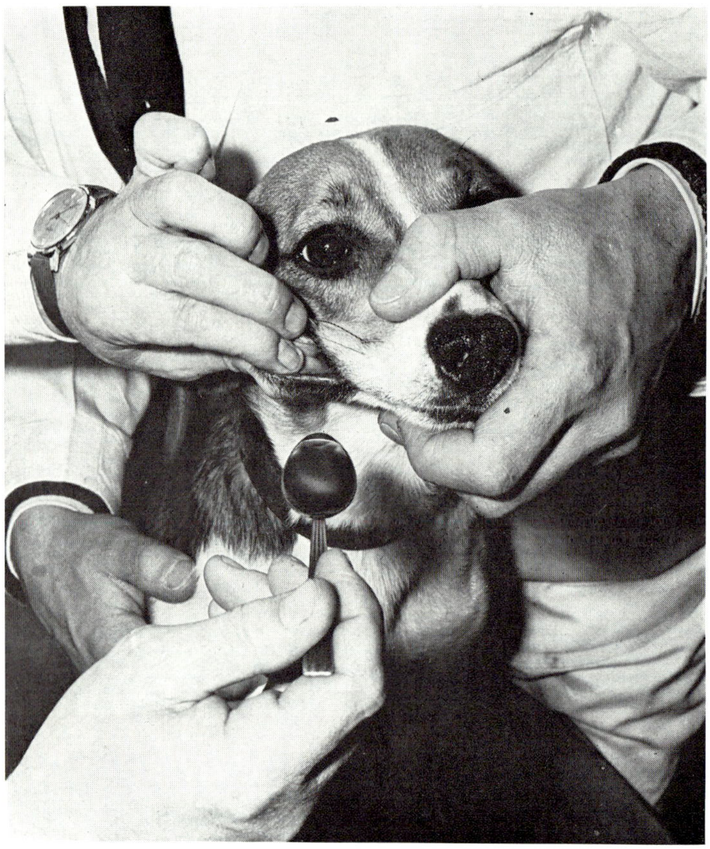

Fig. 5.7. Dosing dog with fluid. (Photograph by courtesy of Burroughs Wellcome & Co.)

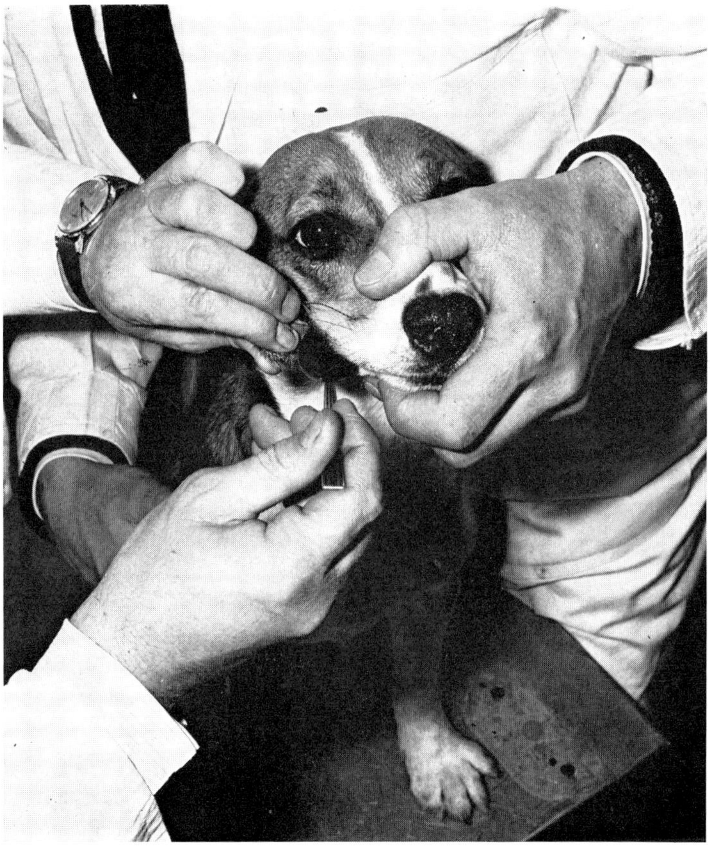

Fig. 5.8. Dosing dog with fluid. (Photograph by courtesy of Burroughs Wellcome & Co.)

The recurrent bandage

This is used for the paws, the tail and the pinna of the ear (prior to bandaging it flat against the head). A length of bandage is laid along the long axis of the appendage, over the end of it and up the other side. This procedure is repeated until the end of the structure is well covered (the claws may poke through a foot bandage if insufficient turns are made). The bandage is then twisted, and a single spiral used to secure the first layers. When bandaging the feet, it is important to place small pieces of cotton-wool between the digits and under the dew claw, to prevent pressure necrosis and absorb sweat and exudate. When bandaging the tail, two series of spirals should be made, in opposing directions, and some hair should be enclosed in the bandage to help keep it in position.

The many-tailed bandage

This is of cotton, crepe or flannel and is rectangular in shape, with parallel strips cut along the two short sides. Four holes are made in it to accommodate the legs. The strips should be rolled in the same way as a roller bandage. The many-tailed bandage may be applied with the ties along the back for protection of a ventral wound or with one tie under the belly for the protection of a dorsal one. In the latter case, since the leg-holes cannot be used one pair of ties should be knotted in front of the chest.

The tubular bandage

This is made of relatively fine material and therefore does not provide a great deal of support to the tissues, nor is it very suitable for use as a pressure bandage. Applicators are usually supplied with lengths of tubular bandage. A generous quantity of the latter is pulled on to the cylindrical applicator and cut off the roll. The applicator is passed over the area to be dressed (foot, tail or head), a short length of stockinette pulled off the applicator on to the animal, and the applicator is twisted. This has the effect of causing the bandage to grip the tissues lightly. The applicator is next passed down to the end of the appendage, rotated again and the whole procedure repeated. If it is required to create pressure, the applicator may be rotated continually during application of the dressing. A length of adhesive plaster is used to hold the bandage in place.

The RANA: Personal Appearance and Hygiene

It is of great importance that a RANA (or indeed anyone working with sick animals) should achieve, and maintain, a very high standard both of personal appearance and cleanliness.

On the standards which she sets herself will depend:

1. The health of her patients.
2. Her own health and that of the people amongst whom she works.

3. The prestige that she achieves in the eye of the public.

A tidy appearance and good grooming will improve the RANA's working efficiency and help to keep up her own morale as well as that of the practice in which she is employed.

Hair should be worn short or at least contained by either a cap or a head-band. Long finger-nails have no place in a veterinary practice if for no other reason than it is not possible to "scrub up" properly unless nails are well trimmed. Equally, long nails will break when handling animals, and can perforate sterile rubber gloves when these are worn.

Jewellery should not be worn whilst on duty. Footwear should be sensible, preferably washable, and should be standardized to some degree throughout the nursing team. Rubber boots can be worn for outside work and a separate pair may be kept for operating-theatre duty. Boots should be washed and disinfected after each session. Wooden "exercise sandals" have been recommended by medical operating teams for use in the theatre, but the rubber soles should be kept in good repair.

Ideally uniforms should be worn, and those suggested by the BSAVA have many advantages. Gradually the public is becoming used to the ANA trainees' and RANAs' uniform, and the more observant amongst them can now recognize the qualified RANAs' and the first- and second-year trainees' uniform. Aprons particularly should be clean, and a plentiful supply should be available to change into when working in the consulting room; there is nothing worse than the effect of a soiled apron on an otherwise efficient and tidy-looking RANA.

In the hospital, a RANA's hands constitute one of the potential disease vectors. The hands should be cleansed in an efficient disinfectant between treatments and this is especially important when dressings are being carried out.

It is advisable for a RANA to change clothes before leaving the premises in which she works. If items of clothing become "infected", they can safely be soaked in a weak solution of cetrimide or benzalkonium chloride, although the latter will dissolve nylon if used in concentrated form. A good deodorant disinfectant is required to remove the smell of undoctored male cats' urine from the clothes.

Further Reading

Canine Surgery (1st Archibald edition).
The Merck Veterinary Manual.
Handbook on the Handling of Animals and First Aid.
Veterinary Applied Pharmacology and Therapeutics.

(d) MEDICAL NURSING

JOAN O. JOSHUA, FRCVS

Introduction

The duties and responsibilities of the animal nursing auxiliary in medical nursing will be almost entirely concerned with in-patients, i.e. those animals admitted to veterinary hospital kennels for a variable length of time; only very occasionally will she be required to nurse out-patients and in such rare circumstances she will be acting under very specific instructions.

Anyone who enters upon the ANA training will be a person deeply interested in animals—the writer abhors the term animal-lover—and it is therefore almost superfluous to say that nursing implies caring for the well-being of the patient in *all* respects, not merely the physical aspects. In order to do this some understanding of the problems posed by animal hospitalization is essential and again this is not solely related to disease problems, but must include a knowledge of the reaction both of different species to hospital routine and of special categories within a particular species. Since animal in-patients largely comprise dogs and cats this section will be written with these in mind; unusual problems presented by the occasional exotic or other small animal pet admitted to hospital must be dealt with on an *ad hoc* basis.

Dogs as In-patients

The vast majority of dogs settle down remarkably well and quickly to hospital life. As a rule there is so much activity throughout the day in kennels that the dog has more to interest it—provided it is not too ill—than it usually has at home. At the same time a small proportion of dogs *do* fret and the nurse must learn to recognize these and report them to the veterinary surgeon who must then decide whether such an individual is better discharged sooner than was intended. The different types of temperament and consequently differing reaction to hospitalization must be recognized and so far as possible catered for. The extrovert friendly dog to whom every human being is a friend is no problem at all. The one-man or one-family dog (of which the Chow Chow is the prime example) poses considerable problems. Any dog with well-developed guarding instincts, especially trained guard dogs, may become possessive over their own bit of territory, i.e. their kennel or cage, and become aggressive when approached in the cage no matter how friendly outside.

The submissive breeds—Alsatians and working Collies are good examples (although the Alsatian may mix this with intense territorial guarding!)—normally respond well to firmness of approach and handling. It is the introspective individual which can be met in any breed which is possibly the most difficult to manage; it lies huddled miserably in a corner of its cage not responding to any outside stimulus at all; such patients demand a high degree of sympathetic skill from the nursing staff if they are to adapt satisfactorily as in-patients.

The very young dog, especially infants of 4 to 10 weeks of age, presents several problems quite apart from marked susceptibility to infectious disease. Not only do they require frequent small meals of specially prepared food but it is extremely difficult to cater for the alternating play and sleep periods characteristic of this age group. Young pups are extremely resilient and if responding to treatment they very quickly want to revert to a normal way of puppyhood. The screaming, yelling puppy is extremely irritating—it is also intensely bored and even 2 minutes' play with a nurse is very valuable; they also require long periods of undisturbed sleep, which is most difficult during the busy routine of kennels.

At the other end of the scale the old dog has special problems and in judging age the average longevity of different breeds must be borne in mind. The Boxer or Bulldog of 8 years must usually be regarded as an old dog, whereas for a Cairn Terrier or Yorkie it may well be the prime of life. The very old dog is like a very old person and is completely adapted to his home environment; change his environment and he can become seriously disorientated with slow mental reactions to ordinary stimuli and often very rapid physical deterioration too.

The dog with impaired kidney function can be a serious risk if hospitalized and even comparatively young dogs *can* have damaged kidneys. Many dogs with renal disease have achieved a remarkable degree of balance on their home regime but the change to kennel routine may precipitate a rapid and serious deterioration in their condition which may be totally unrelated to the reason which has made them in-patients. Owing to controlled, brief and usually infrequent exercise periods the normal pattern of urination for an individual, especially if a male, is drastically changed; water intake is usually changed as well and either of these factors can alter a chronic nephritic from a state of balance to one of profound uraemia which is rapidly fatal; when both factors are changed, as is usually the case, the risk is very great indeed. Many nephritic dogs die in kennels quite unexpectedly but an understanding of the situation should at least make it an anticipated hazard. The veterinary surgeon will always advise the RANA of known nephritics but the prudent RANA may well inquire when an old dog is admitted for the first time if anything is known about its renal function.

Cats as In-patients

Cats adapt less well to kennel routine than dogs. They are usually more introvert by nature and less inclined to be interested in the daily routine. Even if appetite is not impaired by the condition causing their admission, many cats refuse all food and drink for several days. They are less ready to respond to the cajoling of attendants. They have a very strong sense of territory which will be referred to again later. They are particularly fastidious in excretory habits and may be even more difficult than house-trained dogs to adapt to hospital conditions.

Other Pets

Occasionally it becomes necessary to admit other species to hospital, the management of some of which may not be well known to veterinary surgeon or RANA. The commoner small pets such as budgerigars, mice, rabbits, guinea pigs and hamsters, seldom present serious problems but in the case of the more exotic cage birds and less usual small mammals it may be wise to accept both food and cage from the owner. It is particularly important to provide daytime seclusion for nocturnal species.

General Precautions

Once an animal is handed over to the care of a veterinary surgeon in hospital premises, that veterinary surgeon becomes responsible for its safety in several respects, of which one of the most important is security, i.e. ensuring against escapes.

Whilst it is true that the veterinary surgeon is responsible in law for errors committed by his employees no RANA will wish to cause her employer worry or even risk of litigation by a too casual attitude to safety and security.

Certain precautions will reduce escapes to an absolute minimum. Exercising areas for dogs should be entered only through double gates or doors as many dogs will make a bolt for freedom when a single door is opened. RANAs should pay particular attention to the behaviour of dogs during exercise periods and in addition to the very important duty of observing excretory patterns and the excretion itself, should try to recognize the dog which is an inveterate "escape artist"; such dogs are best exercised only on a running chain.

It is a wise rule to have two doors between any cat and freedom, i.e. the door of the room and the door of the cage; the latter should not be opened unless the former is securely shut. When cats need to be transferred from room to room this should always be done in a proper basket or cage; the carrying of loose cats to theatre, X-ray room, etc., is to be deplored.

Bitches admitted at short notice, possibly in emergency, may prove to be on heat, a fact which a distressed owner may omit to mention and which may not be noted during clinical examinations which are undertaken under stress; RANAs should, therefore, make it a routine to glance at the bitch's vulva to detect any sign of swelling or discharge.

Other points a nurse admitting a new patient should note are presence of any abnormal discharges from eyes, nose, vulva, or prepuce, any skin lesions or obvious signs of parasite infestation (notably fleas or lice).

Infectious and Contagious Diseases

The vast majority of veterinary hospitals do not admit infectious cases as in-patients with the possible exception of certain skin infections such as sarcoptic mange; indeed the bugbear of all hospital premises is the inadvertent introduction of infection. It may be asked how can infection ever be introduced inadvertently? Unfortunately this is all too easy, mainly in one of three circumstances. (1) New patients may be in the incubation stage of an infection, i.e. the interval between an infective agent gaining entrance to the body and the appearance of first clinical signs; no matter how careful the clinical examination of such an animal no evidence of disease can be found. (2) The carrier animal; this is possible in only a few diseases of which feline respiratory disease is one. In this case the carrier itself remains perfectly well but harbours the causal organism in its body which it sheds either constantly or intermittently. (3) The animal which *must* be admitted to hospital regardless of its state of health, e.g. the unvaccinated puppy with a fracture requiring open fixation.

To understand how to minimize the risk of infection in kennels some understanding of the behaviour of infective agents is essential.

First of all the commoner infective agents themselves. These are:

(a) *Bacteria.* Very small living organisms which cannot be seen by the naked eye but can be seen through a microscope. They do not pass through certain specialized filters whereas most viruses can pass through similar filters.

No ordinary living animal is devoid of bacteria and all carry in their naso-pharynx and intestine, for example, certain bacteria which under normal circumstances do no harm to their host and may even have a vital function, e.g. certain bacteria in the gut synthesise vitamin B. Under certain circumstances, which may be quite varied, normal bacteria can become pathogenic, i.e. disease producing; furthermore, organisms which are harmless to their own host may be harmful to another, hence the problems which can arise in a surgical ward.

Bacteria vary considerably in their susceptibility to heat, dryness and disinfectants and the nurse requires to know some of the exceptionally resistant organisms which can be very difficult to eradicate from wards, instruments and dressings.

(b) *Viruses.* These are ultra-microscopic organisms which can only be seen with the aid of highly specialized microscopes and techniques and which usually can pass through the filters which hold back bacteria. Viruses cause some of the most serious animal diseases. Whilst they may be difficult to tackle in the animal body most viruses are fairly easily destroyed outside it, although as is well known the virus of foot and mouth disease can be quite a problem to eradicate from farm buildings.

(c) *Ectoparasites.* These are multi-celled parasites which live on, not in, the animal host. Some can be seen with the naked eye, i.e. are macroscopic, but some, e.g. sarcoptic mange mites, are microscopic. Some are easy to eradicate but some, such as the mite causing follicular mange (*Demodex folliculorum*), are very difficult.

(d) *Endoparasites.* These are also multi-celled organisms which inhabit some internal organ of an animal. The commonest endoparasites are the intestinal worms but other organs such as lungs and heart can be parasitized.

To understand how infectious disease may be minimized the various methods of transmission of infection must be recognized.

SPREAD OF INFECTIOUS DISEASES

These can be transmitted in a variety of ways but not necessarily including contact, direct or indirect, between the infected animal and another. In this section bacterial and viral diseases are most important but fungal and yeast infections should also be included.

Modes of transmission include:

(a) Infected secretions and discharges, e.g. saliva, nasal secretion, ocular and nasal discharges and occasionally sputum, e.g. canine distemper, feline virus diseases.

(b) Excretions: in some cases urine and faeces contain the infecting organism, e.g. leptospirosis, bacterial gastro-enteritis.

(c) Air-borne spread, droplet infection. The exhaled air from an animal is moist having come from the lungs and bronchi and the myriad droplets of moisture contain infective material, especially virus particles and these will contaminate the atmosphere which can then infect other occupants of the same ward unless they are kept quite a distance apart. Obviously any disease of which sneezing is a feature will be disseminated more widely due to the propulsive force of the sneeze.

(d) Indirect transmission. Here there is no direct transmission of infected material from one animal to another but there is an intermediary substance.

Examples of indirect transmission are:

(a) Infected material remaining in an inadequately disinfected kennel or cage.
(b) Infected discharges in the exercise area.
(c) Infected excretions, i.e. urine, faeces, in the exercise area. Infection can persist even after removal of the mass of faeces or hosing down after urination.
(d) Infected material on attendants' clothing; one of the commonest and least-well-recognized methods and, although theoretically easy to prevent, is not always so in practice. An unusual source of indirect infection is the virus of canine distemper which is excreted from the foot-pads often long after apparent recovery; this naturally contaminates surgery and ward floors and streets.

In some cases transmission of an infective agent requires an intermediate host, either for its full development to the stage when it can infect its final host, e.g. the commonest dog tapeworm, *Dipylidium caninum*, which has to pass part of its life cycle in a flea or louse, or as a vector, i.e. some living agent, which mechanically transfers the infecting organism, e.g. mosquitoes transmitting the protozoan parasite which causes malaria.

Obviously, direct contact between animals suffering from infectious disease will spread such infection.

ADVANTAGES AND DISADVANTAGES OF HOSPITALIZATION

Having made brief reference to infectious conditions, it is probably appropriate to refer to both sides of the question of whether to hospitalize or not. It must be said at the outset that since the Second World War the circumstances of the average family have greatly changed. It is commonplace these days for every member of a household to be out at work for the whole or part of the day, making the proper nursing of a sick animal difficult or impossible. This is not the place to debate the propriety of such households keeping pets, particularly dogs. The effect, however, is to make hospitalization of many animals wellnigh essential which hitherto would have been nursed at home.

Some of the advantages of hospitalization of patients are:

1. Regular attention, including administration of drugs at proper intervals. Some expansion of this point is desirable. The efficiency of many drugs, especially antibiotics, is dependent on the maintenance of a therapeutic blood level. This means a concentration of the drug in the blood (and to a lesser extent other tissues of the body), which will kill or prevent reproduction of the infecting organism; if the concentration is allowed to drop below a certain level, not only is treatment ineffective but can be positively dangerous in the sense that it may simply produce a state of drug resistance in the pathogenic germs. Most drugs when administered are absorbed into the blood and some tissues of the animal where they do their work; both the speed and degree of absorption are extremely variable. It can therefore be realized that while a single injection of certain drugs can result in a therapeutic blood level being maintained for 24 or even 36 hours, in other cases the duration is as little as 4 hours. Some people believe that this problem can be overcome by doubling or trebling the dose in the expectation that a therapeutic blood level will persist for longer. This is simply not true. Drugs *must* be administered at the correct intervals and for a sufficient number of consecutive days, regardless of intervening week-ends, Bank Holidays and God wot.

2. Control of diet and administration of nutrients by special routes.

3. Regular dressing of surgical wounds and other lesions.

4. Confinement to kennel or cage which will prevent an animal damaging itself, particularly post-operatively, or will provide rest in cases such as fracture of the pelvis.

5. Regular observation for any significant change in an animal's condition. It is popularly supposed by owners that there is much advantage in having an animal in "for observation". The author's view is that this exercise is seldom as valuable as is believed. The change of environment and management often has so much effect on an animal that the symptoms of which an owner complains may be completely masked. Most veterinary surgeons are familiar with the dog which, according to the owner, is refusing all food but on admission to kennels proceeds to eat vigorously, also the dog said to have a persistent cough which may never be heard to cough in a period of 3 to 4 days in kennels. Furthermore, excretory habits of the average house-trained dog are so drastically changed that no useful information is obtained.

6. Obtaining of faecal, urine and blood samples at convenient times is much easier.

7. Removal of a dog from an over-anxious owner. There is unquestionably a strong emotional bond, call it telepathic if you wish, between owner and dog, more rarely between owner and cat; whilst this can be utilized to great advantage in

nursing, an over-anxious owner may, in certain circumstances, have an adverse effect on the patient and can delay recovery. This is especially true in cases of paraplegia or paresis (paralysis or weakness of the hind limbs) and the following true example illustrates this point: a Sealyham sustained a disc protrusion episode ("slipped disc" is a bad and incorrect term anatomically speaking) and was apparently making a rapid recovery but he would not walk although clinical examination suggested he should be able to do so; his devoted owner was an anxious type and it was decided to transfer the dog to kennels where he was left one evening still not using his hind legs; he was visited next day and trotted briskly out of his kennel, tail wagging! Once his owner was assured he could walk she relaxed and all was well.

Some of the disadvantages will have become obvious from the preceding text; temperamental difficulties, change of habit, masking of symptoms, risk to nephritics amongst others. Rather more specifically some disadvantages are:

1. Risk of cross-infection. This may be of virus or bacterial diseases (e.g. distemper, leptospirosis, feline enteritis), skin diseases (e.g. sarcoptic mange, ringworm, fleas and lice) or the build-up of bacteria, such as Staphylococci, in a surgical ward. In the last case, organisms which were not originally pathogenic may, by passing through different hosts, become disease-producing themselves or bacteria which are harmless in one animal may be pathogenic in another. This type of cross-infection is the bugbear of human hospital wards and can be very serious; it is rarely so serious in veterinary hospitals but even so care is needed and the regular thorough cleansing of rooms used to house patients is essential.
2. Disorientation. Already discussed and commonest in old animals.
3. Variation in response to owner or hospital nursing. In most cases household pets respond better to nursing by their owners than by strangers; this is particularly true of long-stay cases such as paraplegics. The exception is, as previously mentioned, the over-anxious owner.

In most cases, no matter how well staffed is a veterinary hospital, an animal can receive far more attention from its owner, in terms of time especially, than in kennels.

The decision as to whether a particular case will be hospitalized or not will naturally rest with the veterinary surgeon as will the duration of its stay in kennels.

Most veterinary surgeons have fairly decided views on certain types of case which need hospital treatment. The author has always preferred to hospitalize aural resections and all cases in which any part of the alimentary tract has had to be surgically opened whilst being quite happy to discharge pyometras as soon as they were fully conscious and very definitely wishing to discharge caesarian bitches and puppies at the earliest possible moment.

Routine in Hospital Kennels

The routine will naturally vary to some extent with the circumstances of each establishment in the sense that the times for feeding, cleaning, exercising, routine dressings and injections will be suited to the particular practice.

The following are suggestions for essential routine procedures:

1. *Observation.* RANAs should quickly observe each patient as soon as the ward is opened each day. Newly admitted animals may still be shy and distressed but after a few days in kennels behaviour becomes more relaxed and changes of posture, brightness, etc., can be noted. The kennel or cage is rapidly observed for signs of haemorrhage, vomit or abnormal urine or faeces. Any marked change must be reported as soon as feasible.

2. *Temperature taking.* Routine daily temperature taking is a must in all cases and this must be recorded on the in-patient card. Temperature should, as far as possible, be taken in the resting animal; exercise, feeding or agitation during dressing, etc., can cause a transient rise in temperature.

3. *Cleaning and exercise.* These two are considered together since it is easiest to clean the kennel while the inmate is in the exercise run. It is easier for the nursing staff simply to transfer a patient to an already clean cage and then clean the previous one at leisure. The writer believes this to be bad practice since it destroys the sense of territory and thus security, which an animal very quickly acquires after admission. This is especially important in cats. Every effort should be made to keep a patient to its own cage throughout its stay. In cases where any infectious discharge is present it is essential to keep the patient to its own cage. Obviously circumstances will arise, e.g. unexpected admission of a large dog, which will necessitate a "general post" but this should be regarded as exceptional.

House-trained dogs are often reluctant to use a hospital kennel or run for urination and defaecation; watching them makes matters worse but when a reluctant dog *is* seen to have performed, a word of praise and encouragement helps to establish the habit. In hospital kennels it is usual to exercise one animal at a time unless the kennels have individual runs.

4. *Feeding.* The actual time of feeding can be varied to suit the individual hospital but it is highly desirable that those animals on normal diets should be fed at approximately the same time each day.

Most dogs adapt readily to the routine diet but cats are less easy and it is a wise precaution to ask the owner of a sick cat if it has any particular food-fads.

In special cases the dietary regime will be laid down by the veterinary surgeon but certain general principles apply. Little and often for the very young and very old, and food and drink to be offered in very small quantities only to all animals which have had major surgery in the previous few days.

The special diets required in certain categories of medical case will be given in more detail later. Although more properly the sphere of surgical nursing, it is useful to comment here that all patients which have had any part of the alimentary tract surgically opened must be most carefully dealt with for the first 5 to 7 days post-operatively; in some cases nothing whatever is permitted by mouth for 24 to 72 hours, nutriment being provided by suitable parenteral fluid therapy supplemented by multi-vitamin preparations and/or hydrolysed protein solution. When oral feeding is commenced, only material which is absorbed from stomach and upper small intestine is allowed, e.g. glucose water, hydrolysed protein, meat essence or pre-digested milk; a gradual return to normal feeding over the next 4–6 days follows, starting with low-residue foods such as lean meat, egg, fish or pre-digested milk (milk not pre-digested leaves an indigestible curd in stomach and bowel).

Patients with diarrhoea are usually put on to a low protein diet, excluding flesh foods, for 24 to 48 hours; easily digested carbohydrates are in order—these will include bread and milk, rice puddings, custard, cereals, arrowroot and cornflour. When repeated vomiting is a major symptom, complete starvation for 24 to 36 hours may be ordered; if fluids are permitted by mouth they should be given in small quantities frequently, i.e. every hour. If oral fluids are forbidden, subcutaneous infusion may be needed.

In certain conditions dogs and cats drink excessive quantities of water and part of the treatment routine may be to limit (never entirely to withhold) water intake. It is often easier and more efficient to make an animal limit its own water intake voluntarily by rendering the fluid less palatable. This may be done by one or a combination of the following methods:

(a) Boil the water.
(b) Add glucose to the boiled water; approximately one teaspoonful per pint.
(c) Add cooking salt to the boiled water; only a very small pinch to a pint is required. To use more could result in a water-crazed animal getting salt-poisoning!
(d) Make barley water.

All these measures render water less acceptable to animals and, whilst they will be obliged to take sufficient fluid to maintain existence, they will seldom drink more than is essential; this is far more effective than giving measured quantities of ordinary water, which the patient mops up and demands more.

5. *Bedding*. The type of bedding selected will vary according to the type of kenneling and the individual circumstances. Newspaper has much to commend it in almost all circumstances.

It should be a general rule that any soiled bedding should be changed as soon as practicable after it has been noticed. Many house-trained dogs are very miserable if left in a kennel with bedding they have been obliged to foul.

Warmth is normally best provided by a warm atmosphere, i.e. the ambient temperature should be correct, whether this be by room heating or underfloor heating of the kennels. Rugs and blankets are not required for the average in-patient but are essential in certain circumstance, such as during recovery from general anaesthesia when the heat loss from the animal's body is not fully counteracted by a high ambient temperature. "Chilly mortals" such as Whippets, Italian Greyhounds, Chihuahuas (smooth) and Smooth Dachshunds feel the cold intensely, even in warm surroundings, and many of these breeds will appreciate a blanket over them. Nylon fur fabric has recently received favourable comment as a material for dog blankets.

The recumbent patient requires special consideration. Some dogs, whether due to multiple fractures or paraplegia, remain in a lying position for several weeks and contact of bony prominences with the hard surface of a kennel soon produces bed-sores (decubital ulcers). Foam rubber covered with plastic has much to commend it in these circumstances but great care must be taken to ascertain that the patient is not an inveterate "chewer", which ends up with obstruction of the intestine due to foam rubber in addition to its other ills!

SOME IMPORTANT DISEASES OF DOGS AND CATS

Diagnosis is the province of the veterinary surgeon, not the RANA, but some understanding of certain aspects of the common canine and feline diseases will make the RANA better able to co-operate in management and the application of treatment. A superficial acquaintance with immunity to disease, natural and artificial, will also help the nurse not only to understand some of the problems inherent in infectious disease but to give logical explanations to telephone inquiries regarding vaccination.

IMMUNITY

The animal body reacts to invasion by an infectious pathogenic organism by producing antibodies, substances which act against the specific germ concerned and which prevent its multiplication or kill it. Generally speaking, antibodies are not produced until some 10 days after initial infection. Antibodies are quite specific as relating to one particular disease only, an animal which has adequate antibodies circulating in its blood will be immune to that disease.

Antibodies are acquired in different ways:

(a) Passive

1. *Maternal.* Some antibodies are acquired from the mother's blood or milk so that the newly born animal is resistant to some diseases for a variable time after its birth. This is maternal immunity. The concentration of any one antibody and also the number of diseases against which maternally transmitted antibodies are acquired will depend upon and vary with the dam's own immune status. For example, puppies born to a bitch which had recovered from an attack of canine distemper 6 months before their birth would "inherit" a high concentration of distemper antibodies but pups from a bitch which had neither been in contact with, nor been vaccinated against, distemper would get no antibodies at birth at all. The persistence of maternal antibodies in the young will vary due to several factors of which the two most important are the concentration of antibodies (expressed technically as a titre) and the disease concerned. The veterinary surgeon must know all about the second one but the first can only be determined by complex scientific tests which are costly and time-

consuming; the timing of vaccination depends largely on the stage at which maternal antibodies drop below a certain level. If the level is too high, the young animal will not respond to vaccination, i.e. it will not "take", yet if vaccination is delayed too long it may become susceptible and contract infection before being vaccinated. A difficult problem which causes veterinary surgeons much concern.

2. *Hyperimmune serum.* Passive immunity can be conferred on an animal by the injection of serum containing a high concentration of antibodies against a particular disease. The techniques involved in producing hyperimmune serum need not concern the RANA.

(b) Active or acquired immunity

This means the development of antibodies by the individual animal itself, i.e. it does not receive them ready-made. These are:

1. *Natural.* This is always the result of an infectious agent entering the host's body; it may not always cause obvious disease and in these cases a subclinical infection is spoken of. When disease is caused antibodies are also produced, often to a higher level, and, if the animal recovers, it is left with a pretty good share of antibody. The duration of both natural and acquired active immunity will be discussed later.

2. *Artificial.* This is an active immunity produced by administering a substance which will cause the animal's body to produce antibodies; such a substance is known as an antigen and is usually given in the form of a vaccine. A vaccine is essentially a modified form of the virus or bacteria causing each particular disease but it must be in such a form that, whilst it acts as an antigen, it does not cause serious disease. This state of affairs is achieved by a variety of methods. The infecting organism may be killed, e.g. by adding formalin to the culture, and this would result in a dead vaccine. Live vaccines may be produced by propagating special strains of, say, a virus, which are antigenic but not virulent. The virulence of a virus may be modified by passing it through a series of animals which are not its normal host or by growing it on an artificial medium such as one of the membranes of fertile hens' eggs or in cultures of certain tissue cells. Canine distemper virus will grow in hens' eggs and for many years an egg-adapted distemper vaccine was widely used; most present-day distemper vaccines are produced in tissue cultures, which have marginal advantages. Canine virus hepatitis vaccine is usually produced in a culture of pigs' kidney cells.

Duration of Immunity

A number of factors affect the duration of immunity.

1. *Naturally acquired immunity.* Following an attack of a disease, the animal becomes immune as described previously. Broadly speaking, immunity following a virus infection is life-long, *but* there are exceptions: canine distemper, canine virus hepatitis and infectious feline enteritis are examples of diseases which nearly always produce life-long immunity in recovered animals; it is very rare for these diseases to occur a second time in the same animal. On the other hand, the feline respiratory virus

complex results in very temporary immunity only, often a mere 6 weeks, and thus resembles human influenza and the common cold. It is very important to know this when taking the previous health history of new patients. If a dog has had distemper or a cat had enteritis one can usually feel fairly sure it is safe from reinfection; not so the cat which has had so-called "cat flu".

2. *Artificial immunity*. The immunity conferred by a dose of hyperimmune serum is very transient, some 2 to 4 weeks, but may be enough to protect an animal over a short period of high risk, e.g. a dog or cat show.

Vaccination confers longer immunity if the vaccine is of good quality, and the receiving animal is in good health and of the right age. Live vaccines give a much longer duration of immunity than killed ones.

Some common examples include:

Canine distemper vaccine. Usually a live tissue culture vaccine. In theory confers life-long immunity when used correctly. Some people believe that, with the decreasing incidence of canine distemper and therefore the lessened chance of a dog "boosting" its immunity by repeated natural contact, the degree of immunity does wane and booster doses are advisable. Views on the periodicity of these boosters are very varied.

Canine virus hepatitis vaccine. May be living or dead. The former confers very long-lasting immunity, the latter much less so. When dead vaccines are used, annual booster doses are usually recommended.

Leptospira vaccines. These are dead vaccines conferring limited immunity. Annual boosters are required.

Feline infectious enteritis. Nowadays usually a living, attenuated tissue-culture vaccine, giving a long immunity.

Autogenous vaccines. These are vaccines specially produced from an animal's own germs or from material from an outbreak in an establishment, e.g. feline respiratory disease in a cattery. They are usually killed vaccines and these give only brief immunity. They are sometimes used in treatment rather than prevention.

Use of vaccines

Vaccines must be used only under optimum conditions and this includes many factors:

1. *Storage*. The manufacturer's directions as to storage *must* be carefully followed and they must be kept in the appropriate part of the refrigerator or, in some cases, a cool room. They must *never* be kept in hot places, e.g. the mantelpiece over a fire or the back window of a car.

The shelf-life must be noted and vaccine ordered appropriately so that it does not go out of date. Out of date vaccine must not be administered. The RANA should keep note of stock, and expiry dates.

2. *Administration*. It must be given cleanly and efficiently. It is usually injected

subcutaneously; oral vaccines are not used for animals and one which is instilled into the conjunctival sac of the eye has not found wide favour. Syringes and needles (if not in pre-packed sterile form) must be sterile; spirit must not be used in the syringe or needle as it may kill the fragile vaccine as may a hot syringe removed recently from a sterilizer. Syringes and needles should have been autoclaved or boiled and allowed to cool in a sterile container. Care must be taken over cleansing the site of injection as any strong antiseptic may also affect the vaccine.

3. *Fitness of the recipient.* The animal to be vaccinated must be healthy, not recently exposed to infection and of the correct age. The veterinary surgeon will instruct the RANA as to the inquiries she should make on the latter points.

Young animals to be vaccinated should not mix with patients in the waiting-room. Whether vaccinations are better done at the surgery or at home is controversial. The author prefers the former, with the vaccinee being kept by the owner in the car and then carried through and placed directly on a carefully disinfected table. The veterinary surgeon's clothing can so easily become infected by discharge from a patient seen on a round prior to the visit to vaccinate; with the best will and organization in the world this can happen and one cannot return to the house for a complete change of clothing between visits but at the surgery a clean coat can be quickly donned.

By organizing her side of the practice work efficiently, a RANA can do much to promote effective vaccination.

(e) SOME COMMON DISEASES OF IMPORTANCE TO THE RANA

JOAN O. JOSHUA, FRCVS

Ectoparasites

PARASITIC SKIN DISEASES

As has already been emphasized, all patients admitted to hospital should receive a quick routine check for evidence of gross parasitism.

1. *Fleas.* Dogs and cats are often infested with fleas; most commonly it is the dog or cat flea *Ctenocephalides* spp., sometimes the human flea, *Pulex irritans*, and occasionally bird or hedgehog fleas *Ceratophylus* spp. One surprising fact is that some animals can tolerate a heavy infestation and only show the most minor clinical signs whereas others get a really severe reaction from a few parasites.

Infested dogs and cats show irritation by both scratching and nibbling at the affected areas, especially the posterior part of the back. Fleas are seen as brownish elongated insects which run through the fur rather than jump; they are best looked for just above the base of the tail, down the back of the thighs and in the thinner hair of the abdomen; hedgehog fleas often infest the head. If the parasites themselves are not easily seen the typical excreta is looked for; this is in the form of shiny blackish/brown spherical specks which, when dropped into water, give it a reddish tinge due to the ingested blood. Infestation is commonest in summer and early autumn.

Fleas do not complete their life cycle on the host but in such places as bedding, baskets, chairs, etc., so whenever flea infestation is diagnosed, treatment must include thorough cleaning of all places where the animal sleeps.

Treatment is by application of suitable parasiticides by bathing or powdering; common agents in use are derris, gamma benzene hexachloride, pyrethrum, pybuthrin and—rarely—Dieldrin. Gamma BHC must be used with care on cats and DDT (Dicophane) should *never* be used. Owing to the tendency for cats to lick themselves all excess dressing should be removed from the surface of the coat. Dressings are repeated at least once at an interval of 7–10 days; this ensures that all adult parasites are destroyed at the first application and the second one is designed to kill the next generation before they reach breeding age.

Fleas are important as an intermediate host in the life cycle of the tapeworm, *Dipylidium caninum*.

2. *Lice.* Common enough but less common than fleas, especially on cats. They are unlike fleas in several respects; they do not move perceptibly, they complete their life cycle on the host and the eggs (nits) can be seen on the hairs. Lice may be light brown or greyish/blue in colour. Scratching is the main clinical sign and is of a particularly well-directed type; anaemia may be seen in severe chronic infestations in dogs as lice are blood feeders. The parasites are mainly seen on the ear flaps and body, especially round the shoulders; a hand lens will help a great deal in identifying them. The typical elongated whitish eggs are easily seen glued to the hairs.

Treatment is as for fleas but bedding, etc., is seldom contaminated in the same way as with fleas, although bedding into which lice have fallen can reinfest the same host or transfer infestation to others. Lice also act as intermediate hosts for the tapeworm *Dipylidium*.

3. *Ticks*. Both dogs, cats and tortoises (!) can harbour so-called "sheep" ticks. These ticks are usually of *Ixodes* spp. and, in fact, often have hedgehogs as the natural host, which accounts for their appearance in domestic pets which have never been within miles of a sheep. They are small when first becoming attached to a new host but over a few days become rapidly engorged with blood and attain a size of some 0·5 cm, by which time they are obvious. Ticks are of comparatively little significance to the nurse but she should always report their presence so that appropriate treatment, if considered necessary, can be prescribed.

4. *Harvest mites* (*Trombicula autumnalis*). Common in some localities, absent in others. These are very small parasites, orange-red in colour, just visible to the naked eye especially when in clusters. They can often be seen in the depths of the space between the toes. They cause intense irritation. Again, if these are seen they must be reported to the veterinary surgeon who may prescribe a medicated bath such as gamma benzene hexachloride or sulphur.

Mange Mites

These are usually not visible to the naked eye (*Otodectes*, the ear mite of cats *is* just visible) and are thus known as microscopic. Many of them cause quite serious skin disease in domestic pets and some even have a public health significance in that they can cause skin infections in human contacts.

The actual morphological difference between the various mites is largely a matter for the diagnostician but RANAs should be able to recognize mange mites in a prepared skin scraping although the final identification is rarely their responsibility. Great patience is often needed to find *Sarcoptes scabei* (the cause of sarcoptic mange) and many microscopic fields may have to be examined before a mite is found; contrariwise *Otodectes* (the ear mite) is very easily found in material from cats' ears.

The mange mites all have a similar life cycle which is completed on the host animal. The eggs are laid on the host and these hatch in some 3–7 days to become larvae; these mature quite quickly and become nymphs; there may be more than one nymphal stage before the fully mature breeding adult develops.

Periodicity of treatment is based on this life cycle, the object being to kill off new generations of mites before they become sexually mature; once-weekly treatment is the usual rule for a period of not less than 3 and preferably 4 weeks. The secret of treating mange cases is *thoroughness*, whether the prescribed treatment is by bathing, local application of suitable lotions or even by the now old-fashioned (but very effective) method of clipping out and rubbing in sulphur and oil; rushed baths or dressings are quite useless and will merely result in an unnecessary prolongation of treatment.

Whilst mange mites cannot survive long off the host they can persist in cages or bedding (especially if the floors are wooden) for a sufficient time to infect the next inhabitant, so very thorough disinfection must be the rule.

The following are brief notes on the principal characteristics of some of the common mange mites:

(*a*) *Otodectes cynotis*. The mite causing ear disease in cats and occasionally in dogs. Is largely confined to the ear canal but may spread locally around the ears. When present in large numbers, as is common in the cat, can be seen in the ear canal as whitish dots moving in the mass of dried brown waxy material which characterizes these cases.

It is wise always to look at the ears of newly admitted cats and, if a heavy infestation is seen, report to the veterinary surgeon, who will usually want to prescribe cleaning and dressing; in most cases once-weekly dressing is sufficient. If a preparation containing gamma benzene hexachloride is used care should be taken not to swamp the cat's head in it; quite safe if used discreetly but can be toxic if used to excess.

(*b*) *Sarcoptes scabei*. Causes sarcoptic mange in dogs and other mammals, including man. The cat is pretty resistant to it. Is not visible to the naked eye. Causes intense irritation with persistent scratching; pruritus (itching) is so severe that an affected dog may stop in the middle of a meal or walk to have a good scratch.

Ear edges, axillae (arm-pits) and inside thighs are most commonly affected but the whole body can become involved in severe cases.

The susceptibility of humans varies greatly; some get scabies almost by looking at a case, others never contract it no matter how many cases they handle. The disease in humans is mild and very easily treated but should the RANA get itchy spots on her forearms or thighs she should report it at once.

(*c*) *Psoroptes communis cuniculi*. Causes ear mange in rabbits; the ears become filled with a flaky or cheesy exudate.

(*d*) *Cheyletiella* spp. This parasite can infest dogs, cats and rabbits, often without causing any lesions in these hosts, but can, and often does, cause a very irritable rash in humans. If any signs are seen it is usually the presence of excessive flaky scurf, frequently on the posterior surface of the back.

Follicular or Demodectic Mange

This differs from the above types in many respects. The parasite concerned (*Demodex folliculorum*) is microscopic and can perhaps best be described as resembling a carrot with stumpy legs. The skin condition caused can be exceedingly difficult to treat but this is the province of the veterinary surgeon. Although infection can be transmitted by prolonged bodily contact, e.g. puppies sleeping in a basket together, for all practical purposes in a veterinary hospital the nurse can regard it as non-infectious.

Endoparasites

These are parasites living in the body rather than upon it as in the previous section. These include the intestinal worms, some of which are common in this country. Although other parasites, such as the heart-worm of dogs, *Dirofilaria immitis*, and the hook-worm, *Ancylostoma caninum*, may be seen in dogs undergoing quarantine they are not widespread in indigenous British pets, hence merit only the briefest mention here; RANAs working in quarantine kennels will receive special instructions from the supervising veterinary surgeon to enable them to cope with alien situations.

The following are some of the intestinal parasites occurring regularly:

THE DOG

1. *Round worms (Ascarids), Toxascaris leonina and Toxocara canis.* In both species the adult worm inhabits the intestine and if present in very large numbers can cause severe ill-health and even obstruction in young puppies. The larval stages are passed in other tissues, including lungs, liver, brain and eye; larvae can pass through the mother's tissues and invade foetuses which are in the uterus, thus pups are born already infested with round worms. The worms in the intestines are fully developed 4 to 5 weeks after the pup is born, hence serious disease due to Ascarids is confined to the young puppy, usually between 4 and 8 weeks of age.

Larvae of *Toxocara* can invade humans, especially children, and on rare occasions can cause symptoms, so there is a public health angle to be considered.

2. *The Hookworm, Uncinaria stenocephala,* is occasionally seen in British dogs. Infestation with this worm is seldom serious. Infestation with *Ancylostoma* is more serious and can cause anaemia; it is virtually only seen in imported dogs.

3. *The whipworm, Trichuris vulpis,* has been met in this country and may become more widespread.

Ascarid worms are large (3–6 in. long) and can easily be seen in the faeces but in all the above cases diagnosis is usually based on microscopic examination of a faeces sample and recognition of the eggs which are characteristic for each type of worm. Hookworms and whipworms are not normally visible.

4. *Tapeworms.* The mature segments of tapeworms can usually be seen quite easily in the faeces or in the hair round the anus where they may dry and be rather like rice grains. The whole worm may reach several feet in length. All tapeworms have an intermediate host in which part of the life cycle takes place. Effective treatment therefore includes elimination of the intermediate host as well as removing adult worms from the dog.

The commonest tapeworm of the dog is:

Dipylidium caninum: The adult worm can be up to $1\frac{1}{2}$ ft in length but individual segments are small and oval in shape (cucumber-seed shape) and have the ability to move; they may resemble small maggots in the hair round the anus. The intermediate hosts are fleas and lice, therefore effective treatment will include examination and treatment for either of these two ectoparasites.

Other tapeworms also occur which have their intermediate stage in rats, mice, rabbits, hares and sheep; eating of small rodents or raw viscera from rabbits, hares and sheep causes infestation.

Treatment for tapeworms is not always easy and in resistant cases it may be necessary to give an enema. In any case it is highly desirable to watch the dog carefully after treatment, examining the stool to make sure if the worm has been passed intact, i.e. with the head (scolex) attached; this is recognized as a small round blob on the end of a narrower "neck".

THE CAT

The cat can be infested with the roundworms *Toxascaris leonina* and *Toxocara mystax;* there is very little evidence that the latter is a public health hazard.

Tapeworms, especially *Dipylidium* and *Taenia* spp., having their intermediate stage in rats and mice are occasionally seen.

Cats are also subject to infestation with the lungworm, *Aleurostrongylus abstrusus* but the RANA will seldom be concerned with this except that she should report any kitten or young cat showing a cough or respiratory abnormality.

COCCIDIA

These are protozoal parasites which can infest the small intestine of both dog and cat; the species involved are *Isospora* and *Eimeria.* They are seldom a problem in veterinary hospitals but could cause trouble in closed communities such as breeding kennels and catteries. Diagnosis is by microscopic examination of faeces.

The RANA's main duty with internal parasites is to report seeing any specimens in a patient's faeces or on its hair, to retain a specimen of the adult worm for examination and also a sample of fresh faeces for microscopy; secondly, to supervise treatment, if this is given on the veterinary premises, giving enemata as necessary and examining specimens passed.

Virus Diseases

CANINE DISTEMPER

This is a common infectious disease of dogs and some other animals such as ferret and mink. In many areas widespread vaccination has considerably reduced its incidence, but in some of the larger cities where uncontrolled dogs, owned by owners who neither care about nor can afford vaccination, roam free, the infection persists and is known as endemic—more correctly enzootic when referring to animals—i.e. it is always present in the animal population concerned.

Canine distemper is due to a virus which has a particular property of invading and multiplying in tissue of the nervous system, i.e. it is neurotropic. Nerve tissue heals poorly or not at all and therefore serious symptoms such as fits, chorea (a twitch in muscle—St. Vitus's Dance), and even paralysis may arise and are seldom curable. It is for this reason that canine distemper is regarded as a very serious disease of dogs and cannot be dismissed comparatively lightly as are the childhood fevers such as chicken pox and measles.

As has been emphasized before, diagnosis is not the province of the RANA but familiarity with some of the common signs of canine distemper is essential if cases which develop in hospitalized dogs are to be quickly recognized and reported. It may well be added that the conclusive diagnosis of canine distemper is not easy, despite the commonness of the disease, and for all practical purposes diagnosis is based on a suggestive symptomatology.

The incubation period, i.e. the time lapse between the virus entering the body and the first clinical signs, is variable, on average around 10 days; under certain experimental conditions it can be as short as 5 days and under natural conditions may be as long as 28 days.

The response of an animal to infection is often marked by a rise in body temperature; canine distemper is no exception to this rule but it follows a curious pattern known as di-phasic. There is an initial temperature rise which lasts only 24–36 hours during which time the dog may miss a meal or pass a loose stool; this phase is seldom detected except by unusually observant owners or regular temperature taking; this fever quickly subsides and the dog becomes apparently normal but some 10 days later the "typical" signs of distemper appear; this is the stage of secondary bacterial invasion. Certain systems may be affected more than others, e.g. in the alimentary form there will be vomiting and/or diarrhoea, in the respiratory form there will be a cough and discharge from the eyes and/or nose.

Any susceptible dog which has any one or more of the following signs should be promptly reported:

Vomiting.
Diarrhoea.
Cough.
Sneezing.
Inappetence.
Discharging eyes and/or nose.
Half-closed eyes with reddened membranes.
Loss of brightness and energy.
A persistently hard, dry nose.

In most circumstances nursing a distemper case will not be part of normal hospital work and in the few specialized veterinary hospitals which cater for infectious cases, and they are *very* few, the nursing staff will receive specific instructions. Golden rules for distemper cases are rest, isolation and cleanliness. Exercise should be forbidden and the dog only allowed out into the owner's garden to urinate and defaecate; play must not be encouraged. Discharge must be cleaned from eyes and nose regularly using moistened cotton-wool; the nose will benefit from the application of Vaseline. In cases of copious nasal discharge medicated inhalations give relief.

The symptoms of distemper may persist for several weeks necessitating prolonged nursing. The depressing feature is that nervous symptoms may develop several weeks after apparent recovery.

The RANA must always be very conscious of the risk of transmitting infection to other patients after handling, perhaps inadvertently, a distemper case. A protective plastic or rubber apron which can be easily removed and disinfected can be a great safeguard. Surgery coats, etc., should be changed frequently and especially after handling a suspicious case.

It is better to be over-cautious in reporting clinical signs, disinfection and cleanliness than to adopt a wait-and-see attitude which can result in disaster.

CANINE VIRUS HEPATITIS

This is another virus disease of dogs which is widespread, especially in certain localities, but its exact incidence is not easy to ascertain. The reason for this is that the disease can exist in a variety of forms from the hyperacute, in which the dog is either found dead without symptoms having been observed or dies after a very short illness of a few hours, to a subclinical infection in which no sign of illness is detected. The midway house, the acute form, is the type when diagnosis is usually possible and lasts 2 to 7 days. It is the subclinical form which causes confusion as to incidence and it is also an important factor in spread of infection; dogs which have had such an infection can only be detected by specialized laboratory techniques which demonstrate antibodies to CVH.

The RANA is only likely to be concerned with developed clinical cases which develop in hospitalized dogs. The symptomatology is varied but the sudden onset of profound dullness and/or a very high temperature, →41·6°C (107°F), should arouse suspicion; such a dog should be promptly isolated. Most vaccinated dogs will have had CVH included in their immunization programme and as the vaccine appears to be pretty efficient it is reasonable to assume such patients are resistant.

Infection is spread mainly via urine and this is the crunch. Urine of recovered dogs remains infectious for a long time after clinical recovery and sub-clinical cases also excrete infective urine. Routine swilling down of exercise yards is adequate in ordinary circumstances but if there is any ground for suspicion that CVH infected urine is being passed by an in-patient the use of a very hot, strong solution of washing soda should be substituted.

During the recovery phase of CVH some patients develop a "blue eye". If a dog is noticed suddenly to have a dense opacity affecting one or both eyes it should be reported to the veterinary surgeon who may decide that this indicates a CVH case and special care regarding urine, etc., will be needed.

FELINE INFECTIOUS ENTERITIS OR PANLEUKOPENIA

This is a severe, acute disease of cats with a high mortality rate. Most well-cared-for cats are vaccinated and many catteries require evidence of vaccination before admission. It is probably the most dreaded infection in cat kennels. Although described as enteritis (inflammation of the bowel *is* a regular post-mortem finding) diarrhoea is not the most typical feature of the illness; vomiting, depression and very rapid weight loss due to dehydration (within 24 hours of onset) are far more typical; thirst is shown by the cat hanging its head miserably over a saucer of milk or water but ability to drink is very poor.

When a case is diagnosed in a cattery all admissions must be stopped and the ward concerned rigidly isolated; if possible one RANA should look after cats in this ward single-handed, should wear complete protective clothing which can be washed down every time she leaves the room concerned and should walk through a bath of disinfectant at the door.

The most important feature of nursing is to maintain hydration and this often means repeated infusions of glucose-saline or other fluid therapy as prescribed; anything which can be done to boost a patient's "morale" is valuable.

In some practices it is customary to suspend all routine feline surgery such as castrations and spays during a local epidemic of feline enteritis.

FELINE RESPIRATORY VIRUS DISEASE (SYNONYMS CAT INFLUENZA, CAT DISTEMPER)

This is a complex subject and it is not necessary for the RANA to know in detail the various virus entities which have been recognized. What she must know is that, as with human influenza, there are many strains of virus involved and none gives a long-lasting immunity. Very few owners of catteries, whether veterinary or purely boarding, can claim never to have experienced an outbreak of feline respiratory disease on their premises. The first—and ominous—sign is a sneeze; the observant auxiliary will note a sneeze virtually subconsciously and will report it instantly. Immediate isolation of the sneezer *may* do something to prevent spread but the incubation period is short and it is usually too late. Once again the infected ward must become a self-contained isolation unit.

A carrier state definitely exists and apparently healthy cats shed the virus for years; after several outbreaks it is often possible to identify an individual cat whose admission has each time been followed by an outbreak of disease; the observant RANA may be a great help in pin-pointing the offending carrier.

Once disease has broken out good nursing is of the essence. Full protective clothing drill is again required. Affected cats develop a variable degree of oculo-nasal discharge and some become really miserable, streaming objects and are profoundly depressed. Specific treatments are of comparatively little avail although antibiotics are usually prescribed to reduce the risk of secondary chest infection. Regular, frequent cleaning away of discharges, even medicated inhalations or the use of steam kettles may be needed for symptomatic relief. The temperature of the ward must be kept stable but adequate ventilation is essential; the air must never be allowed to become dry. Some cats continue to eat reasonably well but many lose their appetite and this in large measure is due to inability to smell due to the copious discharge.

It is useless offering such cats typical invalid foods such as steamed plaice in milk! Appetite must be titillated by offering pungent smelling foods such as kippers, sardines, salmon, giblets, etc. Recovery and convalescence is often a protracted business and it is usually several weeks before the last patient can be discharged.

After any outbreak of infectious disease, especially feline, closing of the room concerned, fumigation with formaldehyde gas and subsequent thorough swilling down of cages, floors, walls and ceiling is routine. The ward should be left empty for a minimum of 1 week after the above measures are completed.

Bacterial Diseases

Although bacterial diseases may be infectious they are usually not quite so easily transmitted as virus infections. Some people find it difficult to understand that a disease can be described as infective and yet is not necessarily infectious. The former term denotes a condition caused by an infective organism which could be, but often is not, passed on to other animals whereas the term infectious implies a likelihood that it will be passed on. It must also be understood that some bacteria which are normally found in certain sites in animals, e.g. *Staphylococci* in dog skin, *Pasteurella* in the cat naso-pharynx, and in such sites do not cause disease, can do so if change in their habitat occurs.

Pustular dermatitis can be due to a dog's own *Staphylococci* if they gain entrance to deeper layers of the skin following injury, even such slight damage as may follow clipping; similarly Pasteurellas lie harmlessly enough in the nose and throat of cats but usually cause severe septic infection if planted in human or animal tissues following a cat bite.

Examples of bacterial disease are tonsillitis and bacterial gastro-enteritis (mainly in dogs) and septic infection in cats following bites; the former conditions may be transmitted to other dogs especially in closed communities, the latter is in the form of local lesions and is not infectious. Obviously in the case of tonsillitis infection will most likely be transmitted by saliva, hence great care should be taken over cleanliness of feeding utensils whereas gastro-enteritis will be transmitted by vomit or faeces so that it is the exercise area which matters.

LEPTOSPIROSIS

Bacterial diseases deserving special mention are those caused by two species of *Leptospira*.

1. Leptospira icterohaemorrhagiae

This organism is harboured by rats and is passed in their urine. It can cause a serious disease in man, Weil's disease. In dogs it also causes a serious, often fatal, illness mainly affecting liver and kidneys; jaundice—a yellow staining of the tissues—is often seen and the disease is often called leptospiral jaundice. It is commoner in rural areas.

From the RANA's point of view the knowledge that rat urine transmits infection is important; any evidence of rat infestation of kennels, especially food-storage areas, must be vigorously dealt with. Feeding-stuffs should be stored in rat-proof containers.

Should the RANA be required to assist with the nursing of a case of leptospiral jaundice she must remember the infectious nature of the urine and take suitable precautions, e.g. wear rubber gloves. Areas where infected dogs urinate must be thoroughly cleansed; a hot solution of washing soda is excellent as leptospiras are very fragile and cannot survive in an alkaline solution.

2. Leptospira canicola

The infection caused by this organism is commoner in urban dogs. It causes nephritis (inflammation of the kidneys) and leptospiras are present in the urine of primary cases and also intermittently in the urine of some apparently recovered dogs. This organism can, rarely, cause a mild illness in man, canicola fever. Nursing precautions resemble those already mentioned but the disease is much less of a public health hazard.

An important point to remember is that if a urine specimen is required for microscopic examination it must be *fresh*. Dog urine quickly becomes alkaline when stale and any leptospiras which may have been present die and disappear so that false negative findings could be made.

Many dogs are vaccinated against both types of leptospirosis but, remembering that this is a killed bacterial vaccine, annual boosters are required and not all owners are punctilious in this respect.

Cats are not subject to clinical leptospirosis.

Nutrition in Relation to Disease

It is comparatively rarely that the RANA will be concerned with nutritional disease as most patients are not in hospital for a sufficient length of time to cause problems, but in certain circumstances, e.g. hospitalization of big breed puppies, problems could arise.

Most adult dogs and cats on an average mixed diet are unlikely to suffer gross deficiences but some points need to be remembered.

1. BONE

For the development of sound, healthy bone and for the prompt repair of fractures, certain nutritional factors must be present; these are calcium and phosphorus in *correct ratio*, vitamin D and to a lesser extent vitamins A and C.

Large breed puppies detained in hospital may well require mineral and vitamin supplements and in any case should receive ample fresh milk. Obviously calcium and phosphorus are in the correct proportion in bone so the best method of giving the necessary minerals is by adding sterilized bone flour or bone meal to the food; 1 to 2 teaspoonsful daily is usually adequate. Bone meal so readily available as a garden fertilizer is unsafe for feeding.

Since excess vitamin D can be as harmful as a deficiency the veterinary surgeon will usually prescribe exactly what is required. Common sources of both vitamins A and D are cod liver oil or halibut liver oil.

It is wise for the RANA to inquire as to whether any special feeding or supplementation is required for each orthopaedic case.

2. DIARRHOEA

The type of low protein feeding usually recommended for animals with diarrhoea has already been referred to. Another important point is to recognize what can happen in patients where prolonged antibiotic therapy, especially if given orally, is necessary. The bacteria which are always present in the intestine, the normal flora, have several functions of which one is to synthesize vitamin B; if an animal is maintained on a broad-spectrum antibiotic for long periods (in excess of 7 days or even less) many of the normal bacteria are killed off and the animal may become vitamin B deficient which can itself cause diarrhoea! It is therefore customary to administer some form of vitamin B—this may be by something as simple as yeast—when broad-spectrum antibiotics are used.

3. SKIN DISEASES

The actual diagnosis of nutritional skin disease is a matter for the veterinary surgeon but some animals, both dogs and cats, suffer severe dermatitis due to an allergic response which may be to something in the diet. Recognition of the actual item of diet involved is a highly specialized matter but the important point is that, once identified, that item must be totally excluded, reduction of amount is not sufficient.

Fat deficiency, which is sometimes seen, can often be corrected by addition of margarine or pure linseed oil to the diet.

4. URINARY CALCULI (STONES IN THE BLADDER OR URETHRA)

Although stone formation can occur in the kidneys it is those in the bladder and urethra which cause trouble in dogs and cats. There are various chemical types of stone. The commonest is the phosphate stone. Phosphates remain in solution in an acid medium but precipitate out in certain circumstances when the urine is less acid. Although dog urine is classically described as being acid, routine examination of specimens from dogs on average mixed diets shows that the urine pH is around the point of neutrality; part of the treatment for dogs liable to produce phosphate stones is to keep the urine acid and this is done by the regular administration of acidifying agents such as sodium acid phosphate or ammonium chloride in the hope of preventing or at least delaying recurrence. An adequate water intake is also desirable so that urine does not become too concentrated; if essential, drinking can be encouraged by adding a very small pinch of salt to the food or water but not sufficient to make it unpalatable, as described earlier in the chapter.

Cysteine stones are also common and these are more soluble in alkaline urine, hence sodium bicarbonate is given to prevent the urine becoming acid; this is less effective than the acidifying regime.

In occasional cases of urinary stones it may be recommended that flesh protein be reduced or eliminated; in these cases cheese and eggs are the normal substitutes.

Some Categories of Medical Disease requiring Special Care

HEART DISEASE

In most veterinary practices heart cases are treated at home but a few specialized centres are being established and any RANA employed in such a place would receive very careful instruction in care of cardiac patients. Sometimes, however, heart cases are admitted for a few days to get a patient stabilized on digitalis or one of its fractions. The basic thing to remember with any animal with faulty cardiac function is that the heart is not fully capable of pumping blood round the body to keep the organs and tissues adequately oxygenated; a heart that is capable of maintaining circulation in the *resting* animal may not be able to do so under any form of stress. From this statement it follows logically that rest is of the utmost importance and in severe cases, which may present as apparently acute, a few days' confinement to kennel or cage can work wonders. It is not only physical exercise which produces stress; any form of excitement, pleasurable or the reverse, can also make sudden increased demand on the circulation and cause worsening of the patient's condition, whether temporarily or permanently, thus the cardiac case must be handled with extreme care when giving necessary attention such as administering drugs by mouth or injection; forcible restraint is highly inadvisable and is to be avoided if at all possible; unfortunately, owing to poor blood supply to the brain, heart cases are often extremely irritable and resent even minor interferences. On the other hand, prescribed drugs *must* be given at the correct intervals. Excitement and playing must be minimized. Large bulky meals are to be avoided as the distended stomach causes pressure on the diaphragm and may impede still further the action of a failing heart.

Heart failure is not, as many believe, a sudden fatal episode; it is the state which arises when the faulty heart can no longer keep vital organs supplied adequately with oxygenated blood so that they, in their turn, cease to function; this state may last some time.

Heart attacks, although nothing like so common as in man, do occur in animals, especially dogs. They may take the form of a faint, when the brain suddenly ceases to receive adequate blood, and the animal just collapses unconscious and is quite limp when handled; this type of episode usually lasts only a matter of seconds—although it may seem much more to the observer!—and recovery is nearly always spontaneous; the state of complete physical rest which occurs during a fainting type attack is enough to allow blood supply to the brain to resume and consciousness returns. No positive action is required in this type of case other than to ensure adequate ventilation both from environment and by removal of any obstructions to the animal's own respiratory effort, e.g. a tight collar. Careful note should be taken of the colour of the mucous membrane during the attack, i.e. are they cyanosed (having a bluish tinge) or are they very pale. Pulse volume and rate may be checked. The form of stress which provoked the attack should be noted with a view to future avoidance if this is possible.

Heart attacks may also take another form in which cramp appears to be a feature. Since it is impossible to obtain subjective evidence of pain this can only be deduced from observation; the dog often looks apprehensive before showing signs of collapse; the collapse may be total or partial—in the latter case affecting one or more limbs. The limbs appear rigid as compared with the faint type attack. Sometimes the dog cries out prior to the attack. In this type of attack consciousness is not always fully lost as the failure is of circulation to limbs rather than brain; for this reason gentle massage of the limbs during an attack may accelerate recovery.

It is very difficult indeed to differentiate a heart attack from a fit as so much reliance has to be placed on the owner's description; it is therefore most important for the RANA to observe closely during an attack and report in minute detail to the veterinary surgeon. Urine and/or faeces may be voided involuntarily during either a fit or heart attack. One useful point is that whereas the cardiac patient appears completely normal in behaviour as soon as consciousness returns, the fit case often does not; there is a phase during which the dog wanders aimlessly and does not respond to normal stimuli such as being called by name. The actual differentiation of heart attacks and fits is for the veterinary surgeon but the RANA's observations may be crucial in arriving at a decision.

The basic treatment of cardiac disease is obviously for the veterinarian but occasionally first-aid measures may be called for; the obvious requirement is for more oxygen so that some form of oxygen administration will always help—this has been dealt with in more detail elsewhere. The administration of stimulants such as alcohol is usually better deferred for professional advice.

RESPIRATORY DISEASE

Antibiotics and sulphonamides have revolutionized the treatment of most serious and acute respiratory disease, and nursing, whilst still important, is seldom the vital factor it was.

Diseases of the respiratory system include those affecting the nasal chambers, larynx and trachea, bronchi and lungs, as well as less usual organs such as the soft palate.

Respiratory disease is characterized by a change in respiration which may be reflected in rate, depth, noisiness and distress; coughing, sneezing, snorting and gasping may also occur. Animals whose lung tissue has become partially consolidated by pneumonia or tumour deposits have a greatly reduced oxygen exchange level and show "air hunger"; in the dog a characteristic puffing out of the lips and cheeks at every respiratory effort is very typical—it is a very serious sign. Collapse of lung tissue will occur from any pressure within the thorax but outside the lungs, e.g. air or blood in the thorax of the dog (pneumo- or haemo-thorax) and pus in the chest of the cat (pyothorax); the signs seen in such cases are exaggerated respiratory effort, the animal making an obvious conscious effort either to draw in or expel air (inspiratory or expiratory dyspnoea); affected animals often stand with elbows abducted and find difficulty in lying down and sleeping.

Any extra effort induced by struggling, etc., may precipitate a fatal crisis; great care must be taken when positioning such patients for radiography and a careful check must be kept on respiration, pulse and colour of mucous membranes.

The RANA must note the type of respiration and the character of any cough. In dogs which have a productive cough it is usual for a spasm of coughing to end in a retching effort and owners often, mistakenly, describe this as vomiting. The noisy, harsh cough of "kennel cough" is loud and non-productive. Any sudden change of temperature, excitement, barking or pulling on a lead may provoke an attack of coughing.

Although it is unlikely that dogs and cats with a respiratory infection will be admitted for nursing, an outbreak of such disease in kennels or cattery often does occur and the nursing staff becomes involved willy-nilly.

Some good general rules for nursing respiratory cases are:

Maintenance of good ventilation without draughts (if electric heating is used, see that the air does not get too dry).

Regular and frequent cleaning of the nose (and eyes) when nasal discharge is a feature; Vaseline smeared on the nostrils helps to avoid drying and cracking.

Avoidance of sudden change of temperatures (e.g. at exercise) and of excitement or struggling.

Care to be taken when administering drugs by mouth.

Presentation of appetizing food with an attractive smell.

HEAT-STROKE

This merits special mention as first-aid treatment may save a life. Heat-stroke occurs in dogs fairly regularly, mainly in hot weather and under conditions of stress such as dog shows or being shut in an inadequately ventilated car; the breeds with short faces and poor airways are the most prone. The animal is panting and salivating and may be collapsed; temperature is usually 41·6°C (107°F) and upwards, often "over the top", i.e. above 43·3°C (110°F). The dog must be put in a cool, shady, airy place, *not* shut in a kennel. Temperature *must* be reduced rapidly if irreversible brain damage is not to occur and this is best done by sousing the dog in cold water, under a tap or from a hose. The rectal temperature should be taken every 10–15 minutes and as soon as it is obviously dropping steadily the cold-water treatment may be stopped. Chlorpromazine (Largactil) by injection is useful but should not be given without reference to a veterinary surgeon.

DISEASES OF THE DIGESTIVE SYSTEM

The special nursing related to surgery of the alimentary tract has been dealt with elsewhere. Non-surgical abnormalities include inflammation and changes secondary to other conditions, e.g. nephritis.

Vomiting and/or diarrhoea are common symptoms.

Vomiting

Dogs vomit easily and quickly whereas cats vomit less often and the retching efforts often seem distressing and even painful. Anything which causes repeated vomiting in the dog may quickly result in establishing a "habit" of vomiting—this can happen within a few hours—and in such cases it is often necessary to give a drug which has a depressant effect on the vomiting centre in the brain. In the majority of cases of acute vomiting it is customary to withhold all solid food for 24 hours; since dehydration results quickly from loss of fluid in the vomit it is essential to administer fluid by some route. Vomiting dogs are naturally very thirsty and if left unchecked will drink large quantities of water which they promptly return. Fluid by mouth is valuable if it can be retained; it is therefore given in small quantities frequently, 7–25 ml at $\frac{1}{2}$- to 1-hourly intervals; boiled water or normal saline with glucose added is frequently prescribed. The old-fashioned remedy of beaten egg-white, glucose and brandy can still be very useful in the severe vomiting case; since egg-white is albumen this must not be given to any animals with any kidney disease. Failing retention of fluid by mouth parenteral fluids will normally be ordered. Once vomiting is under control the next step is a gradual return to normal diet and this change should occupy 3–4 days at least. Foods must be of a demulcent (soothing) type so that the sensitive mucous lining of the stomach is not further irritated. Plain milk leaves a heavy and somewhat indigestible curd in the stomach and so is best avoided for the first 24 hours. Predigested milk foods such as Bengers, or complete diets such as Complan, are useful at this stage. Hydrolysed protein, invalid meat extracts and sieved baby foods are the next stage. After this milky cereal-type food such as Farex, milk pudding, cornflour, etc., can be introduced. Protein is reintroduced gradually in such forms as fish, chicken, veal, rabbit or tripe (dressed) and the return to normal feeding is attained between days 4 and 7.

When vomiting is due to some underlying pathological condition such as pyometra or nephritis attention is primarily directed to treating these.

Diarrhoea

Diarrhoea implies the frequent passage of faeces of abnormally soft consistency; it is not genuine diarrhoea if an animal merely passes unformed stools once or twice daily. Diarrhoea is a symptom of many diseases and often it is the underlying illness, e.g. canine distemper, which has to be treated. Diarrhoea is a feature of bacterial gastro-enteritis and it is not uncommon to get outbreaks of diarrhoea in hospital kennels. Whilst in an individual case this may be due to change of diet, if several animals are scouring it is more likely to be of an infectious nature. Such episodes should be reported without delay. Modern antibiotic and/or sulphonamide treatments usually check bacterial enteritis very quickly.

In cases of diarrhoea the RANA should note the following points:

Frequency, consistence, colour, presence of blood and/or mucus, any undue straining during defaecation, change of odour and consistence after an interval of 1–2 hours from the time of being passed.

Great care is required in cleanliness of feeding and drinking utensils and in disinfecting exercise areas. Dogs and cats with profuse coats may need attention to soiled "trousers". Ulceration of the anus is common in cases of prolonged diarrhoea, gentle washing and powdering with talc will help.

Some animals with diarrhoea continue to eat well but it is customary to withhold flesh protein foods for 24–72 hours in acute cases. Easily digested carbohydrates are substituted, cereals, rice, milk puddings, arrowroot, cornflour, plain sweet biscuits and plain cake (e.g. Madeira) may be offered. Gradual return to normal diet is again the rule.

Dogs and cats with liver disease may show vomiting, usually of bile-stained fluid, and/or diarrhoea; faeces are often orange or yellow in colour. Many liver patients are dull and off food but when possible diet should include readily available carbohydrates such as glucose and good-quality, lean protein. Fats must be avoided. When milk is used the cream should be discarded.

Cases of pancreatic deficiency often pass unformed, bulky and greasy stools. Treatment has to be specific following confirmatory tests and diet should initially exclude fat.

Miscellaneous causes of digestive disturbance include colic due to eating windfall apples—dogs surprisingly often do this. Indigestion following eating of mutton bones and impaction of the large bowel after excessive quantities of any type of bone. Dogs and cats with impaction (in cats the cause is usually hair) strain a great deal and often pass small quantities of fluid only, thus giving rise to misleading reports of diarrhoea; after a few days they go off food and start vomiting. Treatments, according to the severity of the case, include bulk laxatives (e.g. Isogel, All-Bran) *not* purgatives; salines such as Epsom salts, enemata or even manual relief under anaesthesia.

DISEASES OF THE URINARY SYSTEM

The commonest diseases of the urinary system which the RANA is likely to encounter are nephritis (inflammation of the kidneys), cystitis (inflammation of the urinary bladder) and urinary calculi (stones).

Nephritis

Whilst primary leptospiral nephritis can be a severe and acute disease it may also occur in subclinical form which passes unnoticed. The type of nephritis seen most commonly in the dog and cat results in scarring of the kidney tissue and progressive decrease in function. It is often seen as a chronic disease in the older dog and cat but even so the animal's state of health may vary from apparent normality to quite severe illness. Because kidney function is impaired waste products are not so efficiently excreted and to compensate for this a greater volume of dilute urine has to be produced if urea is not to reach a dangerously high concentration in the blood and other tissues; because an increased volume of urine has to be produced water intake likewise has to be increased so that thirst is a very common feature of nephritic animals. Indeed the cardinal signs of nephritis are reduced appetite, increased thirst, vomiting and weight loss and any hospitalized dog or cat showing any or all of these signs should be reported at once.

Many older animals which have never been suspected of having kidney disease have attained a state of balance or compensation; change of routine such as occurs on admission to hospital rapidly upsets this delicate balance. The main factors are the altered water intake and opportunity for urination, either of which can precipitate an animal from an apparently healthy state to obvious nephritis; both factors in combination are very likely to do so.

Dogs and cats with advanced kidney disease may become uraemic and often an ammonial or urinous odour can be detected on the breath; should the RANA note such an odour or should she see ulcers in the mouth she should at once report it as this will signify a very sick animal.

It is customary in cases of renal disease to put the patient on to a low protein diet; the purpose of this change is to reduce the part of the diet which results in the greatest work for the kidneys, viz. excretion of the breakdown products of protein, especially urea. It is very nice and easy to say that a given dog or cat must be fed a diet containing little or no protein; dogs and cats are essentially carnivorous and normally prefer protein foods; nephritic animals have a reduced appetite in any case and to transfer them to a less palatable diet is often easier said than done. It is rather futile to insist that a patient has no protein and make it starve itself in consequence! This may sound absurd but is often true, especially of cats. It is therefore necessary to strike a balance between maintaining adequate nutrition and amending the diet as recommended. Protein may be provided in the form of the hydrolysed product whereby essential amino-acids are absorbed without involving kidney function, but to maintain animals on these for long periods is both time consuming and costly. Complete invalid diets such as Complan are invaluable but are not particularly appetising and again are costly. Carbohydrates are usually freely permitted but again it may be difficult to get the patient to accept adequate amounts; cereals, rice, bread, plain cake such as Madeira and the plainer sweet biscuit are in order; milk and glucose are valuable. If protein as flesh products has to be fed to maintain basic nutrition it is customary to supply the more digestible high-quality foods such as chicken, veal, tripe, fish, rabbit and, if necessary, lamb; red meat is best omitted. Once again the preferred regime is little and often; it is useless to confront a nephritic dog or cat with one bulky meal daily.

Water intake should be limited by the methods detailed earlier. Water should never be totally withheld from animals with renal disease but the amount taken at any one time should be controlled to avoid causing vomiting.

Cystitis

This is common in both dogs and cats; bitches are more frequently affected than male dogs. The inflammation may be due to bacterial infection or to mechanical irritation from the presence of stones. Animals with cystitis have a desire to urinate frequently; they usually pass only small amounts at one time and considerable straining may be noted. Blood may be seen either mixed with the urine or being passed as drops at the end of urination. Any sign of increased frequency, undue straining or blood associated with urination (haematuria) should be noted and reported. The urine voided should be carefully inspected for the presence of blood, mucus, small stones or gravelly material; whenever possible collect a specimen in a clean container while the animal is urinating. The RANA should make sure that the animal does succeed in passing urine as cases of obstruction to urine flow are urgent.

Diagnosis and treatment are matters for the veterinary surgeon but animals with cystitis should usually be encouraged to drink plenty of water so that urine may be kept as dilute as possible.

Urinary Calculi

These are common in the dog (both sexes) but in the cat tend to occur as a sandy material rather than actual stones.

They are sometimes found in the kidneys of dogs but they rarely cause clinical signs; they occur in the bladder where they often cause cystitis. In male dogs and cats obstruction of the urethra is a frequent problem, in the former due to lodging of smallish stones, often just behind the os penis; in the latter due to accumulation of a sandy type of debris.

Urethral obstruction is a serious condition requiring prompt attention; it causes great discomfort so that early relief is required on humanitarian grounds, it is also necessary to prevent serious and possibly fatal sequelae.

Dogs attempt repeatedly to urinate and although usually cocking their legs in the early stages they soon revert to the straddled stance of puppyhood. Cats squat and strain and the penis may be seen protruding from the prepuce; it can be difficult to differentiate attempts to urinate or defaecate in the cat and when an owner reports that the cat is constipated it should not be dismissed lightly with telephone advice to administer laxatives; any cat reported as constipated should be examined as soon as feasible by the veterinary surgeon to ensure that it is not a case of urinary obstruction.

Diet in relation to formation of urinary calculi has been dealt with previously.

ENDOCRINE DISEASES

The RANA is most likely to be concerned with cases of diabetes mellitus; most other endocrine diseases will be more the concern of the diagnostician than the RANA.

Diabetes mellitus is due to failure of certain specialized cells in the pancreas, the islets of Langerhans, to produce sufficient insulin; this results in defective carbohydrate digestion with consequent abnormally high sugar levels being found in the blood and, in the later stages, degenerative fatty changes occur in the liver. Diabetes occurs in both dogs and cats although the latter species is often, mistakenly, regarded as not being prone to the disease.

Most diabetic dogs are, or have been, overweight or even frankly obese but they lose weight when the disease is fully developed and severe. Increased thirst is the most significant early clinical sign. In severe cases sugar can be detected in the urine; in milder cases the urine is sugar free but the blood glucose levels are abnormally high. Diagnosis therefore depends on the detection of glucose in blood or urine and the RANA will be asked to assist by obtaining specimens at the right time.

For an accurate estimation of blood glucose the sample is best examined within a few hours of being taken and it should be obtained not less than 5 hours after the last meal, i.e. it will be a "fasting" blood-sugar. This may mean some change in feeding routine to fit in with laboratory requirements. The last meal before blood sampling should not have contained a large quantity of carbohydrates, especially sugar, as a false positive result *can* be shown by even a normal dog which has recently eaten a rich carbohydrate meal!

Urine samples must be obtained with great care as even the smallest trace of sugar (in any form) will give a false positive reaction.

Insulin by injection is undoubtedly the most efficient treatment for diabetes. The dose has to be established for each individual animal as also has the particular type of insulin to be used; depending on the type of insulin injections may have to be given as often as twice daily although once may be sufficient with certain types. It is sometimes decided to admit a patient to hospital kennels for "balancing"; this term implies working out the dose of insulin which will reduce or eliminate sugar from the urine and stabilize the animals's condition as regards appetite, thirst and body-weight; when easily available repeated blood glucose estimations are included in the balancing regime. The diet must also be adjusted to reduce or even eliminate carbohydrates. A diet of lean meat and vegetable is often prescribed but after balancing on insulin and diet a small proportion of carbohydrate (not more than 25% of the total ration) may be permitted. The RANA will be responsible for controlling the diet, giving injections of insulin at the correct times (this is often suggested just before or even during a meal; in the latter instance dogs often continue feeding without even noticing the prick!) and carefully watching for signs of hypoglycaemia, i.e. an abnormally low blood sugar caused by too much insulin and/or too little food; the signs of hypoglycaemia are restlessness, trembling and eventually leg weakness, collapse and coma. Should severe hypoglycaemia occur and the veterinary surgeon not be available some glucose water should be given by mouth or, if the animal can and will swallow voluntarily, a knob or two of sugar may be offered.

SKIN DISEASES

Some veterinary hospitals admit cases of contagious skin disease for treatment, some do not; most will admit non-contagious skin cases for attention.

It is neither possible nor necessary to go into the problems of diagnosis of canine and feline skin disease but certain general principles will apply.

Firstly the RANA must know if the condition can be transmitted in any way, e.g. is it sarcoptic mange, ringworm, flea or louse infestation? If so appropriate steps must be taken to eliminate infection on the patient according to prescribed treatment, to isolate it from contact with other patients and to deal appropriately with bedding and kennel structure.

If it is not contagious, is self-mutilation a problem, i.e. is the patient making matters worse by biting or scratching affected areas? If it is, steps may need to be taken to prevent self-damage although the prime concern is always to remove the cause of the irritation; even so biting and licking can become a habit and it may be necessary to keep an area permanently covered or to prevent the patient being able to reach the lesion by providing a restraining type of collar such as a plastic bucket fitted over the head and neck. Some dogs are very cunning and are never *seen* to bite or lick a lesion but careful observation shows that they are doing so when they think they are not being watched.

The RANA must also have some idea of whether the dressing being used is in any way toxic; if it is, great care must be taken to ensure that the patient cannot ingest it by licking. In the case of dusting powder applied to the whole body surface it is always wise to remove excess from the surface of the coat by wiping the animal down with a duster or chamois leather; this is especially necessary in cats.

Medicated baths are often prescribed and common-sense precautions must be observed. The therapeutic agent must be used in the correct dilution—too concentrated a bath could be toxic and too dilute it will not do the job. The bath must be of appropriate temperature; a useful guide is that the water feels pleasantly warm but not hot to one's own hands. Rinsing, if prescribed, must be thorough. Care must be taken not to get the medicated fluid into eyes or ears; a smear of Vaseline along the eyelids will assist, so will a small piece of cotton-wool introduced into the ear canal but *not* put in too deeply as it *must* be removed immediately after the bath. Thorough drying is a must, whether by towels, paper towels or hair-dryer; change of temperature should be avoided for several hours after a bath.

If local dressings are to be applied to a circumscribed area this should be done carefully; an excess of ointment, cream or lotion should be avoided and care should be taken not to spread it over adjoining normal skin.

It is often necessary to clip hair from a suppurating lesion such as a patch of wet eczema or around an infected bite wound; sedation may be necessary to do this efficiently and humanely. Blunt-ended curved on flat scissors are best used and an area around the lesion should also be clipped. Bathing with diluted hydrogen peroxide often helps in dealing with suppurating skin lesions. The aim is to remove all hair, exudate and scab and the resulting area should—surprisingly—look very red and raw; healing will take place from the edges; clipping may need to be repeated every few days.

DISEASES OF THE NERVOUS SYSTEM

There are numerous pathological conditions of both the central and peripheral nervous systems, most of which pose problems of differential diagnosis to the veterinary surgeon but are not very likely to be encountered as nursing problems. Two important categories with which the RANA will come into contact are fits and paraplegia.

Fits

The term fit denotes an episode arising from the central nervous system, directly or indirectly, characterized by spasm of muscles, loss of consciousness, often salivation and sometimes urinary and faecal incontinence during the attack. Sometimes the signs of any or all of the above are so slight that they are barely noticeable. The term convulsion is often used synonymously.

Broadly speaking fits may be due to epilepsy; inflammatory change in the brain or its coverings (encephalitis and meningitis); degenerative changes in the brain due to an infection, especially canine distemper; pressure from an abnormal mass in the brain such as tumour, cyst or haemorrhage; some of the modern organic poisons; heavy round worm infestations in very young puppies; occasionally during the teething phase in pups; sudden drop in blood sugar (e.g. during acute virus hepatitis), i.e. hypoglycaemia and occasionally due to stress in neurotic subjects, e.g. a poodle shut in a car. This is not an exhaustive list of the causes of fits but covers most of the common ones.

A fit can vary from a prolonged convulsive seizure during which the dog falls to its side, shows galloping movements of the limbs, champs the jaws, salivates, urinates and/or defaecates and consciousness is lost; to the mildest of episodes when the dog may do no more than draw up one limb and/or turn its head to one side; the latter is usually a very mild manifestation of epilepsy. Once the convulsive phase has passed most patients go through a phase lasting anything from 30 seconds to 1 hour during which they tend to wander aimlessly, may bump into obstacles and do not recognize or respond to the owner; this is the one period when the patient may be aggressive if handled or restrained.

The RANA's main duties in connection with fits fall into three categories: (1) management of the patient during a fit, (2) first-aid measures and/or telephone advice when the veterinary surgeon is not available and (3) close observation of patients suspected of having fits.

1. *Management.* There is, in effect, very little which can be done. If it is possible to ensure quietness, reduced light and freedom from all danger from furniture, etc., this should be done but it is not wise to handle and move the animal during the convulsive phase so the necessary adjustments should be made to its environment at the time. On no account should physical restraint be applied to a convulsing dog or cat. Neither should the patient be handled or restrained during the post-convulsive phase of automatic behaviour; no handling should be attempted until the animal itself makes some obvious sign of recognition and normal response.

2. From the above it will be realized that first-aid measures are virtually nil and may simply be removal of the patient from the distressed owner; if the veterinary surgeon can be contacted by telephone instructions may be given to administer a sedative injection. Because of the wide range of causes of fits it is not possible to recommend any injection which can routinely be used in all circumstances. Tranquillizing drugs are ineffective in controlling convulsions.

More often the RANA will need to give telephone advice to an owner whose dog or cat is having a fit for the first time. It is imperative to ensure that the owner does not attempt to restrain the dog but advice to subdue the light, reduce noise and remove all possible objects from the room are both useful and keep the owner occupied. As previously stated the owner also must be advised not to handle the animal until it clearly recognizes them.

Reassurance is also required. Owners need assuring that the patient is not suffering as it is unconscious and therefore unaware of its condition; it is the onlooker who is distressed. Owners often ask if a dog subject to fits is dangerous; the owner can safely be assured that such dogs will not be aggressive *unless* forcible physical restraint is attempted during the convulsive or post-convulsive period when it may bite in resisting restraint; it will not attack. The exception, of course, is the rabid dog but this problem does not exist in Great Britain outside quarantine kennels.

3. *Observation.* Occasionally a patient may be admitted to hospital for observation of episodes reported by the owner. Unfortunately change of environment often results in fits ceasing for the time being! The RANA should closely observe all

physical signs shown by the patient, try to decide how long consciousness is impaired and note any factor, e.g. noise, which precipitates an episode. These observations may be of critical importance in assisting the veterinary surgeon to arrive at a diagnosis.

PARAPLEGIA

This term implies paralysis of the hindquarters. In small animal patients the commonest cause is disease of the intervertebral discs of the dog. Accidents resulting in fracture and/or dislocation of the vertebral column may also cause paraplegia. It is unlikely that the RANA will encounter the dog which is paraplegic due to canine distemper other than at consultation in the surgery.

The nursing of a paraplegic dog, whatever the cause, is both time-consuming and demanding if the patient is to be maintained in a reasonable condition. Recovery may take weeks or even months.

In the early stage the dog may suffer physical and/or mental distress. Pain is controlled by the use of appropriate analgesic drugs; mental distress and anxiety is controlled by tranquillising drugs.

Rest is of vital importance, hence confinement to the smallest cage compatible with the patient being able to lie stretched out should be the rule. Once the early pain has passed dogs will drag themselves around quite briskly on their forelimbs. In the early stages (10 to 21 days) at least this is highly undesirable.

If the patient is totally recumbent, i.e. unable to raise itself by its forequarters, it should be turned from side to side at regular intervals, not less than twice daily, to reduce the risk of bed-sores and hypostatic congestion of the lungs.

Foam rubber pads or doubled nylon fur fabric is excellent for bedding provided the bored patient is not able to make a meal of it! Newspaper or blankets must be changed frequently.

If the dog is incontinent great care is needed to keep the coat and skin sweet and clean. Frequent washing, drying and powdering is essential.

Food should be light, of good quality, low residue and given in several small feeds daily. Water drinking should be encouraged to keep urine dilute and reduce the risk of cystitis.

Many paraplegic animals lose the ability to urinate and defaecate; the former is infinitely more important than the latter although the laxative-loving British public take a lot of convincing! It is essential that the bladder be emptied at least twice daily. Catheters are sometimes used but if the bladder can be effectively emptied by pressure alone—and this is usually possible—risk of introducing infection is reduced.

Bladder emptying is usually achieved by applying pressure by both hands to the abdomen; supporting the dog in a standing or squatting posture will help as will taking it to a place it associates with urination. It is important to empty the bladder as completely as possible as persistence of residual urine predisposes to cystitis.

Bowel emptying is far less important and if faeces are passed every second or third day this may well suffice. Sometimes stimulation of the anal area will result in passage of faeces; a small sliver of soap inserted into the rectum often has the desired effect but in obstinate cases a warm soapy enema will be required.

Anything which the nurse can do to amuse and occupy the patient's attention will be most helpful—time permitting.

In dogs recovering from paraplegia various methods may be employed to assist this process.

Infra-red irradiation to the spine, massage, passive movement of joints and assisted walking, e.g. by supporting the hindquarters with a scarf, may all be prescribed. Warm or hot baths are occasionally recommended.

The case of the paraplegic is exacting, sometimes depressing, but very rewarding when evidence of returning function is at last seen.

(f) DISPENSING

J. Stratton

Introduction

Dispensing is the science and art of compounding and preparing drugs for administration to the patient. Today the manufacturing chemist performs most of the operations which were formerly in the province of the veterinary dispenser. However, the RANA is expected not only to be able to measure or weigh out the correct amount of a preparation from a bulk container but also to be able, if necessary, to make simple preparations.

The Dispensary

The door of the dispensary should have a lock and the room should be fitted with a work bench, with water tap and sink, gas tap and electric plug. Shelves should be arranged to avoid stretching or bending when reaching for stock bottles. A cupboard fitted with a lock should be reserved for poisons (see below). Those items in common use should be arranged conveniently to hand. Only stock for the day-to-day running of the animal hospital need be carried, and drugs may be stored elsewhere in bulk. Some system of stock control should be used so that, on the one hand, supplies are adequate for any emergency at any time and, on the other hand, excessive stocks are not carried or allowed to deteriorate through prolonged storage. A refrigerator is required for the storage of vaccines and sera.

EQUIPMENT

Dispensing balance class B (accurate to 12 mg)* with set of weights 50 mg to 50 g.
Domestic or commercial balance with set of weights 50 to 500 g or 1 kg.
Glass measures—10 ml, 100 ml, 250 ml and 500 ml or 1 litre.
Graduated pipette, 0·1–1·0 ml.
Funnels—glass and plastic, various sizes.
Spatulas—large, medium and small.
Glass stirring rods.
Pestles and mortars—large and small.
Dispensing paper, labels, bottles and corks, ointment boxes, tablet envelopes, etc.

Reference books: *British Veterinary Codex*; *Pharmaceutical Handbook* (published by the Pharmaceutical Society); Manufacturers' catalogues and price lists; Dispensary book.

* Class A balance (accurate to 3 mg) only used for weighing small quantities of toxic drugs and not required for normal dispensing operations.

PRESCRIPTIONS

A prescription is simply a written request to the dispenser in the following form:

Address of Prescriber
Date

℞

Make }	*Names and amounts of drugs or preparation*
Supply }	*Instructions to dispenser*
Label	*Title*
	Instructions to client
	FOR ANIMAL TREATMENT ONLY

Client's name and address

Prescriber's signature and qualifications

If the prescriber's intention is not quite clear the dispenser should immediately contact him to discover what is required.

The animal nursing auxiliary is rarely called upon to dispense a formal prescription; more often a simple written instruction is given. An animal nursing auxiliary should *never* dispense from verbal instructions, except under the *direct* and *immediate* supervision of the veterinary surgeon.

ROUTINE

1. Read the prescription and check the doses.
2. Record the prescription in the dispensing book.
3. Write the label.
4. Place stock bottles required on the work bench and check the labels with the prescription. Weigh or measure out the amount required and replace each stock bottle on the shelf as it is used. Poisons should be added last.
5. Perform the appropriate operations.
6. Check the label and the prescription, label and wrap.
7. Clean dispensing equipment and bench.

The purpose of this routine is to avoid errors. The dispenser must be accurate. When weighing or measuring poisons a witness should always check the operation.

LABELLING

The label should have a title. It must bear the words "For animal treatment only" and the name and address of the veterinary surgeon. The instructions to the client should be quite clear. Normally printed labels are used and it is only necessary for the dispenser to write in the title and the instructions, for example:

> FOR ANIMAL TREATMENT ONLY
>
> *The tablets for Mrs. Smith's Boxer dog*
> *One tablet to be given every 8 hours*
>
> A. N. Other, BVetMed, MRCVS,
> 42 Main Street, Any Town.

If the preparation is to be handed to the client it may be wrapped in dispensing paper and sealed with sealing wax or adhesive tape.

OPERATIONS

Weighing. The dispensing or pharmaceutical balance has a closed pan on the left for the weights and an open pan on the right for the powder. Powders are only added to the open pan or removed from it with a spatula when the beam is in the down position. Before using a balance check that it is clean and properly adjusted. Take care not to spill drugs on the balance or the weights.

Household or commercial balances are used in the same way.

Measuring. Liquids are measured in the appropriate sized glass measure. The measure is designed to be read at eye level and the bottom of the meniscus is employed. A measure is calibrated to measure not to deliver, so it should be rinsed after use and the rinsings should be added to the preparation.

Pipettes are calibrated to deliver so the question of rinsing does not arise.

Manipulations. Solids and semi-solids are manipulated with a spatula of convenient size. Solids are reduced to a finer state in a mortar by pounding with a pestle. The pestle and mortar are also used for mixing powders and the preparation of suspensions and emulsions. Solutions are made in a glass beaker or measure and the process is speeded by the use of a glass stirring rod.

Preparations for Administration by Mouth

Capsules. The medicament is enclosed in a gelatin or other suitable envelope. Although capsules are usually purchased ready filled, it is possible to obtain empty capsules and to fill them by hand, but this is only necessary or economical in exceptional circumstances.

Electuaries. The powdered medicament is mixed with treacle or honey and smeared on the animal's tongue. As it is difficult to divide the electuary mass into doses accurately, it is better to supply individual doses of the medicament in powder form with instructions for the client to mix each dose with treacle or honey. Some ready-made electuaries are available, particularly those designed for the treatment of coughing in horses (often termed cough pastes).

Emulsions. An emulsion is a combination of two immiscible liquids (e.g. oil and water) the one being dispersed in the other and stabilized by an emulsifying agent. Preparations which are titled emulsion are fluid preparations for administration by mouth and are oil in water emulsions, e.g. cod-liver oil emulsion, liquid paraffin emulsion. It is possible to make this type of emulsion by hand, but it is most conveniently purchased ready made. Emulsions are dispensed in wide-mouth bottles and labelled "Shake the Bottle".

Mixtures. Mixtures are solutions or suspensions of drugs in water or other suitable vehicles designed to be administered by mouth. Mixtures are divisible into doses. If the bottle contains only a single dose, the preparation is properly termed a draught or drench. Most mixtures are purchased in bulk but they can be prepared by hand. The following system is used:

1. Soluble solids are dissolved. If there is more than one soluble solid in the mixture they are dissolved separately and the solutions are mixed.
2. Insoluble solids are suspended. More than one insoluble solid can be suspended at the same time.
3. Liquids are measured separately and diluted before being mixed.

All these operations are carried out before the mixture is placed in the bottle. It is impossible to make satisfactory mixtures in the bottle.

Colourless solutions are sometimes coloured by the addition of burnt sugar solution.

Suspensions must be labelled "Shake the Bottle".

Pills. Pills are spherical masses for administration by mouth. It is possible but tedious to prepare pills by hand.

Powders. Powders are still dispensed for large animals. They may be supplied in bulk, but usually they are divided into doses and each dose is separately wrapped. When a powder contains more than one powdered ingredient it will be necessary to mix them together. If the ingredients are of the same colour and texture, it will be necessary to incorporate a colouring agent to assist the mixing process. Armenian bole, which is insoluble and inert, is used for this purpose. Innocuous powders are mixed in bulk and then divided into doses. If the powder contains a toxic ingredient this should be weighed out dose by dose so that there is no possibility that each individual powder contains other than the proper amount.

Tablets. Tablets are prepared by compression and are essentially machine made.

Preparations for Parenteral Administration

Implants. Implants are sterile cylinders or discs of medicaments, produced by fusion or compression, designed to be introduced subcutaneously and to be absorbed over long periods. Implants are essentially machine made.

Injections. Injections are sterile aqueous or oily solutions or suspensions. Most injections are purchased but certain of the aqueous solutions used in large volumes in cattle practice may be prepared by hand, e.g. calcium borogluconate, magnesium sulphate, dextrose. The medicament is dissolved in freshly prepared distilled water (prepared by the process described in the pharmacopoeia for water for injection). The solution is filtered into a suitable container and sealed, usually with a rubber bung and metal screw cap. The preparation is then sterilized in an autoclave, at a temperature of 115 to 116°C, which is attained if the steam pressure in the autoclave is 10 lb/in^2 in excess of normal atmospheric pressure.

Containers of	100 ml	should be held	for	30	minutes
,,	250 ml	,,	,,	40	,,
,,	500 ml	,,	,,	45	,,
,,	1 litre	,,	,,	50	,,

Intramammary injections. It is not practicable to prepare intramammary injection by hand.

Preparations for Topical Application

All preparations for external application are labelled "For external use only" and liquids are dispensed in bottles of distinctive shape.

Creams, see *Ointments*.

Dusting powders. Dusting powders used for the control of ectoparasites are conveniently purchased ready packed in sprinkler topped containers or puffer packs.

Eye lotions. Eye lotions are freshly prepared solutions of medicaments in freshly boiled purified water used for the irrigation of the conjunctival sac. Eye lotions are usually dispensed in concentrated form with instructions to dilute with an equal volume of warm water. The final dilution should be isotonic to lacrimal secretion, otherwise discomfort is produced. Rinse the apparatus and a coloured fluted bottle with freshly boiled purified water before dispensing the eye lotion and filter it into the bottle. Close the bottle with a glass stopper or a screwcap with a polythene liner; corks should not be used.

Eye ointments. It is possible but not convenient or economic to prepare eye ointments by hand as they must be sterile and free from irritant particles. It is much more convenient to purchase them ready made and ready packed in collapsible tubes.

Eye drops. Eye drops are aqueous or oily solutions of medicaments. They must be sterile, free from irritant particles and isotonic to lacrimal secretion. While it is possible to dispense eye drops by hand it is far more convenient to purchase them ready made and packed in dropper bottles.

Liniments. Liniments usually have stimulating properties and are massaged into the skin. It is convenient to purchase liniments in bulk. However, it is traditional in large animal practice to prepare a turpentine oil and ammonia liniment by hand usually to a recipe which has been handed down from father to son for several generations. White liniment *BVetC* is a modern version of this traditional liniment. This type of liniment is an emulsion and must be labelled "Shake the Bottle".

Lotions. Lotions are liquid preparations for external application. They may be aqueous or alcoholic solutions or suspensions. They are prepared in the same way as Mixtures (q.v.). Suspensions must be labelled "Shake the Bottle".

Ointments. Ointments are semi-solid preparations for application to the skin. The more fluid preparations are known as creams. Ointments and creams are usually purchased either in bulk or in ready-packed collapsible tubes. It is possible to make this type of preparation by hand. The medicaments can be incorporated into the base by hard labour with a spatula upon an ointment slab, or the base can be heated in a double saucepan and melted when the medicaments are stirred in.

In large animal practice either of these methods may be used for the preparation of strong mercuric iodide ointment *BVetC* (Red Blister).

The usual ointment base is white or yellow soft paraffin. Animal fats may be used, e.g. lard or wool fat (lanolin).

Many modern ointments and cream bases are synthetic emulsions. The oil-in-water type of emulsion base gives the water soluble ointment or cream which can easily be removed from the skin.

Legal Obligations

In Great Britain only registered veterinary surgeons are legally qualified to diagnose animal disease, treat sick animals, or to prescribe for them. Similarly, only registered pharmaceutical chemists are legally qualified to dispense prescriptions issued by registered medical practitioners, dentists or veterinary surgeons.

The RANA or animal nursing auxiliary trainee, and other veterinary aides can only treat sick animals or dispense medicines for them under the direct and immediate supervision of a registered veterinary surgeon.

Veterinary aides must at all times be circumspect in their dealings with the general public. In particular they must not supply medicines to a client without reference to the veterinary surgeon, for the majority of drugs are controlled by law.

There is nothing in the law to stop anyone rendering *first aid* to an animal in need of immediate attention, pending the arrival of a veterinary surgeon.

The Pharmacy Acts control the sale of those substances which can cause poisoning. The veterinary surgeon is concerned particularly with the Pharmacy and Poisons Act of 1933 and the various orders made thereunder. Certain drugs are available to the public on prescription only, including many of those commonly used in animal medicines, e.g.

Antihistamines, such as promethazine (Phenergan).
Barbiturates.

Tranquillizers, such as chlorpromazine (Largactil), promazine (Sparine).
Sulphonamides.
Phenylbutazine (Butazolidin).

The veterinary surgeon can obtain these drugs for animal treatment on a signed order. He can use them for the treatment of sick animals and he can supply them to his clients for the same purpose. Records should be kept and containers should be properly labelled using the system already quoted in these notes. No restrictions are placed on the storage of these drugs other than that the public should not have access to them, but it is obviously advisable to keep them in a locked cupboard, particularly the barbiturates.

The Therapeutic Substances Act, 1956, controls the manufacture and supply of various therapeutic agents. Part Two of the Act controls the sale, supply, dispensing and administration of the antibiotics, e.g. penicillin, streptomycin, chlortetracycline (Aureomycin), oxytetracycline (Terramycin), chloramphenicol (Chloromycetin), erythromycin, neomycin; and the corticosteroids, e.g. cortisone, hydrocortisone, prednisolone, dexamethasone, betamethasone (Betsolan), etc. These substances can be obtained by the veterinary surgeon for the treatment of animals, and they can only be administered to animals by him or by a person acting in accordance with his directions. The Medicines Act, 1968, will eventually replace the above legislation, but at the time of writing no orders have been made under this Act.

The Dangerous Drugs Act, 1965, is designed to prevent the misuse of the drugs which are habit-forming in man, these are the drugs of addiction often referred to as narcotics, e.g.

Opium.
Indian hemp (cannabis—"pot").
Morphine and diamorphine (heroin).
Cocaine.
Pethidine.
Diethylthiambutene (Thamalon).
Phenazocine (Narphen).

Registered veterinary surgeons can obtain these drugs for animal treatment. Records of all transactions must be kept in the form laid down in the Dangerous Drugs Regulations, in a register used for that purpose only. All drugs controlled by the Dangerous Drugs Act must be kept in a locked receptacle and the key must be kept by the veterinarian. Veterinary aides, including RANAs are not authorized to supply, procure or possess drugs controlled by the Dangerous Drugs Act. If in the course of their work they come across such a drug they should at once bring it to the attention of the veterinarian.

The Methylated Spirits Regulations, 1952, made under the Customs and Excise Act, 1952, control the supply of methylated spirit. A registered veterinary surgeon can obtain 4 gallons of mineralized methylated spirit or $\frac{1}{2}$ gallon of industrial methylated spirit at one time for animal treatment. If this is dispensed to a client, not more than 1 pint may be supplied for animal treatment and the container must be labelled "for external use only".

Weights and Measures

METRIC SYSTEM

Mass	1000 micrograms (μg or mcg)	= 1 milligram (mg or mgm)
	1000 milligrams	= 1 gramme (g)
	1000 grammes	= 1 kilogram (kg)
Volume	1000 millilitres (ml)	= 1 litre

Always write the units out in full rather than use abbreviations. The metric system should always be used in prescriptions and for dispensing.

HOUSEHOLD MEASURES

It is convenient, but inaccurate, to use an ordinary spoon to measure the dose of a mixture. There is considerable variation in the capacity of spoons.

A small teaspoon will hold approximately 3·5 ml (a coffee spoon holds rather less than this).
A large teaspoon will hold approximately 5 ml.
A dessertspoon will hold approximately 7 ml.
A tablespoon will hold approximately 14 ml or $\frac{1}{2}$ fl. oz.
A special 5-ml dosing spoon or a measuring glass should always be used to measure the dose of a mixture.

Obsolete Forms

LATIN

In the Middle Ages the universal language for medicine and pharmacy was Latin. The use of Latin in the writing of prescriptions persisted until the early part of the twentieth century. Today prescriptions are written in full in English. However, certain Latin abbreviations are sometimes employed, e.g.:

B.d.d., B.d.s., B.i.d.	twice a day
F., ft., fiat	make
Mitt., mitte	send
N.P., nom.prop.	label with proper name
Non rep., non repet.	do not repeat
Q.S.	sufficient quantity
Sig.	label
T.d.s., T.i.d.	three times a day

APOTHECARIES' SYSTEM

The Apothecaries' System of weights and measures also dates from the Middle Ages.

Mass The Apothecaries' grain is the same as the Imperial grain.
20 grains (gr xx) = 1 scruple (℈)
3 scruples (60 gr) = 1 drachm (ʒ)
8 drachms (480 gr) = 1 ounce (apothecaries) (℥)

Volume 60 minims (♏ x) = 1 fluid drachm (ʒ).
8 fluid drachms (480 minims) = 1 fluid ounce (℥).

IMPERIAL SYSTEM

The Imperial System of weights and measures is still used upon occasion; the grain, the minim and the fluid ounce are the same as in the Apothecaries' System.

Mass 437·5 grains (gr) = 1 ounce (avoirdupois) (oz)
16 ounces = 1 pound (lb).

Volume 480 minims (min) = 1 fluid ounce (fl. oz).
20 fluid ounces = 1 pint (pt).

Equivalents

Mass 1 grain = 0·0648 gramme.
1 ounce (avoirdupois) = 28·350 grammes.
1 ounce (apothecaries') = 31·104 grammes.
1 pound = 453·59 grammes.

Volume 1 minim = 0·059192 millilitre.
1 fluid ounce = 28·412 millilitres.
1 pint = 568·25 millilitres.

CHAPTER 6

Surgical Nursing

(a) GENERAL SURGICAL NURSING

D. G. EARNSHAW, MA, BSc, MRCVS

Inflammation

Whenever the body is injured either by violence (trauma), by bacteria (infection), chemical agents (corrosive burns), or heat (thermal) a defensive response is generally evoked by which the body attempts to curtail the extent of the injury and to initiate reparative measures. This interaction of causal factors and body responses is termed inflammation.

The essential changes occurring in the inflamed region are, firstly, an increase in the number of functioning blood and lymph vessels and dilatation of these vessels. Their walls become more permeable to fluid and cells. Later, cellular changes, such as fibrosis, predominate. The former are defensive measures, the latter reparative.

When the reaction occurs over a short period and is of some severity, the lesion is referred to as acute inflammation, whereas if the causal agent is applied over some time and provokes a prolonged but not such an intense reaction the inflammation is chronic. These terms are not very precise. An intermediate type of lesion is referred to as subacute. We also use the terms mild, moderate, marked and severe to indicate the intensity of the inflammatory reaction.

The picture of inflammation at the cellular level can be followed in more detail if we consider the case where the skin is broken, the subcutaneous tissues slightly damaged, and a number of pyogenic (pus-forming) bacteria enter the gap created. This is what we find in a small infected wound.

Blood vessels, at least of capillary size, may be damaged and there may be a little bleeding. The body defence mechanisms come into play, and at first there is a transient constriction of vessels in the area. Very shortly afterwards the vessels dilate and become more permeable to the passage of fluid and cells. The inflammatory zone becomes inundated by tissue fluid derived from the blood. Cells of various types, particularly polymorphs, invade the area and come into contact with bacteria; later other cells, including histiocytes, play some part in phagocytosis (engulfing bacteria). Pus may be formed from dead and disintegrating bacteria, polymorphs and other cells. In the later phases the outer part of the inflammatory zone is invaded by fibroblasts which produce fibrin and tend to wall off the region.

If early recovery occurs and the bacteria are killed with little or no frank sepsis (pus, suppuration) the products of cellular disintegration, increased tissue fluids, etc., are removed by the increased circulation. In such cases the fibrotic reaction is small and directed to repairing the tissue and everything heals up. Healing is known as resolution.

In the case of chronic inflammation there is a marked increase in the fibrotic reaction, and less evidence of cellular activity.

Inflammation is manifested clinically by "cardinal signs" which may be correlated with the microscopic picture, viz.:

(1) *Pain*—due to pressure on nerve ends by the increase in tension of the area produced by infiltration of serum, dilation of vessels, etc., and possibly also by the action of chemical breakdown substances on the sensitive nerve endings.

(2) *Heat*—due to increased metabolism in the area and increased blood flow.

(3) *Swelling*—due to increase in volume of fluids as indicated in (1).

(4) *Redness*—due to increase in blood in the area. Only seen clearly in animals with non-pigmented skins and where the hairy coat in the area is thin or absent, e.g. ears, under chin, axillae, belly or inguinal region.

(5) *Loss of function*—commonly due to increased pain of moving the injured part; muscle spasm in the area may also occur. Injury to important structures (such as nerves and bones) in limbs will produce marked loss of function.

THE RESULTS OF INFLAMMATION

(1) *Resolution*. The body defences rapidly overcome the inflammatory cause or causes and the tissues heal and become virtually normal within a short time. Generally, there is little or no pus formation, e.g. aseptic surgical wounds.

(2) *Suppuration* (pus formation). Commonly this phase of inflammation ensues where the body defences have not been able to dispose of invading micro-organisms rapidly. Here there is massive cellular mobilization in the area especially polymorphs and other white blood cells. Pus is formed as previously indicated. Pus may also contain bacterial toxins, enzymes and products of chemical disintegration of body tissues such as cells. Pus may be mixed with serum, blood, mucus or other body fluids and is described accordingly. Abscesses are common septic lesions caused by bacteria and consist of a mass of pus surrounded by fibrous tissue wall. They may extend internally and involve other tissues or may "point" to the surface of the body, rupture and discharge their contents (pus).

(3) *Necrosis* (rotting). This refers to the death of tissue on a larger scale and is seen by the naked eye. Necrotic tissue may come away (slough) from the healthier tissue with which it is continuous and this is one of the means by which healing can proceed. Liquefaction of such tissue does not occur to any extent except at the zone of separation from the healthy tissue.

(4) *Gangrene*—refers to gross death of tissue. All the local tissues are affected and they die. The gangrenous region may become extensive unless drastic measures are taken. This phenomenon may ensue when an extremity is deprived of its blood supply, e.g. over-enthusiastic use of tourniquets or when certain bacteria (e.g. Clostridia) invade tissues. The latter case is not common in small animals but often ends fatally. The gross tissue destruction is often accompanied by general systemic disturbance due to toxins from the dead tissues and/or the invading bacteria.

(5) *Ulceration*. Where the skin or surface of epithelium is broken—but the lesion is shallow and more or less confined to the surface. Ulcers show little or no tendency to heal. Frequently a discharge is shed from the surface of the ulcer.

(6) *Granulation* (fibrosis). This is, in essence, chronic inflammation with marked connective tissue reaction. It occurs when the body defences cannot overwhelm the inflammation rapidly or when the inflammation is of low but continuous activity, e.g. continuous rubbing of the skin against a hard object. Pus may be present in pockets in the inflamed tissue. Cold or chronic abscesses are thick walls of granulation tissue enclosing watery sanguineous fluid.

HEALING

Where inflammatory lesions show early resolution and rapid restoration to the normal we refer to it as healing by first (or primary) intention. This is the way in which most surgical wounds heal. The tissues are closely opposed, the small amount of haemorrhage is rapidly organized and the tissues are rapidly knit together with a minimum of fibrous tissue. The surface wound dries, forms a thin, more or less flat linear scab, and is not painful or irritating.

In the case of large wounds with a gap between each side, or in infected wounds, the tissues are not readily brought together. There may be considerable seepage of tissue fluid or actual bleeding, into the gap, and infection more readily gains a foothold. This is what happens with many accidental and neglected wounds.

After cessation of bleeding, the zone of tissue adjacent to the gap of the wound becomes invaded by fibroblasts and new capillaries and a process of organization occurs much the same as in primary healing but far more extensively and, of course, over a longer period. A sheet of smooth but uneven tissue, known as granulation tissue, is produced. If this is healthy it is pink and only very slightly moist; if infected, it may be dark in shade, or grey coloured, and be overlain by a discharge.

Healthy granulation tissue, once formed, is somewhat resistant to infection. It becomes thicker until the wound gap is filled, and then, when the tissue level reaches that of the subcutaneous tissues on either side of the lips of the wound, the skin (epithelium) grows in to cover the surface. This type of healing is by second intention, or by granulation.

Healing by second intention takes much longer and there is much more scar formation. This process may be complicated by producing too much healing tissue which is then known as proud flesh and it often protrudes beyond the wound margins and above the surface of the epithelium.

The healing of specialized tissues varies—some cells do not regenerate, e.g. nerve cells of the brain and elsewhere. Axon, or nerve-cell processes, can heal, but there may be some interference from the general healing process of fibrosis, and one frequently encounters fibrous tissue formation instead of the normal functional tissue which was originally present. In most wounds, this may not matter very much as the animal body is wonderfully adaptable, but sometimes there is a permanent interference with normal function, e.g. in the case of injured brain cells. Muscles can still function fairly adequately even if there is some fibrotic replacement. Other blood-vessel branches can compensate for loss and damage to the circulatory system. Nerve trunks may show some regeneration, especially if adequate surgical therapy is applied immediately after injury. Glands and glandular tissues frequently show good regeneration, and even where their functioning tissue has been replaced by fibrous tissue there is no apparent disability for a very long time. The body is normally endowed with much more of certain glandular tissues than are actually required, e.g. between 20% and 75% of the liver can be removed and a dog continues to remain healthy, and the liver tissue increases almost to the original bulk in about 2 months. A dog has to lose about 60% of its kidney mass before a serious clinical manifestation is apparent.

Haemorrhage

Haemorrhage in plain English means bleeding. There are three main types of bleeding.

1. *Venous bleeding*, where a vein, or venule is opened. In this type the blood flows out in a constant stream, depending on the size of the vessel, but not under obvious pressure unless the vessel is very large. This blood is dark in colour, being deoxygenated. It is a very common type of bleeding but, unless vessels are fairly large, may be of little consequence and can generally be arrested fairly simply.
2. *Arterial bleeding* occurs when an artery is opened. The blood is bright scarlet, and spurts out under pressure in pulsations synchronous with the heart-beat. It is usually treated as serious and should receive early attention.
3. *Capillary bleeding* occurs as a slow or more rapid oozing of blood from an abraded surface. Its colour may be rather bright red. It is not generally of serious consequence, but should be arrested as it may occur from a large area and the total volume become substantial.

In all types of haemorrhage the RANA's function is to assist in the arrest of bleeding, although in some cases, e.g. snakebite, bleeding of the wound should be encouraged during the early phase immediately after it has been inflicted.

The section on first aid will already have dealt with measures to be used in circumstances where bleeding occurs. The veterinarian may require the application of further sterile dressings or compression pads, the local application of styptics such as adrenaline, alum, or the local application of cold water, or ice, or of hot fomentations. He may wish to give drugs to encourage blood coagulation or to ligate bleeding vessels. Ligation may involve putting an animal under an anaesthetic and tying the bleeding point off with plain catgut, linen or other suitable material. It may be necessary to administer oxygen in such circumstances.

Once bleeding has been arrested it is important to give consideration to the restoration of blood volume. This may be done by encouraging the body to replenish its own blood volume by giving haematinics or drugs containing minerals such as iron, copper, etc., and by giving high protein diets and also plenty of fluids with some extra sodium chloride (common salt) in the diet. Certain vitamins, e.g. B_{12}, are of importance in haemopoiesis. Plenty of rest in equable, comfortably warm surroundings is also important.

Extra fluids containing sodium chloride, dextrose and protein-like substances may be formulated and prepared for subcutaneous infusion as part of the short-term measures to counteract loss of circulating blood volume.

In acute blood loss, whole blood from a compatible donor may be given intravenously, though generally whole blood transfusion is better reserved for real emergencies where life is endangered.

Transfusions and Infusions

It is necessary that the administering apparatus be clean and sterile. The term transfusion usually refers to the taking of whole blood or blood plasma from a donor and the giving of such blood or plasma to a recipient.

Infusions are fluids other than whole blood or plasma which may be prepared in the laboratory or under similar conditions and given a recipient either intravenously or by some other route, e.g. subcutaneously. Common infusions are "physiological" saline (this is frequently referred to as normal saline and is a solution of 0·85% sodium chloride in water): dextrose/saline, used generally as 5% dextrose in 0·85% solution of sodium chloride in water. This last solution is isotonic with the blood. There are tablets commercially available which when dissolved in a definite amount of water give solutions of definite concentration depending on the formulation of the tablet. The indications for the foregoing procedures are:

1. Maintaining or restoring blood volume and content. In acute haemorrhage, e.g. where a volume of whole blood has been lost from the division of a large vessel there will be some degree of shock present as well as a lowered blood pressure and volume. A healthy animal can lose up to about 30% of its circulating blood volume before clinical effects are observable. In such a case the intravenous transfusion of compatible whole blood is most beneficial, plasma is helpful though not as effective as whole blood, and saline or crystalloid substances are of little value and if given intravenously may be dangerous.

2. Maintaining the fluid volume of the body. The body loses fluid in dehydrated states, such as often follows diarrhoea, vomiting and conditions where fluid intake may be less than fluid loss. An animal will present clinical signs of dehydration when an amount of body water equal to about 6% of the body weight is lost. In such cases

subcutaneous physiological saline solutions are useful and some of the common compound electrolyte solutions even more so.

3. Maintaining electrolyte content of blood and body fluids. In certain conditions these is an upset in the balance of electrolytes in the blood, although clinically these conditions are not always recognized with precision. Common electrolyte solutions are Ringer's, Hartmann's and Darrow's.

In febrile conditions such as toxaemias, transfusions and infusions are frequently found to be of benefit to the patient. The principle of using these substances in this way is called supportive therapy.

Where a fluid is allowed to pass very slowly over a period into a vein, the procedure is referred to as a "drip". Fluids used for transfusions or infusions should be compatible and "isotonic" with the blood and body fluids as is 5% dextrose in physiological saline.

TRANSFUSION REACTIONS

As in other species, there are definite blood groups in dogs and cats, but incompatibility (i.e. the mixture of blood of one individual with that of another resulting in rapid coagulaton) is weak. The only important antigen in dog RBCs is designated A.

It is considered that there is little risk in provoking transfusion reactions in dogs (*Note:* there are virtually no records of the use of transfusions in cats) where a random transfusion is performed using a donor only once. About 1 in 4 random transfusions would involve giving A-positive blood to an A-negative recipient. Within a fortnight or so the recipient develops anti-A antibodies and a further transfusion when this has occurred would result in a breakdown of the donated RBCs which may produce serious effects on the body. If A-negative donors are available their blood is available for repeated transfusions to the same or other recipients.

As whole blood transfusions are being used more and more it may be wise to cross-match the bloods beforehand, though the test described below is not always infallible.

CROSS-MATCH TEST

A drop of donor's whole blood is mixed with a drop of recipient's serum on a slide and left for 1 hour at room temperature.

On examination under the low-power lens of the microscope it will be seen whether or not there is agglutination, i.e. the RBCs clumping together. A control guide may be set up on another slide using donors blood and a drop of normal saline.

BLOOD COLLECTION

For small quantities, say 10–20 ml, and where the recipient is immediately available for transfusion an easy method is to charge the syringe (preferably one with an eccentrically placed nozzle) with 2·5 ml of sterile 3% sodium citrate solution for every 10 ml of blood, and suck blood gently from the donor's vein and with as much mixing as can be achieved without dislodging the needle. The jugular or radial vein may be tapped, and as large a needle as possible compatible with the size of the vein used. The blood, after further mixing, can be injected directly via a smaller needle into the radial vein of the recipient.

To collect large quantities the only essential difference is to use a large collecting vessel—a standard MRC collecting bottle is often utilized—and increase the amount of sterile 3% sodium citrate solution though still preserving the ratio 1: 4.

The speed of injection is not really important—but should be reasonably slow in case any adverse reaction arises.

A dog can take the equivalent of its own blood volume as a transfusion over 24 hours. Hence overtransfusing will very rarely arise in practice. The best way to judge the amount is to try and estimate the volume lost and inject a little more if it is available. Frequently, injecting "to effect", i.e. until clinical signs of improvement comes about, is a useful procedure. Such signs include return to normal levels of heart-beat, pulse and respiration, more rapid filling of veins, healthy bright pink colour to mucous membrane, increase in warmth of extremities, and disappearance of general depression.

It has been suggested that the citrate solution used as an anti-coagulating agent may produce adverse effects; however, the intravenous injection of calcium gluconate solution at the completion of the transfusion will avoid this.

ADVERSE EFFECTS OF TRANSFUSION

Incompatibility may be shown by the recipient becoming restless with no other cause in view by shivering, vomiting or defaecating. In such event the transfusion must be stopped. The intravenous administration of an antihistamine drug may minimize such untoward reactions.

Shock

This is too complex a subject to deal with in detail and it is necessary to oversimplify. Shock in animals is often not recognized as such. It may be defined as circulatory failure accompanied by depression of vital functions. Shock is most frequently associated with loss of blood either by haemorrhage to the outside or inside of the body, or by neuro-circulatory activity which produces rearrangement of fluids of the circulation resulting in a reduced circulating blood volume.

Shock is associated with injuries, operations and disease. Fright and pain are factors which may initiate shock—but apprehension of pain and emotional trauma are not considered to be as important factors in initiating shock in domesticated animals as they may be in human beings, and in wild animals.

SIGNS OF SHOCK

Capillary stasis.
Reduced circulating blood volume.
Tissue anoxia (peripheral darkening of mucosa).
Reduced blood pressure.
Increased pulse rate.
Haemoconcentration.

Clinical examination may show the following:

1. Weak, rapid and irregular pulse (*Note:* the normal pulse of the dog is somewhat irregular).
2. Paleness of the mucosa and sometimes a blue tinge to mucous membranes.
3. Cold (shivering may occur), clammy skin. Sweating is not a feature in the small animals because of the peculiarity of the arrangement of their sweat glands.
4. Sub-normal temperature.
5. Shallow respirations.
6. Thirst.
7. Fall in blood pressure.
8. Lack of response to stimuli. Disinterest, apathy and weakness.
9. Vomiting.
10. Dilated pupils (they still react to light).
11. Shivering, etc.

Consideration of the case-history should make the RANA aware of the possibility of shock arising. Prevention is very much easier than cure. Shock may be classified as:

1. Impending (threatened).
2. Reversible shock, or developed.
3. Established, or irreversible shock.

Impending Shock

Signs may not be evident; but from the history of the case one might expect a state of shock to develop.

Action

(a) Restore circulating blood volume. Compatible whole blood being the best agent to use.
(b) Restore blood pressure by use of hypertensive drugs (*Note:* this may have the undesirable effect of increasing bleeding where blood vessels have been damaged).
(c) Reassuring the patient. The tone of the voice is invaluable to soothing a frightened animal. Gentle handling is also of assistance.

(d) Alleviation of pain by anodynes, analgesic drugs.
(e) Prevention of loss of heat. It is unwise to make an animal warmer than its surroundings. Hot water bottles, electric blankets may increase cutaneous dilation of vessels and actually permit the animal to lose heat. At most a light-weight insulating cover is required.
(f) Oxygen, given by a method which does not disturb the patient unduly, may assist where there is respiratory depression or cyanosis.
(g) Respiratory stimulants may be given.
(h) Posture. The animal's head should be kept low by raising the hind end slightly but the animal should be kept lying down and generally as flat as possible. The head and neck must not be unduly bent—or airways may be obstructed.
(i) Cardiac stimulants may be necessary.
(j) External cardiac massage by manual compression of chest.
(k) Artificial respiration.

It may be difficult to carry out many of the above procedures in a conscious animal. Gentle handling and sympathetic understanding can be applied especially easily when animals are subjected to elective operations, e.g. spaying, and there is plenty of time for the nurse to get to know the animal and vice versa.

Use of drugs to allay fear and pain, etc., prior to elective operations, e.g. ataractics (tranquillizers), sedatives, helps to prevent shock.

Prior administration of glucose by mouth, a valuable pre- and post-operative measure which can often be undertaken by the owner, also assists in avoiding shock.

Acute Surgical Cases

Prior to surgical or operative treatment, an animal is prepared so as to be in the best possible state to withstand shock, etc., of such an operation.

The best conditions for performing surgery on an animal is when it is fit and healthy and the surgeon can choose his own time. This is what we mean by elective surgery.

However, many patients are presented whose state of health is such as to require early surgical intervention, if not urgent operation. These are often in the nature of emergencies.

The veterinary surgeon will already have made his diagnosis and prognosis (his forecast of the probable outcome of the condition) and it may be that he has advised the owner that it would be kinder to have the animal destroyed.

Veterinarians and owners are often unwilling to save an animal's life if it means that the animal is likely to suffer severe pain thereafter or if there is no possibility of a reasonable restoration of physical and mental integrity. The acid test applied as far as the veterinary surgeon is concerned is usually whether the patient is likely to enjoy life or not. Owners are influenced by different criteria and may wish to make attempts to prolong an animal's life in the hope of some improvement—their acid test possibly being whilst there is life, there is hope. In some cases owners may be self-interested and for complex reasons will not take veterinary advice at the beginning of a case.

The RANA's duty, however, is determined by the veterinary surgeon's instructions:

1. Involving injuries, wounds, etc., e.g. street accidents, dislocated eyeball.
2. Obstetrical emergencies.
3. Obstruction or retention, e.g. some cases of F.B. alimentary or urinary tracts.

The RANA's duty is to prepare instruments, dressings and patient for surgery. She must make arrangements for anaesthesia and to arrange pre- and post-operative measures as instructed by the veterinary surgeon. Some of these cases may need first aid. If the veterinary surgeon is available he will no doubt issue the appropriate instructions. However it may be that the animal nursing auxilliary is on her own.

Early attention will normally be concentrated on stopping bleeding and cleaning dirty contaminated wounds as well as attempting to reduce shock and pain. No anodyne or tranquillizing drug should be administered except under the instruction from the veterinary surgeon. You will have gained some knowledge of the problems involved from the study of the section on first aid. Gentle and sympathetic handling of the patient is essential to reduce anxiety and apprehension as well as to avoid aggravating the damage already done.

One of the most useful solutions for the cleansing of wounds is sterilized warm physiological saline (0·85% or 0·9% sodium chloride in distilled water). This is poured gently over the wound and allowed to drain away into a receiver. The part of the animal not being irrigated should be protected from wetting by a mackintosh of some type. Proprietary antiseptic solutions useful in this field are Hibitane, Savlon and Roccal used according to the manufacturer's instructions. The RANA may assist in preventing or reducing shock by seeing that the animal is comfortable and warm and reassuring the patient by voice, manner and gentle handling. Animals recently involved in accidents are often in extreme states of fear and excitement and may struggle, bite or scratch with little or no provocation. The RANA should avoid provoking such responses by taking time over her approach.

She should observe carefully the presence of wounds, bleeding and deformity and the general state of the patient—if conscious, comatose or unconscious.

It is useful to take the temperature, pulse rate and strength and respiratory rate and also to note the colour of the mucous membrane of the eye and gum.

Gentle palpation of the skull, spine, pelvis and limb bones may yield information, but a RANA needs considerable experience before she is competent to do this without aggravating the patient's condition. Generally it is safer to keep the patient as quiet and still as possible until the veterinary surgeon arrives.

Naturally she will wish to report to the veterinary surgeon at the earliest possible moment, and if this has to be done by telephone she will get more effective advice if she herself can give an accurate report of the patient's condition.

Exposed or raw tissues may be kept covered with a swab wrung out in warm normal saline. A dislocated eyeball can be covered with a layer of sterile liquid paraffin then a swab as indicated in the previous sentence.

In the case of obstetrical emergencies—these are seldom as urgent as the owner assumes, and usually can await the arrival of the veterinarian. This is a case where the owner needs sympathetic and tactful handling. It is helpful if the RANA can obtain as much factual information as possible.

Some owners have very little knowledge, and, unless there is definite evidence that the case is obstetrical, it is as well to find out when the animal was last in season and if she was mated. False pregnancy is a very common occurrence in bitches and gives rise to behaviour and physiological changes simulating the true condition.

Labour—especially in bitches pregnant for the first time—may be fruitless, and in such cases the bitch does require veterinary assistance before she completely exhausts herself. The general condition of the bitch is an important factor in dystokia (difficult birth) and often reflects the local condition within the womb.

Sometimes a foetus (either puppy or kitten) becomes stuck in the birth canals, and this occasions great alarm on the part of an owner or attendant. Most cases can be remedied by an experienced RANA who should also have acquired enough knowledge to know when not to apply active methods. A little waiting will not harm the dam—though it may have adverse effects on the offspring if it is living. Again it is usually a matter of reassuring the person in attendance. Animals in labour are normally better left quiet and on their own—though a few appear to benefit by the presence of a well known and loved human owner.

The veterinary surgeon's actions in the case of obstetrical emergencies will be to examine and diagnose the condition. If uterine inertia is present, medical means of stimulating active uterine movement will be employed. The surgical procedures to be adopted are usually of (1) attempted digital, manual or forceps delivery or (2) caesarean section.

In either case the RANA will need to have ready hot water, soap, towels and sterile instruments. Some form of anaesthesia should also be in a state of readiness so that it can be brought into instant use. The RANA will be instructed on these points by the veterinarian. Anaesthesia is a particularly delicate business at this time.

OBSTRUCTION

Of Anterior Alimentary Tract

Complete obstruction of the pharynx or oesophagus by a foreign body or of the anterior alimentary tract may be an emergency when severe paroxysms of choking and retching occur. The action here is to induce general anaesthesia at once and locate and remove the obstruction.

Tympany (gaseous distension) of stomach or intestines producing signs of severe acute colic and often visible distension of the trunk high in the left paracostal region. The cause may be a twist (torsion) of the gut, obstruction of the intestine, or acute enteritis—an easily fermentable diet may be a predisposing factor, and the very large sized breeds seem to suffer more than others. To save the animal's life the distended organ may have to have a trocar and canula inserted, and the latter tied in place.

Respiratory Obstruction (threatened asphyxia)

Any sudden blockage such as a foreign body, acute swelling of tissue (*vide* insect sting in the tongue), regurgitation of stomach contents whilst under anaesthesia, hypersalivation in Bulldogs (in such cases abnormally voluminous soft palate is an added factor).

Urinary Retention

We have dealt elsewhere with urinary calculi. In the castrated male cat urethral obstruction may result in urinary retention the danger of which is not appreciated by the owner. The patient tends to sit in the same crouching position all the time. He gets very depressed, will not eat, and may cry a little especially if handled. The case is easily diagnosed by palpating a grossly distended urinary bladder. Relief is readily obtained by antero-pubic paracentesis of the bladder with a long fine needle, aspirating urine carefully. The primary condition of urethral obstruction which caused the retention must, of course, be attended to as well.

Post-Operative Care Of Patients

The first phase of recovery from anaesthesia will be dealt with elsewhere. The most important duty of the RANA is to reassure patients who are not recovering too well. Generally animals are left to regain consciousness on their own and any manual interference during this stage may provoke reflex action, excitement or fear. It is wise to look at the patient occasionally to see that nothing untoward is happening and that it is not injuring itself on its surroundings, etc.

Once an animal is again in full control of its senses then it may interfere by licking, biting or scratching with any sutures, dressings, casts, or splints which have been applied and the RANA must discourage this. The following procedures may be of value:

(1) *Discipline.* The stern tone of the voice may be sufficient to stop an animal, and after a few repeated strictures the animal may forget about any transient irritation from sutures, etc., and adapt itself to putting up with them. For very badly trained (or untrained) pets, a stern reprimand accompanied by gentle physical prevention, or threatening a light tap on the muzzle by a rolled up newspaper may be necessary. If an animal will not respond to such methods, then the RANA must proceed further, viz.:

(2) *An Elizabethan collar* of suitable size may be placed around the neck so that the collar is always between the animal's mouth and the wound or source of irritation.

Elizabethan collars are usually of leather or cardboard. They may be purchased, or made by the RANA. They should be fairly rigid but light, easy to clean and to disinfect. Figure 6.1 shows how the collar may be constructed. Chafing by the inner edge may be prevented by padding the collar.

An animal may be prevented from scratching by hobbling the hindlegs with bandage or lamp wick in the form of a figure of eight placed above the hocks.

Measures to protect dressings or casts from being interfered with include painting the outside of the dressing or cast with some nasty-tasting material. Muzzling of the dog with a suitable leather or wire muzzle may be worthwhile, but it is uncomfortable for the animal to wear such an appliance for a long time.

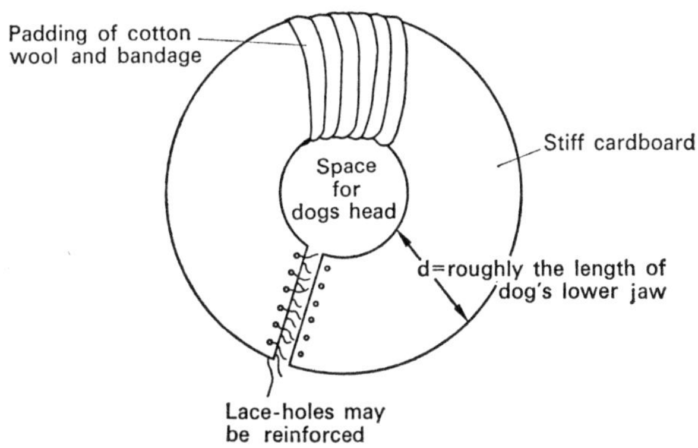

Fig. 6.1. An Elizabethan collar.

Where the region of the eyes has to be protected, special guards of rubber and wire mesh can be made or face-masks such as those used by underwater swimmers may be adapted.

The use of sedatives or tranquillizers may be effective in eliminating self-interference either alone or in combination with the aforementioned appliances.

Wounds, etc., must be kept clean and may require inspection at intervals.

Veterinary surgeons often prefer to leave sutured wounds open to the air and without dressings. Usually some anti-bacterial and drying dusting powder is applied after suturing and this can be renewed at intervals. Dirt must be kept away from wounds and warm saline is used to clean them up if necessary. The wound should be carefully dried afterwards with gauze, or warm air. Gentleness in handling is most important, and when dry a fresh application of antiseptic dusting powder may be applied. All these procedures should be carried out as aseptically as possible.

The general progress of a patient after surgical intervention should be carefully observed. Where a healthy animal has been under a general anaesthetic for a short period with a minimum of surgery, the recovery period is usually short and the patient is fully himself in less than 24 hours. The ability to recover quickly depends on the health of the patient prior to surgery, the type and duration of anaesthesia, the type of surgery performed, and post-operative care.

Many animals are rather obviously depressed during the day or so immediately after operations involving general anaesthesia. During this period they should be kept warm and quiet and care is necessary regarding their diet. If they are continuously lying down, their position should be changed every few hours. Indeed, unless there is some strong reason for not doing so, they should be encouraged to get up and walk around a little from time to time.

Bowel activity is related to the food taken. As animals are generally fasted before operation, and, as they may have little appetite in the 24 hours following, one should not expect them to be concerned much with this function. Blood loss will reduce fluid output, and until the animal is drinking fairly well it will not require to be allowed out to urinate frequently, but careful observation on these points is essential as animals are usually conditioned to passing urine and faeces outside.

Operation wounds should be inspected. There is often some swelling at the suture line for up to about 48 hours after operation; this normally subsides and becomes drier where matters are proceeding favourably and the tissues unite without worrying the patient. Sometimes the swelling increases, the area appears reddened and moist and the patient tries to lick the wound. These are indications that all is not well and the attention of the veterinary surgeon should be drawn to the matter. The temperature for the first 2 or 3 days after operation is often a degree or so above the normal level. The third day is really a critical time and if the animal is going to go on well there is usually a definite improvement in appetite by this time, bowel and bladder functions are fully restored and the animal behaves more normally. If, however, the appetite is still poor, there is apathy, temperature more then 2 degrees above the normal, bowel and bladder functions perhaps suspended, then these are indications that all is not well and the surgeon must be notified.

If these observations are noted and the temperature, respiration, pulse and normal functions (bowel, bladder, appetite) written on a chart, an invaluable reference record is then permanently available.

The veterinary surgeon may order special measures such as antibacterial injections, or a special regimen of feeding during the immediate post-operative period. It is the RANA's duty to carry out such instructions, and if a chart is kept, to record them.

As soon as the immediate post-operative period of 3 to 5 days is over, the patient enters upon a period of convalescence proper. During convalescence appetite should increase, and the animal become brighter and more eager to behave normally. The owner will be informed by the veterinarian with regard to diet, exercise and natural functions, and the RANA should be aware of what advice has been given. Convalescence may last from 1 to 6 weeks as a general rule, though sometimes the period is extended. Usually the veterinary surgeon will wish to see the patient again towards the end of the convalescence period so that he may discharge him properly.

Common Surgical Conditions

A brief description of a number of the more common surgical conditions and the principles of their alleviation is given. It should increase the interest of the RANA and also indicate some of the ways in which she may assist.

Abscesses

Where an abscess is thought to be arising, it may be encouraged to point by clipping and shaving the hair of the skin overlying the abscess and bathing the area frequently with warm water. Painting the area daily with weak solution of iodine has a similar effect. Abscesses may rupture, discharge their contents (pus) and heal. They may repeat this cycle of events and become chronic. It is important that the discharge opening is large so that the contents can drain well, and irrigation with antiseptics carried out. Healing takes place by secondary intention from the depths of the tissue. If toxic substances from the abscess are absorbed into the system, a general condition (toxaemia) occurs.

Toxaemia produces a febrile reaction of the animal's system with accompanying rise in temperature, respiratory and pulse rates, inappetence, urinary concentration and some degree of general depression. The condition usually remits somewhat when an abscess ruptures.

Haematomata

Haematomata (singular haematoma) are swellings which appear fairly suddenly on the body surface after traumatic injury. They are warm and fluctuant and must be differentiated from abscesses. Haematomata contain blood. The commonest site is the ear of both dog and cat and the condition known as aural haematoma is usually secondary to infestation of the external acoustic meatus (or ear canal) with parasitic mites (otocariasis). The mites irritate the lining of the canal, the ceruminous glands of which produce excessive amounts of dark brown wax. The combination of mite plus wax causes the animal to shake its head frequently in an attempt to clear the canal. This head-shaking causes blood to tend to flow towards the tip of the ear-flap which ruptures, and the blood flows under the skin or via some other plane towards the tip and produces the swelling which is so common. Sometimes the animal continues to shake and the condition remains, but usually the animal becomes less sensitive to the irritating factors, and the blood in the haematoma becomes organized and contracts to form a thick contracted cauliflower ear. Veterinary attention is concerned with opening and evacuating the haematoma. The reformation of the haematoma must be prevented and the correct shape of the ear preserved, which is not always easy. Naturally the otocariasis and blocked ear canal—which were the causal factors—must also be attended.

Cysts

These swellings, which contain fluid other than blood or pus, are differentiated from abscesses and haematomata. The common type of cysts is a retention cyst where secretory tissue (gland) produces a secretion which cannot escape through its normal duct because of obstruction. The secretion is therefore retained and the back-pressure causes swelling (the cyst) into the gland which becomes non-functioning. Examples are:

(1) *Sebaceous cysts*—often seen in old dogs. These are generally flattened, situated in the thickness of the skin and the contents are viscous and consequently quite firm.

(2) *Ranula*—a globular swelling seen below the tongue and containing honey-like fluid. Blocking of a salivary gland is the probable cause. Both dogs and cats may be affected.

(3) *Inter-digital cysts.* Some breeds of dogs are affected by these small swellings which appear sporadically on the feet. Their cause is somewhat obscure, but a proportion of them contain a small foreign body (grass seed).

Ulcers

These are often seen in the mouths of cats. They frequently occur on the surface of mammary growths in bitches and involving the cornea of the eye. They may be present where a sick animal has been lying for a long time on a flat surface (bed-sores). Ulcers on mucous surfaces may be cauterized.

Bed sores or decubitus ulcers are best prevented by turning recumbent animals frequently, seeing that they have a soft bed, gently massaging "pressure" points (e.g. outside of elbows, hock and down limb bones), and applying alcohol/alum hardening lotions. Bed sores may produce toxaemia, and in any case are very resistant to treatment once they are established.

Fistulae and Sinuses

These are abnormal openings on the body surface which discharge. Fistulae (singular fistula) are canals which connect a mucous surface to the external surface and the discharge is the same as the content of the site from which the canal takes origin, whereas sinuses are invariably blind, i.e. end in tissue, and their discharge is a mixture of blood, pus and tissue fluid.

Examples of fistula are the not uncommon anal gland fistula of the dog which occurs as a short canal and which remains patent and opens to one side of the anus after an anal gland has become septic, pointed and ruptured on the perineal surface. The discharge is glairy, greyish and malodorous.

Sinuses are often found on the dorsum of the foot of the dog and discharge bloody serum or watery sanguinous pus.

Foreign Bodies

These are a wide variety of solid objects which become attached to animals, embedded in their skins or other tissues, or find their way via natural orifices of the body and are retained within. Foreign bodies may also be swallowed in food, etc. The symptoms and effects depend on the size, shape and nature of the foreign body. The hardness and the character of the surface of the foreign body are important from this aspect as well as its final location within the animal body.

A foreign body (e.g. a grass awn) is often found in association with a sinus. The foreign body being the main factor for the sinus persisting.

Some examples of foreign bodies:

1. *Fish-hook embedded in the skin*. This is quite common (seasonal). The barb must be exposed by pushing on (never pulling back) the hook. It is then cut off and the remainder of the hook can then be pulled out without inflicting further damage.

2. *Mouth*—frequently animals may get a piece of wood or a bone wedged between the teeth. This produces frenzied attempts on the part of the animal to remove it, and marked salivation. Proper restraint is necessary for examination, and a general anaesthetic may occasionally be necessary. It is advisable to consider reducing the size of the foreign body *in situ*, e.g. by cutting it in two with pincers, and also to remove it by the same pathway by which it entered. Once the foreign body has been removed, the site where it was located should be carefully inspected for damage.

3. *Ear*. At certain times of the year, grass awns find their way into the dog's ear canal. This usually produces intense irritation and the dog rubs its ear along the ground. Under proper restraint, which may involve tranquillization or general anaesthesia, the canal may be inspected and the foreign body located and removed.

4. *Ingested foreign body*. Puppies chew all manner of things. They swallow some of them especially when affected with intestinal worms, e.g. coal, earth, cinders, stones, sticks, ladies' stockings, slippers and matting are common objects of their attention.

Foreign bodies in the mouth, oesophagus or stomach tend to produce acute symptoms, and gagging, retching or vomiting may be observed. As the foreign body proceeds along the alimentary tract, the anterior functions become lessened and the posterior functions become affected, producing such symptoms as diarrhoea, constipation and straining without defaecation (tenesmus).

Sharp foreign bodies may penetrate through the walls of the alimentary tract either into the pleural or peritoneal cavities, and the condition becomes more serious. Frequently, though, these sharp foreign bodies, especially if small—such as bone fragments—do arrive in the rectum without doing much damage *en route*. Defaecation then becomes extremely painful and the animal plainly indicates its difficulty by howling or yelping as it attempts to pass the fragments. It may give up trying and the owner then often seeks veterinary aid.

Operative measures may be undertaken at any stage and this is, of course, decided by the veterinary surgeon in charge of the case. If the neck is the site, then the oesophagus must be explored. This may be done via a hollow tube (oesophagoscope) being inserted via the mouth and pharynx of the anaesthetized patient—down the oesophagus to the level of the foreign body. Inspection can be done and sometimes the foreign body can be reduced in size and removed by inserting special instruments down the barrel of the oesophagoscope.

Alternatively, the oesophagus may be approached by a skin incision at the base of the neck (cervical or pre-sternal oesophagotomy) (see Fig. 6.2) just in front of the chest inlet; or by an incision over the chest wall and separating or resecting a pair of ribs (transthoracic); or, by performing laparotomy (incision into the peritoneal cavity), the posterior oesophagus, the stomach, small and large intestine and rectum can be

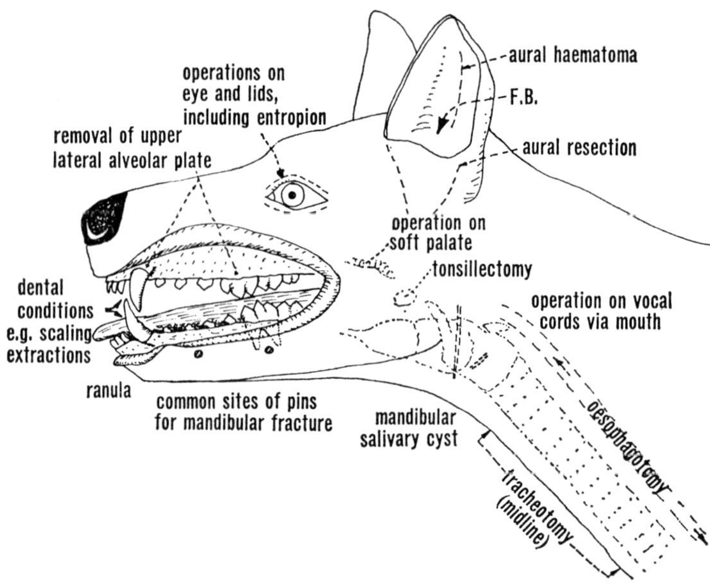

Fig. 6.2. Some points of surgical interest on head and neck of dog.

reached. Where the foreign body is located in the rectum, a rectal speculum or proctoscope can be inserted via the anus and the foreign body removed by instruments, or by irrigation. Very often a gloved finger may be inserted through the anal ring and the foreign body or material removed digitally. The region is then irrigated by warm lubricant enema.

The RANA's duties in connection with the foregoing are fairly obvious from the text. She must consider restraint, anaesthesia or tranquillization requirements, lay out the necessary drugs, needles, syringes, etc., and in some cases administer medication under the veterinarian's direction. For endoscopy she must have oesophagoscope, proctoscope or specula ready and lubricated. For operations, drapes, instruments, sutures, dressings, etc., and the animal must be prepared for surgery. Irrigating solutions such as sterile weak sodium bicarbonate for oesophagus, stomach or intestine and warm soapy enema for rectum and anus may be necessary.

Post-operative arrangements also need thinking about, e.g. the phase during which recovery from anaesthesia takes place and then the few days where the site of the foreign body may be tender or where a special nutritional regimen has to be instituted such as after oesophagotomy.

Special cases of foreign body. Obstruction is the term used to refer to the situation where a tubular organ or conducting passage is blocked. In a number of cases a foreign body is present and we have already dealt with such a situation, viz., foreign body in the alimentary tract, which could just as easily be referred to as alimentary obstruction.

However a number of other factors may be involved, e.g.:

1. *Calculus*—the presence of fine or coarse, discrete or concreted material which have been derived largely from body fluids such as urine, bile, saliva or even faeces. Calculi are often referred to as stones, and they occur most frequently in the urinary tract particularly in the bladder and urethra.

2. *Stenosis or stricture*. This refers to the narrowing of the lumen of tubular structures and is usually due to the formation of scar tissue after operation or injury to the lining or walls of the structure. Scar tissue occurs as part of the repair process and contracts in the course of time, drawing the normal tissue tighter. Hence the surgeon's aim when operating in these sites is to keep scar tissue to the minimum. Calculi may occur as a sequel to stricture, as the later reduces flow of fluids and thus brings about one of the conditions favourable to formation of calculi.

Calculi may cause damage to the wall of the organ containing them, e.g. renal pelvis, bladder or elsewhere. They may also block any passageway in which they become lodged. An obstruction to the flow of liquid or solid is caused and this produces a stoppage. The accumulation of liquid or solid produces increase in pressure within the organ and various secondary effects occur. Urethral obstruction and urinary retention is common in castrated tom cats. Calculi are usually associated with localized inflammation and infection.

It is frequently necessary to relieve the acute symptoms produced by the obstruction though sometimes both diagnosis and treatment are performed simultaneously.

The RANA's function is as usual preparation of the patient and instruments for procedures of relief to be undertaken by the veterinarian.

Neoplasms

These are what lay people commonly call growths or cancer. The causes of this group of conditions are obscure, and the mechanism of their appearance, growth and effect—their pathology—is complex. Neoplasms may appear in virtually any site of the body, but the commoner sites are the skin, the mammary glands (bitch), the alimentary tract (mostly in the region of mouth and pharynx), testicle (dog), bones (especially limb bones of large breeds of dogs such as St. Bernard, etc.), and lymph nodes.

Neoplasms may be termed benign when they grow slowly, are well defined in their shape and extent, and do not exert any serious pathological effects except that of occupying space. Benign growths do not recur when removed.

Malignant growths, or cancer, on the other hand, grow rapidly, infiltrate normal tissue without any well-marked definition of their border, and they have an intrinsic effect on the host in which they are situated, producing wasting. They tend to produce secondary growths and they recur after removal. This terminology used here is not very precise and we have grossly over-simplified the whole subject. However, the RANA should have some idea of their significance. It should not be forgotten that the term cancer is one which has a great effect on many owners—often equivalent to pronouncing the death sentence in their pet, so that it is wise to use a euphemism.

Neoplasms on the external surface of the body may ulcerate, and this is quite common in mammary growths of the bitch. Growths in animals generally appear to be painless.

It may be possible for growths to be removed before they can spread or cause any serious pathological effects. This is the usual line of treatment undertaken by the veterinary surgeon. The RANA will readily appreciate that her role will be concerned with the preparation of the patient for operation, anaesthesia and getting instruments and operating equipment ready. She may have to play some part in reassuring the owner but this should not be undertaken except by very experienced RANAs under the guidance of their employer.

After the growth has been removed it is good practice to send it to a pathology laboratory for examination. From histopathological study a scientific diagnosis may be obtained and an opinion regarding the degree of malignancy present.

Other methods of treatment of neoplasia include drug therapy, desiccation or cauterization by electro-surgery or topical drugs, ligatures where the growth is pedunculated, and radiotherapy. The last named is a specialized field, and for this and economic reasons is not generally available in veterinary practice.

Deformities (Malformations)

These are physical departures from the normal range of an anatomical structure. They may be natural or man-made, congenital (i.e. present at birth), inherited (tendency derived from one or both parents) or acquired during life. Malformations may be external, e.g. extra toes, imperforate anus, or internal such as cleft palate, deformed skeleton.

Many of these cases are detectable at or shortly after birth, some later during puppyhood. As many of them may be hereditary it is probably best to put the patient to sleep. However, many affected animals have owners who are perhaps excessively sentimental and who will not accept this course. The veterinarian is then requested to alleviate the condition which can sometimes be done. Naturally it is important that affected animals should be prevented from breeding and thus perpetuating the condition.

The commoner deformities or malformations which are thought to be hereditary are:

Hip dysplasia	Prolonged soft palate (particularly in Bulldogs)
Patella luxation	Hernia (especially umbilical)
Entropion	
Retinal atrophy	

Others less common include:

Abnormal temperament	Ectropion
Uterine inertia	Trichiasis
Elbow dysplasia	Deafness
Lens luxation	Cryptorchidism

It will be seen that although some of those conditions listed may have a structural or anatomical basis, they do in fact manifest themselves as predominantly functional derangements, e.g. abnormal temperament, uterine inertia and deafness.

Hernia (commonly though inaccurately termed rupture) is a wide group of conditions. The term indicates the protrusion of an organ or structure through its containing wall. Generally it refers to the abdomen, e.g. umbilical hernia—the protrusion of fat-laden omentum through the abdominal wall which has failed to close properly at the umbilicus.

It is generally accepted that there is some heritable predisposition to hernia. Hence affected animals should not be permitted to breed.

A hernia is said to have a sac—which is the peritoneal membrane. The opening through which the sac passes is the ring, and the narrowest part of the sac is termed its neck. The voluminous bulging portion of the hernia—generally away from the neck—is called the fundus. The contents of the hernia varies. The sac may become thickened with tissue, and also develop adhesions within.

The locations of hernia form a basis for classification. Umbilical hernia is frequent in dog puppies and usually contains omentum. It is rarely serious and tends to disappear with time. Inguinal hernia is commonest in the bitch—when it may contain omentum and/or uterus. In the dog and tom cat the testicle and spermatic cord may be retained. Perineal hernia occurring in old dogs is more of a rupture—as the peritoneal membrane is usually broken through. Into this site the urinary bladder may enter producing obstruction since the neck of the bladder must necessarily be retroflexed.

Ventral hernia is the term used for herniation other than via a natural opening, i.e. through muscle wall. When the peritoneal membrane is also ruptured, then the condition should be referred to as eventration. Such a calamity may occur if the stitches closing a laparotomy wound give way.

Another important hernia—known as an internal type—is diaphragmatic hernia which occurs in both dogs and cats where the trunk of the animal is involved in general trauma such as traffic accident or fall from a height. In this type the diaphragm ruptures and some of the abdominal contents such as the stomach may find their way into the thoracic cavity. As there is then a reduction in space, the lungs are unable to expand properly and signs of dyspnoea are evinced. The effect of this category of injury varies, and animals are known to have lived many years after such injury without any signs of discomfort.

The contents of hernial sacs also constitutes a basis for classification: those containing omentum are called epiplocoeles; enterocoeles contain intestine. Hernias are said to be reducible when the contents can easily be returned to the parent cavity, and irreducible when they cannot. Irreducible hernias are of two types: incarcerated where the contents are too bulky to go back through the ring, and strangulated when the contents are under pressure and when the circulation to those contents is impeded. Most hernias are congenital, though ventral and peritoneal types—often resulting from trauma—are acquired.

CONDITIONS AFFECTING THE ALIMENTARY TRACT

Lips

Localized bacterial dermatitis of dogs often appears in skin-folds of those breeds or individuals in which they are present to an excessive degree. The lesion usually affects the lower lip, is foul-smelling and commoner in spaniels and those other breeds with loose lips and who tend to slobber.

Rodent ulcer of the lip of the cat. This term is given to almost any ulcerous proliferation of the lips of the cat. One condition affects the upper lip of the cat. A granulomatous mass erodes into the inner surface of the lip and ulceration occurs. Treatment is by surgical excision (cutting it out) or by the application of caustics such as silver nitrate, or a combination of both methods.

Another condition which is properly fitted by the term rodent ulcer is the basal cell carcinoma of the lip margin. This is, of course, a neoplastic condition.

Canine oral papillomatosis or buccal warts are not uncommonly found in young dogs. The condition appears as a number of small pink–white growths resembling cauliflower heads of different sizes attached to the lining of lips and cheeks. They can spread to unaffected dogs who come into contact with the patient. The condition is self-limiting and disappears usually within a couple of months. Recovered dogs are resistant to any recurrence of the condition.

Teeth

Supernumerary deciduous teeth may have to be extracted to allow the permanent teeth to erupt in their proper positions. This occurs principally in dogs of the smaller breeds, especially miniature and toy varieties.

Tartar deposition on teeth. The teeth of dogs and cats, especially, as they grow older, become encrusted with pale deposits of solid material. This tartar may erode into the surrounding gum and produce gingivitis. Bacteria may become active in sites of gum erosion and extend their activities to the alveolar periosteum—the membrane which anchors the tooth in its alveolus, or socket. Thus the common dental condition —alveolar periostitis—arises. It may occur independently of the cycle of events narrated above. Dental caries is very rare in the dog and cat.

Frequently periodontal disease, i.e. disease of the tissue supporting the tooth, is associated with unbalanced diets and continuous sloppy feeding. It may be so serious as to extend into the bony structure of the jaw and when the region of the root of the 4th upper premolar is affected necrosis and sepsis increases to form an abscess, and by pointing and rupturing on to the face there is ultimately produced the not uncommon condition of dental fistula.

These disorders can be prevented by attention to diet and to the teeth at an early stage. However, dental conditions in cats or dogs are usually quite advanced when presented for veterinary attention. Early on, tartar may be removed (scaling), and gums cauterized. In late stages the teeth will probably have to be extracted and supportive therapy given to patients who are often suffering from a toxaemia by reason of their bad dental conditions.

A pet can survive quite well even though its teeth are extracted providing its food is cut into pieces which can easily be swallowed.

The RANA's function in dental cases is to prepare patient, anaesthesia, instruments, drugs and other necessary apparatus. Veterinary dentistry is usually carried out most conveniently under short acting non-volatile anaesthesia such as intravenous thiopentone. A gag to keep the mouth open is very useful. Scalers of different patterns should be available to assist in removing tartar. Molar, incisor and root forceps should be on the dental tray. Forceps, apart from their primary function to extract teeth, are useful to crack brittle tartar deposits. Wooden applicators with cotton-wool wrapped around one end are used for applying solutions after which they may be thrown away. Solutions for cautery or astringent use are silver nitrate, weak solution of iodine and chromic acid. A special spray-gun, which gives a fine jet, is of value in washing out crevices, etc. Pumice powder or dental paste is very useful for the final polishing of teeth.

Teeth may be fractured—this can allow bacteria into the periodontal tissue, thus extraction of the fractured tooth is often indicated. Dental fistula commonly arises as a result of such fractures. Exposure of the pulp cavity does not appear to be painful in the dog and cat.

Epulis

This is the clinical term used for any small warty excrescence on the gums. It occurs in dogs and cats and can easily be removed by excision. They are usually benign but are occasionally recurring.

Tonsils

These are well developed in dogs and cats, and in the former especially may become inflamed in infective conditions of the mouth and pharynx. The tonsils may also become the seat of neoplastic changes. Tonsils may be surgically removed if medical treatment is ineffective. If the tonsillitis is a local manifestation of a more generalized condition, the inflammation can be expected to die down as the generalized condition remits.

Tongue

Necrosis of the surface of the tongue is not uncommon in cats—either alone or as part of a wider condition involving the upper respiratory and alimentary tracts. The ulcers may be painted with iodine or silver nitrate. Wasp or bee-sting of the tongue, with its consequent swelling, is an emergency in brachycephalic dogs such as Boxers, Pugs, Bulldogs. Unless the airway is kept open, the animal is in danger of asphyxiation.

The sting, if still present, is removed, and neutralization of the local area undertaken initially. Wasp-stings are alkaline and can be neutralized with vinegar or lemon juice; bee-stings are acid and are neutralized by baking and washing soda or very dilute ammonia (caution). If the case is attended early enough, injections of an antihistamine or corticosteroid drug may prevent swelling. If swelling occurs and cannot be relieved by incisions, then an endotracheal tube will have to be inserted under general anaesthetic, and if this is impossible an opening into the trachea (tracheotomy) is the only course.

Reference has been made already to ranula; and rodent ulcer may also involve the tongue.

The oesophagus may be completely or partially obstructed by a foreign body. In the stomach, a foreign body is probably the most important condition.

The Abdomen

Surgical opening into the peritoneal cavity (which is not quite the same as the abdominal cavity though for practical purposes we need not differentiate) is referred to as laparotomy. This is probably the commonest surgical technique practised by veterinarians.

Laparotomy may be carried out in the flank or via the ventral midline (Fig. 6.3). Once the abdomen is opened, then access is obtained to the other organs, viz. stomach, small intestine, colon, bladder, uterus and ovaries (in the female), kidneys (these are technically outside the peritoneal cavity but within the abdominal cavity—often said to be situated retroperitoneally), spleen, and urinary bladder.

Foreign bodies obstructing the intestine may necessitate laparotomy rather than enterotomy (opening into the intestine). If the intestine is telescoped into itself (intussusception) or has undergone local necrosis for some reason (sometimes a sequel to long-standing obstruction), then a portion may have to be excised (partial enterectomy) and the open ends re-sewn together (end-to-end anastomosis).

Enlargement of the spleen (splenomegaly), perhaps as a result of neoplastic change, may necessitate splenectomy. The presence of calculi or stones within the bladder

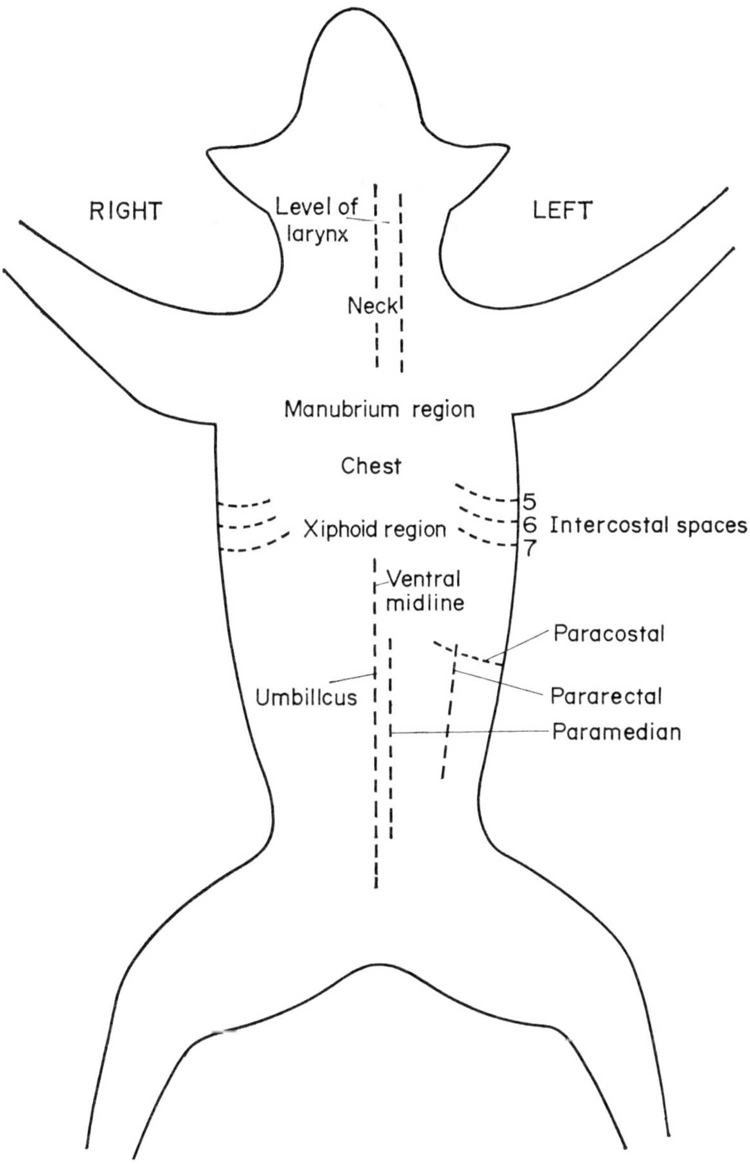

Fig. 6.3. Some surgical landmarks and lines of incision on the ventral aspect of the dog.

(i.e. cystic or vesicular calculi) may require opening of the bladder wall (cystotomy). The common elective operations of spaying entails removal of the ovaries (oophorectomy or ovariectomy) or of the ovaries and a major part of the uterus (oophorohysterectomy or ovohysterectomy).

Imperforate anus is a condition where there has been abnormal development, and the terminal canal of the alimentary tract has no opening to the outside. In mild cases it is as if there is a fine membrane occluding the anal opening, and it is sufficient merely to rupture the membrane. More severe cases require more complicated surgery. The principal patient is the puppy just after it has been weaned.

Another very common condition in this region involves the para-anal sacs of the dog. These may become distended in individual dogs and require their contents to be expressed. Sometimes they are the seat of abscess formation and they may also fistulate. Thus for several reasons they are often removed surgically. Also in the vicinity of the above-mentioned structures are, in the male, the testicles. Removal of these paired organs to prevent breeding, or where they have become severely injured or involved in neoplastic changes, is termed castration or orchidectomy.

EYE AND EAR CONDITIONS

The Eye

The eyelids are frequently affected with in-turning (entropion), less frequently with out-turning (ectropion) in the same breed. Trichiasis is a condition common in the Pekinese in which the eyelashes turn inwards and may exist alone or in conjunction with entropion. The Cocker Spaniel is a frequent sufferer from this group of conditions.

In the first and last-named conditions (entropion and trichiasis) the surface of the cornea becomes irritated and a keratitis arises, and blood vessels proliferate from the edge of the cornea. Corneal ulceration often appears and sometimes erosion is so marked that Descemet's membrane (one of the elastic inner layers of the cornea) bulges through the eroded area. This is occasionally referred to as herniation of Descemet's membrane (keratocele). It is also referred to as a prolapse of the structure. If Descemet's membrane ruptures the aqueous fluid can escape and this permits the structures within the globe to move forward. Generally the iris prolapses and becomes trapped in the rupture with ultimate adherence there (anterior synechia). Usually the veterinarian sees the case before this cycle is fulfilled and he can carry out operations to align the eyelids or lashes correctly and thus prevent the train of events described.

The lacrimal puncta which carry away tear secretions from the conjunctival sac are sometimes absent or become blocked. Tear furrows on the face are then produced as a result of overflow.

Harder's gland is sometimes displaced or inflamed. It can be examined and treated under local anaesthetic.

Dislocation of the lens is a condition at present considered to have a high heritability in Wire-haired Fox Terriers. The lens may be displaced so that it becomes situated behind the iris (in the posterior chamber) or in the anterior chamber. Dislocation may be preceded or followed by glaucoma, in which the pressure within the globe rises as a result of blocking of the drainage vessels. The whole matter is very serious and, unless it can be relieved within a short period of occurrence, the patient will lose the sight of the affected eye and it will have to be removed. Not infrequently the opposite eye is affected though perhaps not simultaneously.

Cataract—where the lens becomes opaque—generally occurs in old dogs. The transparent media (cornea, lens and vitreous) of old dogs often appears rather hazy or cloudy. This change should not be confused with cataract, which may, however, co-exist. Some forms of inflammation of the cornea (keratitis) are confused with cataract by lay people.

The Ear

We have already referred to foreign bodies in the ear canal and to aural haematoma as a consequence of otocariasis. When the condition of the ear canal is chronic and continues to discharge, a veterinary surgeon will often perform aural resection. This involves incision and replacement elsewhere of part of the cartilaginous lateral wall of the canal and establishing better drainage as well as allowing aeration of the exposed canal. An important factor in achieving success by surgery is in the healing which should, ideally, be by first intention. A good technique in applying post-operative dressings to the ear region is of considerable help in getting good results.

Classification of Fractures

The varieties of fractures that might occur have been considered in the section dealing with first aid (see page 200). The following additional terminology will be of assistance to the nursing auxiliary.

1. With reference to the extent of damage, viz. where there is total discontinuity of bone cross-sectionally, the fracture is complete; where it is less than total it is partial (see greenstick). A hair or fissure fracture is also of this type. Damage to important local structures such as nerves or large vessels makes the fracture complicated.

2. Fractures are classified according to the pattern of the actual discontinuity.
   (a) They may be transverse, oblique, spiral or (rarely) longitudinal. These patterns more commonly seen in the longer limb bones.
   (b) Where there are more than two fragments (*Note:* a simple transverse fracture of the shaft of the femur provides two fragments: an upper or proximal one and a lower or distal one) the fracture is said to be comminuted.

3. According to position of the ends of the bone fractured, viz.:
   (a) Where the ends remain in their normal relationship the fracture is undisplaced or is said to be in good apposition.
   (b) Where the ends are apart and there is an appreciable gap at the fracture site but the general alignment of the long axis of the fragments is more or less undisturbed, the fracture is said to be distracted.
   (c) Where the long axis of the fragments is not aligned nor parallel, "angulation" has occurred.
   (d) Where the axis has lost its alignment but remains more or less parallel and the fracture ends overlap each other, is called overriding.
   (e) Where one bone is driven into the other so that one fractured end is virtually pushed into the other, the fracture is impacted.

(f) Where a portion of the surface of a bone is fractured and then pushed in towards its own medullary cavity a "depressed" fracture is produced. This is also a type of partial fracture.
(g) A compression or crush fracture occurs when a bone or part of a bone is pressed down into its own cortex, e.g. an articular head, or where the shaft in a portion of the bone more or less totally disrupts due to crushing pressure directed from either end towards the middle, e.g. crush fracture of a vertebral body. As a result the longitudinal dimension of the bone is reduced.

It can now be appreciated that the classification of fractures is somewhat arbitrary, but it is a convenient basis on which to discuss them. A number of other terms are available in this study but are not in general usage. The RANA should be capable of consulting a medical dictionary if an unfamiliar term crops up.

4. A fracture may also be described according to the actual anatomical site of the discontinuity, viz.:

(a) Shaft (diaphyseal) fracture.
(b) Epiphyseal fracture—this is perhaps more of a separation at the epiphyseal plate than a true fracture.
(c) Articular fracture—where the joint involving the bone is involved. Here the articular surface is split.
(d) Intracapsular fracture—where the fracture line involves the articular extremity and is situated within the joint capsule, e.g. femur.
(e) Extracapsular—similar to (d), but here the fracture line is situated outside the line of attachment of the joint capsule, e.g. femur.

Healing of Fractures

As an example we may consider a simple transverse fracture of the shaft of a long bone in a healthy dog, of Collie type, having suffered, say, a moderate hit by a motor car. When the fracture occurs, the blood vessels of the medullary cavity, endosteum, bone, periosteum and in the local soft tissue are ruptured or lacerated. The shaft of the bone breaks more or less straight across, endosteal and periosteal membranes being ruptured in the process. The adjacent muscles usually suffer at least slight damage. In other words a number of different cells will have been damaged, and those closest to the line of trauma will die, releasing enzymes, etc. A general reaction of shock will appear and we have discussed this elsewhere (see page 343).

The muscles aligned along the fractured bone go into spasm and, as is often the case in the example cited, the ends of the fracture separate and there is overriding. The potential space or actual gap between the fracture ends allows blood to collect there and this constitutes the so-called fracture haematoma. This blood clots and becomes organized within a short time in the same way as the clot of a wound. Cells invade the area, capillaries sprout and the blood supply to the zone is increased. Fibroblasts also collect there and build a framework of granulation tissue. During this early period, which is initiated soon after the trauma ceases and goes on for at least several days to perhaps several weeks, dead cells at the edges of bone, periosteum, vessels, etc., must be removed by osteoclasts and other phagocyte types of cells. One of the most noticeable (radiologically) features following increased blood supply to the zone is the demineralization (decalcification) of the bone in the vicinity of the fracture.

After the clot is organized and a granulation framework is advanced, the zone is invaded by osteoblasts and other cells which lay down cartilage then osteoid tissue to form an increased mass of firm connective substance which unites the fractured ends sufficiently well to allow the patient a good deal of use of the limb. This callus is initially radiolucent but can be palpated. Callus formation is complete in from 4 to 8 weeks. There is usually fairly good fixation of the fracture ends after about a fortnight following injury providing no displacement has occurred after reduction. As the callus gets older it becomes consolidated by the deposition of mineral (calcium) salts and becomes harder and increasingly radiopaque. Ultimately this stage is completed and resculpturing of the bone occurs so that its original form is re-established. This process of consolidation and resculpturing may take between 3–8 months or even longer depending on age of the patient and other factors.

FACTORS INFLUENCING HEALING OF FRACTURES

There are many.

1. *Age*. Fractures of young animals generally heal at a faster rate than those of older animals, other things being more or less equal.

2. *Type of fracture*. The better the blood supply the better (sooner) the fracture heals, e.g. spiral fractures expose more endosteal and periosteal vessels and therefore more rapid healing is encouraged.

3. *Blood supply*. This factor is partly linked with the above section. The blood supply to the bone is generally better in the vicinity of large muscle masses. In some locations there is little except relatively avascular structures such as tendons, and thus the blood supply to the bone may be poor and this is a factor in the healing rate, e.g. distal third of the tibia. Again if large vessels in the vicinity of the fracture are lacerated (i.e. the fracture is complicated), then the blood supply and drainage is affected. It is possible for gangrene of a limb to supervene as a result of the main blood supply being severely damaged.

4. *Type of bone*. Spongy or cancellous bone heals quickly because of the better blood supply. Compact bone, being denser and relatively not so well supplied with blood, accordingly heals more slowly. Hence also fractures heal quicker the further away from the middle of the shaft they are located.

5. *Poor reduction*. If the fracture ends are not close to each other (i.e. if distracted), callus formation will be more extensive and thus takes longer. This extended healing time is referred to as delayed union. Sometimes callus formation does not occur at all, and we have a case of non-union. There may be intervening fibrous tissue in the non-union gap, and a false joint occasionally forms.

6. *Immobilization.* If the fracture ends of the fragments are not virtually held still in relation to each other, then movement occurs and this provides a stimulus for the protraction of the inflammatory reaction with a consequent increase in the extent of fibrosis and the size of the callus.

Treatment of Fractures and Dislocations

First aid in these conditions has been dealt with previously (see page 201). An account of orthopaedic therapeutics will help the RANA to understand what is being attempted and thus enable her to assist more intelligently and with greater interest.

GENERAL

Fractures should be immobilized as soon as possible to prevent further damage. Surgical treatment should be undertaken as soon as the patient's general condition permits. An animal in a state of shock must be allowed to recover before undergoing perhaps general anaesthesia, manipulation or other orthopaedic procedures, many of which are somewhat traumatic.

General anaesthesia for orthopaedic surgery has to be deep; muscle relaxants are often of great value; and blood or plasma for transfusion can make a great difference to the patient. In treatment the aim is to reduce the fracture, i.e. bring the fracture ends back into the position which they occupied before the fracture existed; then to maintain them in the reduced position (immobilization); all this with a minimum of trauma.

Methods of Treatment of Fractures

Treatment is non-operative when reduction is achieved by manipulation, involving principally extension, and where immobilization is obtained by the use of externally applied splints or casts. It is operative when reducing apparatus is applied directly or indirectly to bone either for reduction or immobilization. Generally non-operative measures are "closed" methods and operative measures are "open". These concepts, whilst not entirely accurate, will enable the RANA to get a practical understanding of some of the problems. A number of methods have features common to one or other of the above-mentioned main types.

NON-OPERATIVE METHODS OF TREATMENT

Reduction

Overriding fractures may be reduced by extending the limb in the direction of its long axis. Considerable tension has to be exerted and the base of the limb must be fixed in position. The simple method is to have the patient anaesthetized in lateral recumbency with the affected limb uppermost. The operator places her knee or foot in the patient's groin and exerts a steady continuous pull without jerking by grasping the distal part of the limb and leaning back. Another method of doing much the same is to fix the pelvis in position by a roller towel or sling on to a table then by broad bandages or adhesive plaster attach weights (or a bucket of water) to the distal end to exert continuous traction. An alternative is to use a Gordon extender in conjunction with adhesive plaster. Traction has to be maintained for between 20 to 30 minutes before muscle fatigue sets in and spasm overcome sufficiently to allow manipulation in the fracture region to achieve successful reduction. One type of operative method of reduction is essentially similar. A Gordon extender is employed in conjunction with a pair of ice-tong calipers, the pins of which are driven into the cortex of the distal fractured fragment itself as far as possible away from the actual fracture zone.

Another method of operative reduction is by use of the Ehmer reduction gear, and this is employed in conjunction with the Kirschner splint (q.v.).

Immobilization

Non-operative measures

1. Simple external splints can be made from flat or guttershaped pieces of wood, metal or plastic. These are padded and then bandaged into place. Meccano strips may be employed. Stiff corrugated cardboard is useful and light. Elastoplast strapping is very helpful in binding splints together. Special made-up splints, e.g. Cramer wire, are available commercially.

2. *Plaster-of-Paris cast.* This is a handy and effective method of treating fractures, i.e. distal to the elbow and stifle. POP bandages are commercially available. These are soaked in water, wrung out, and arranged longitudinally to form layers which are built up into a slab which is moulded to the limb for some distance on either side of the fracture site. The limb is not completely encircled but a small gap left. When the slab part is dry and firm a layer or two or encircling POP bandage is made around the limb to complete the cast. Padding may be arranged between the limb surface and the cast and a better "bed" is then formed which is less likely to undergo adverse effects from undue localized pressure of the cast. If the foot is included, the interdigital spaces and paw generally should be padded, but otherwise unpadded casts are still commonly used. Casts should fit closely to achieve good immobilization, but there is always a danger of localized pressure necrosis or even gangrene. Their successful application therefore requires practice, judgement and experience. Casts should not be too heavy as this will increase the degree of muscle atrophy which occurs when the affected leg is not in actual use. If POP casts are applied to swollen limbs soon after the occurrence of fracture, then a fresh cast may have to be applied when the original one becomes loose as the swelling subsides.

The RANA will be called to assist in preparation of the patient, general anaesthesia being most desirable when applying casts. She will have to assemble the correct size of POP bandage, arrange the water, plaster shears, etc. During the application of the cast the limb may have to be fixed or supported in a definite position, and she may also have to assist in moulding the surface of the cast.

POP casts should be examined after 24 hours to check that they are hard, well fitting, that the patient is not in undue discomfort and not interfering with the cast. It is essential also to ascertain there there is no likelihood of pressure necrosis arising. If the foot is exposed at the lower end of a limb cast it should feel normal, be of the same size as its opposite fellow, and at the same temperature. Departures from the normal should be immediately notified to the veterinarian, and until he can act the distal part of the limb held in elevation (by putting the patient on his back). Subsequent examinations of the cast should be made at weekly intervals. POP casts may be removed at periods between 4–8 weeks depending on the patient, fracture, and progress made. Casts may be softened with water (this being a disadvantage during the period when it is required to be rigid) and then cut by special shears. An electrically operated oscillating plaster saw is useful, but an ordinary hand tenon-saw can be employed. It is important not to injure the patient during removal procedures.

3. *The Thomas splint.* This is a padded wire framework built on to a limb for the purposes of keeping the fractured ends aligned and in a state of extension. The device is arranged to exert continuous traction. It is light, wounds can be easily dressed, but unless closed off by bandages, etc., it may get caught up on fixed objects. It is not a widely used method nowadays. The wire is bent to form a basal ring with linear pieces extending down the limb. Distally the limb is extended and fixed by extension plaster (closed or non-operative method), or Kirschner wire or ice-tong calipers (open or operative methods) to the lower part of the wire.

Open or operative methods of fracture treatment

1. *Half-pin splints.* The most useful apparatus in this category is the Kirschner referred to above. There are several half-pin assemblies and they differ slightly. The principle is to insert a pair of converging pins on either side of the fracture zone and by linking them with a long rigid rod, the fracture is immobilized. The pins are driven through skin and soft tissue into the bone, and for secure fixation should emerge a little way through the opposite cortex. Some seepage may occur where they enter the skin and infection may also get in at these points. Local treatment and systemic antibiotic cover is usually given for at least a period after insertion. When the fracture is clinically strong enough, the pin assembly can easily be removed. This technique is quite useful; pins are light, inspection is easy, there is no interference with circulation, and the limb is rapidly brought into use thus obviating disadvantages of muscle atrophy. Some patients interfere with the pins, and generally they must be covered to prevent them getting caught up in fixed objects.

2. *Internal fixation.* This includes a variety of methods by which the fracture zone is usually completely exposed.

Pinning consists of inserting a metal rod into the medullary cavity or attaching a fractured segment of bone on to the parent body by driving a pin through. Apparatus includes the Steinmann pin, Rush pins, Jonas splint, and Leighton shuttle pin. All these types require different techniques for their insertion. Some of these intramedullary pins are removed when the fracture has healed, others may be left *in situ*.

The most commonly used pin is probably the double-ended Steinmann indicated for mid-shaft femoral fractures. It is made of inert metal, commonly a particular specification of stainless steel. To avoid certain reactions and corrosion leading to breakdown within tissues, all metal devices, splints, tools, screws, etc., should be of the same specified chemical composition. Every effort should be made—and here the RANA can play an important part—to avoid scratching, denting and any other injury to the surface of metals used in orthopaedics whether as implants, prostheses or instruments.

Plating is the attachment of a metal plate via screws across the fracture zone. Although the Sherman plate is widely used, the Venables plate is probably the best available at present for general use. Screws should penetrate both cortices as in the half-pin assembly technique. Plates may be left in permanently unless they become loose or when they bridge the epiphyseal line in young, growing animals, in which case they should be removed at the correct time. Screwing is undertaken when smaller fragments of bone require reattachment, e.g. fixation of a condyle, fracture of olecranon process or os calcis.

Wiring may be used in fixing fragments and is also useful in special cases, e.g. patella, mandible.

Methods of Treating Dislocations (see page 207)

Generally, manipulation under deep anaesthesia aided by muscular relaxation is the method of choice. Dislocations have a better chance of being restored to normal and maintained there if they are reduced within a short time of their occurrence. Where the maintenance of reduction is unsuccessful a false or secondary joint is often formed and the patient adapts itself fairly well to the disability. Occasionally, dislocations must be treated by open reduction which entails opening into the joint cavity.

After reduction (repositioning) it may be necessary to resort to fixation in order to maintain the integrity of the joint. The methods by which splints, casts, pins, etc., are used in fracture treatment can be employed in this field.

Recurrent dislocations, e.g. hip dislocations, patellar luxation, usually require special orthopaedic techniques.

(b) ANAESTHESIA IN THE DOG AND CAT

W. B. Singleton, MRCVS

Introduction

A frequent duty of a RANA is to assist in the anaesthesia of patients under the direct supervision of a veterinary surgeon.

In connection with general anaesthesia so many methods exist that it is difficult to learn them all; also every veterinary surgeon has a personal preference, and, although in the hands of one person a particular drug may be eminently successful, in the hands of another it may give poor results. Whatever methods are adopted they should become standardized and if completely satisfactory it is unwise from the point of view of veterinary practice to deviate from strict routine.

Owing to the range of size and species of patients, most veterinary surgeons adopt two or three different techniques to meet the varying requirements. The RANA should become proficient in each and have a confident and positive approach, for a quick decision on her part may save life. When an animal is anaesthetized it is rendered insensitive to touch, pain or other stimulation. This may be limited to a *local* area; or it may be *regional* (part of the body) or *general*. Anaesthesia is necessary for humanitarian reasons and to facilitate the technical efficiency of the surgeon.

The agents which are used for producing local and regional anaesthesia are usually synthetic substitutes of cocain, e.g. procaine hydrochloride. When used to produce local anaesthesia the drug is injected into the tissues and infiltrates through a limited area rendering the area insensitive. When injected over a nerve or nerves (perineural) the region of the body supplied by the nerve(s) is rendered insensitive. In both instances the drug has a limited period of effect.

General anaesthesia may be induced by the administration of certain volatile substances which enter the body by inhalation (e.g. ether) or by the intravenous injection of non-volatile drugs, e.g. thiopentone sodium. Certain non-volatile drugs may be administered by routes other than intravenous, e.g. oral, per rectum or intraperitoneal.

Certain drugs known as narcotics (e.g. morphine and its derivatives: subject to the DDA) can be used to induce varying stages of insensitivity, and although full anaesthesia can be induced by the administration of large doses such practices are fraught with danger, and it is usual for narcotics to be used in conjunction with and supplementary to local, regional or light general anaesthesia.

Tranquillization is frequently used in place of narcosis. The drugs used are less toxic, and less depressing. They are useful adjuncts to any form of anaesthesia, e.g. chlorpromazine, promazine.

Local Anaesthesia

The drugs which are commonly used are frequently known under proprietary names, e.g. Xylocaine, Planocaine, Novocaine, etc. Almost all have a selective temporary interference (reversible) effect on the transmission of impulses of sensory nerves and nerve endings. Usually the local anaesthetic solution contains 1 in 10,000 adrenalin hydrochloride which has the effect of constricting small blood vessels (arterioles and capillaries). This slows down the rate at which the local anaesthetic is carried away from the area into the circulation thus prolonging the duration of anaesthesia. Other substances may be added to a local anaesthetic solution to assist in the wider distribution of the drugs into the tissue, e.g. hyaluronidase.

Administration may be by (a) surface application, (b) epidural and subarachnoid infiltration, (c) field anaesthesia (blocking an area of skin by infiltrating the drug in a line which encircles the site of incision).

Surface Anaesthesia

This is achieved by spraying highly volatile substances on to an area, e.g. ethyl chloride. The rapid evaporation from the skin surface produces freezing and localized anaesthesia. This method is not often used in veterinary practice as there is a chance of tissue damage and even necrosis if the preparations are used too freely. Some of the more powerful local anaesthetic agents, e.g. Xylocaine, may induce anaesthesia if applied in the form of a cream or jelly to a surface, and they are often used on endotracheal tubes (see General Anaesthesia) for this purpose. However, their value in this connection is debatable.

Infiltration Anaesthesia

This is achieved by the injection of a local anaesthetic by means of a hypodermic syringe and record needle (size 2 or 5-ml syringe with 13 mm × $\frac{6}{10}$ needle) or if relatively small areas are involved a Waite's dental syringe is preferable.

The injections can be made in two ways:

1. The use of a long needle which is inserted subcutaneously to its fullest extent and the injection made as the needle is withdrawn.
2. The use of a short record or dental needle which is inserted intra- or subdermally and small injections made which can be seen to bleach the skin in weals. The injections are made progressively along a line. This method is perhaps the least painful.

Regional Anaesthesia

This depends upon the introduction of an anaesthetic solution over the route of a nerve trunk in the premedicated patient. Such techniques require considerable skill and an advanced knowledge of anatomy. Consequently the veterinary surgeon will invariably carry out this procedure.

Before commencing a perineural injection of the dental nerves of the dog a dental syringe is used to anaesthetize a small weal through which the main injection is made.

For the nerve block a 22-gauge 5-cm-long needle is preferable and each nerve should be anaesthetized by an injection consisting of 2 ml of a 2% solution of procaine or similar solution.

For an epidural injection an insensitive weal is first produced over the site of injection and a 21-gauge needle 4–5 cm long is employed for the actual injection. The amount of anaesthetic solution injected will depend upon the extent of regional anaesthesia required and upon the size of the dog. The following is a guide and the amounts quoted should be effective from a point a little in front of the umbilicus to the tip of the tail:

Pekinese	2–3 ml
Fox Terrier	7 ml
Airedale	9 ml
Larger breeds	11 ml

For operations involving only the anus, tail or vulva, half the above dosage is sufficient.

General Anaesthesia

General anaesthesia is defined by Hall in *Wright's Veterinary Anaesthesia and Analgesia* as a state of unconsciousness produced by a process of controlled, reversible intoxication of the CNS in which there is a lowered sensitivity to stimuli from the environment and a diminished motor response to such stimuli. Thus an anaesthetic agent may be defined as a substance which produces in a controllable manner both loss of consciousness and an absence of motor response to noxious stimuli.

General anaesthetics may be volatile or gaseous agents inhaled into the lungs (e.g. ether) or water soluble non-volatile substances (e.g. thiopentone sodium, or pentobarbitone sodium) administered intravenously, but some may be given by the mouth, per rectum, or by intraperitoneal or intramuscular injection.

The action of anaesthetic agents on body tissues is not fully understood. Although they become widely distributed, it is their effect upon the CNS which is most significant so far as anaesthesia is concerned. Inhalation anaesthetics reach the CNS in three phases:

(1) the transference of gases from the upper respiratory tract to the alveoli of the lungs which are lined by epithelial cells;
(2) the passage or diffusion of the gases through the epithelial cells of the lung alveoli, through the endothelial cells lining the capillaries and into the blood stream;
(3) diffusion of the anaesthetic agent from the blood into the tissues. The actual distribution into each type of tissue depends upon several factors, notably the blood supply and lipoid content. The brain being highly vascular and having a high lipoid content accepts a high proportion of the circulating agent available.

The whole process of gaseous absorption depends upon the laws governing the diffusion of gases through membranes. Elimination of the agent depends upon the same principles acting in reverse. Thus it will be appreciated that although the structure of the brain enables rapid and relatively high concentration of gases to accumulate in the tissue, this is governed by the concentration in the blood and in turn the blood depends upon the concentration built up in the alveoli; therefore if anaesthesia is transient the concentration built up in the CNS will fall rapidly due to the transference of the agent back from CNS tissue into the blood and either its ultimate elimination from the body or absorption into other tissues. Consequently to maintain a satisfactory and prolonged stage of anaesthesia, generalized tissue saturation has to be achieved and maintained.

Non-volatile anaesthetic agents if not given intravenously must be absorbed into the blood stream and thence to the body tissues, their absorption into CNS tissue being dependent upon similar factors already referred to in connection with gaseous anaesthetic agents. Whereas the latter are eliminated almost entirely through the lungs and out into the atmosphere, the non-volatile anaesthetics have to be broken down mainly in the liver and excreted via the kidney. Such a process may be slow and depends greatly upon the health of the liver and kidney. For these reasons recovery from inhalation anaesthesia is invariably much quicker than in the case of non-volatile agents.

The transition from consciousness to full surgical anaesthesia is divided into four stages, and in order to understand the whole process it is necessary to recognize each stage, although in practice several methods used, notably induction with thiopentone sodium and other barbiturates, cause the patient to pass through stages I, II and the early part of III so quickly and smoothly that the stages are difficult to recognize. On the other hand, induction and anaesthesia using ether usually enables each stage to be recognized with ease.

STAGE I. *Stage of voluntary excitement*

Signs: (a) consciousness; (b) visible fear and forcible efforts to escape; (c) breath-holding; (d) increased respiratory and pulse rates; (e) pupillary dilation; (f) eye and pedal reflex present.

STAGE II: *Stage of involuntary excitement*

Signs: (a) loss of consciousness; (b) exaggerated reflexes; (c) violent limb movements; (d) vocal noises—dogs whimper loudly and cats hiss; (e) irregular respiration; (f) coughing, swallowing and even vomiting may occur; (g) eye and pedal reflexes present.

All or only some of these signs may be seen in stages I and II, but many can be avoided by premedication using tranquillizers such as promazine. For the peace of mind of the anaesthetist and safety of the animal, premedication is advisable.

The signs in stage II gradually abate as the animal reaches stage III.

STAGE III: *Stage of surgical anaesthesia*

First plane (light anaesthesia). Signs: (a) regular, deep and rapid breathing; (b) limb movements cease; (c) eyeballs move from side to side and finally fix; (d) eyelid reflex absent; (e) pedal reflex present.

Some minor surgery may be carried out at this stage.

Second plane (medium anaesthesia). Signs: (a) regular but slower and shallower respiration; (b) eyeball may be fixed or may move downwards; (c) muscular relaxation apparent; (d) pedal reflex sluggish or absent.

This plane of anaesthesia is correct for all but intra-abdominal surgery and certain orthopaedic operations requiring greater muscular relaxation.

Third plane (deep anaesthesia). Signs: (a) rate of respiration increases but depth decreases; (b) pause between inspiration and expiration; (c) chest movements become slight but abdominal movements maintained; (d) eyeball fixed again; (e) pedal reflex totally absent; (f) muscular relaxation greater.

STAGE IV: *Overdose*

Signs: (a) thoracic movements absent; (b) abdominal contents rise and fall due to movement of diaphragm only—movement irregular; (c) pulse rapid; (d) pupils dilate; (e) "glass eye" appearance.

The irregular and gasping respirations become less frequent and eventually stop. Cyanosis followed by an ashen grey colour, lack of pulse, dryness of cornea indicate death.

The pupils are widely dilated during stages I and II and again when an overdose has been reached.

Before passing to the properties of volatile anaesthetics and their methods of administration, it is important to learn and fully appreciate the significance of two basic physical laws.

Boyle's law. At any given temperature the volume of a given mass of gas varies in inverse proportion to the pressure exerted upon it.

Charles's law. The volume of a given mass of gas at constant pressure varies directly with the temperature.

PROPERTIES AND GENERAL CONSIDERATIONS OF ANAESTHETICS DURING USE

Chloroform: colourless, heavy, highly volatile—a very powerful anaesthetic. 0·035% in the blood produces anaesthesia, 0·06% is fatal.

Disadvantages of chloroform involve the risk of cardiac failure during induction and the toxic effect of this drug upon the myocardium, liver and kidneys which can cause a delayed poisoning. This may become apparent 24 to 48 hours after anaesthesia, the predominent signs being severe vomiting, acetonuria (positive ketones in the urine), albuminuria (positive +++++ albumen in urine) and jaundice which is often fatal particularly in the dog and cat.

Because hazards in its use chloroform is rarely used as an anaesthetic agent today. Chloroform should only be administered through an open mask.

Diethyl ether (ether): colourless, volatile.

ETHER IS HIGHLY INFLAMMABLE AND WHEN MIXED IN CERTAIN PROPORTIONS WITH OXYGEN OR AIR MAY BE EXPLOSIVE. The vapour of ether is twice as heavy as air and may creep along the ground where an explosion can be sparked off by static electricity, a faulty electric switch or an open electric or gas fire in an adjoining room.

DIATHERMY CANNOT BE USED TOGETHER WITH ETHER ANAESTHESIA. NOR SHOULD ETHER BE USED IN THE VICINITY OF AN X-RAY MACHINE.

These points are emphasized because ether due to its continued popularity will be one of the first anaesthetic agents which many RANAs will use and *because serious accidents still occur due to carelessness.*

Due to the effect of ether upon the mucous membranes of the respiratory tract, larynx, pharynx and mouth causing excessive production of mucus and saliva, it is necessary to precede anaesthesia with an injection of atropine sulphate, 0·3 mg to 1·3 mg in the dog and 0·3 mg in the cat. Due to the wide margin between anaesthesia and toxicity, ether remains one of the safest anaesthetics and is considerably more so than chloroform.

The degree of excitement during stage I and early part of stage II may be quite considerable unless premedication has been given, but the effect of the drug upon the heart is much less than chloroform and if a toxic level is approached warning is given because respiratory failure always precedes cardiac failure.

A disadvantage of ether may be observed as the third plane of stage III is reached, the movement of the intercostal muscles becomes very slight and in an effort to compensate, the diaphragm shows increased movement which may be short, jerky and rapid and considerable interference may be caused during intra-abdominal surgery.

Ether may be administered by open, semi-open, closed or semi-closed methods. (These methods are defined and explained later.)

Trichloroethylene (Trilene): heavy colourless liquid with a low volatility at room temperature. It is non-explosive and non-inflammable. A blue dye is added to the drug to differentiate it from chloroform which it resembles in smell.

Trilene is much less potent than chloroform and less toxic. Like ether there is a wide margin between anaesthesia and toxicity. Unfortunately, although Trilene will produce a smooth induction it is very difficult to maintain anaesthesia without rapid respirations and cardiac irregularity. Therefore in practice the analgesic effect of Trilene is utilized in conjunction with nitrous oxide (administered as oxygen: nitrous oxide 1:3 over Trilene). Adrenaline or adrenalin derivatives should be used with caution with Trilene as ventricular fibrillation can be initiated. Intravenous thiopentone sodium injected in minimal amounts is sometimes used in conjunction to produce deep anaesthesia. Trilene cannot be used in closed or semi-closed circuit with a soda lime CO_2 absorber as toxic products including phosgene may be produced.

Halothane (Fluothane): heavy liquid with a characteristic smell. It is non-inflammable and non-explosive. It remains stable in contact with soda lime. As an anaesthetic agent it is twice as potent as chloroform and four times as potent as ether; 2–4% concentration in O_2 or air is satisfactory for induction, and maintenance can be achieved by concentrations of 1·0–1·2%. Adequate premedication will reduce the concentrations required by approximately 40%. When skilfully used, halothane is one of the best anaesthetic agents as there is a wide margin of safety due to the fact that the time interval between respiratory and cardiac failure is relatively long (3–4 min). Recovery from halothane anaesthesia is smooth and quick (5–15 min in the non-premedicated animal).

Special equipment is required to vaporize halothane and O_2 or a combination of O_2 and N_2O is passed *over the surface* of the liquid—never bubbled through. Consequently in the absence of agitation of the liquid by bubbles passing through halothane vaporization is even more sensitive to room temperatures than ether; 18·3–20°C (65–68°F) is ideal, and anaesthesia should not be attempted in rooms with lower temperatures. The advantages of halothane properly administered makes deep anaesthesia safe and even desirable as the muscle relaxation produced has surgical advantages. Even if respiratory arrest occurs this is easily reversible after artificial respiration for a few minutes. Blood pressure falls but on a maintenance level this is not great or dangerous.

Halothane suppresses bronchial secretions and consequently aids gaseous exchange in the lungs—this is particularly helpful in cases of shocked or toxic patients when mucoid congestion of lung alveoli often occurs.

Adrenalin or adrenalin derivatives should not be used in conjunction with halothane as ventricular fibrillation (fine, rapid quivering movements of the ventricular muscles that replaces the normal contractions) may occur.

Methoxyflurane is a clear colourless liquid with a fruity odour, non-explosive and non-inflammable. It is chemically stable and does not decompose in air, light moisture or alkali such as soda lime. It is not possible to induce anaesthesia satisfactorily with methoxyflurane due to the low vapour pressure concentration obtainable in normal working conditions, consequently it is used to maintain anaesthesia after induction with a short active barbiturate. It is a very safe anaesthetic agent and although respiratory depression is linked with the depth of anaesthesia, blood pressure remains remarkably stable and in dogs and cats breathing spontaneously toxic levels seldom arise.

The anaesthetic agent is placed in a vaporizer and administered with O_2 or O_2 and N_2O mixture. The recovery period is larger than with the use of halothane.

Note: Chloroform, ether, Trilene and halothane all decompose in sunlight producing various toxic substances, therefore they should be stored in dark amber bottles in a cool place.

Nitrous oxide is a colourless gas non-inflammable and non-explosive. It is supplied in a compressed form as a liquid in cylinders and vaporizes on release. The weight of the cylinders gives an indication of the amount of nitrous oxide remaining.

The gas flow must be governed by a reducing valve attached to the cylinder and accurate flow administration by the use of a flow meter.

Nitrous oxide is a very weak anaesthetic and in the small animal is seldom used alone but usually in conjunction with oxygen and Trilene in a semi-closed circuit. It can also be used in conjunction with morphine or its derivatives (thiambutene) or in conjunction with thiopentone sodium.

Cyclopropane is a colourless gas with a characteristic smell—*it is highly explosive* and must be administered in closed circuit with oxygen in proportion of cyclopropane: $O_2 = 1:4$. It is a highly potent anaesthetic agent and induction and maintenance is smooth and effective; recovery rapid and uncomplicated. It is non-toxic and has many advantages in experienced hands although special equipment is required for administration.

Basic Anaesthetic Equipment

(incorporated in the Boyle's anaesthetic equipment)

Cylinders (commonly used sizes)

Oxygen is supplied in cylinders available in the following sizes:

24 ft^3 48 ft^3

Nitrous oxide is supplied in liquid form in cylinders in the following sizes:

200 gal 400 gal

Carbon dioxide is supplied in gaseous form in cylinders in the following sizes:

2 lb 4 lb 7 lb

Cyclopropane is supplied in cylinders in the following sizes:

8 gal 20 gal 40 gal

Pressure gauges are attached to the oxygen cylinders and when the stopcock on the cylinder is opened the gauge indicates the quantity of gas in the cylinder.

Reducing valves are attached to the gauges and reduce the pressure of gas leaving the cylinder when the latter is opened fully, thus the pressure of gas flow from the combined unit (i.e. cylinder, gauge and reducing valve) is constant.

Gases leaving the reducing valve are led by means of a narrow bore tubing to the:

Flowmeter. This equipment gives further control to the flow of gas and two basic forms are used:

(a) One of the oldest and simplest flowmeters conveys gases down a tube which is contained in a sealed bottle with separate outlet. The bottle is almost filled with water and the tube which leads to the bottom of the bottle is perforated by a series of small holes. Depending upon the pressure of gas passing down the tube, bubbles emerge through a varying number of holes, thus at the lowest pressure through one hole, at higher pressure or rate through two to six or more holes.

(b) A bobbin-type flowmeter. Gases enter at the bottom of a narrow tube through a regulated aperture. In the tube a bobbin about $\frac{3}{4}$ in. long has free movement. The tube is graduated in 1-, 2-, 3-, 4-, 5-litre marks ascending the tube and the bobbin is floated upwards, depending upon the rate of gas allowed entry through the bottom of the tube.

These give a rough indication of flow rate but are far from accurate.

Rotameter. This functions on the same principle as (b) but the tube and cone are very carefully manufactured so that highly accurate flow rates can be achieved ranging from 50 ml/min to 10 litre/min. Although expensive this type is necessary for most closed and semi-closed systems.

Rotameters are designed specifically for each gas and are not interchangeable.

Vaporizing bottle. Gases leave the flowmeter or rotameter and pass to a vaporizing bottle. These vary in pattern from a simple bottle having a tube passing to the bottom and a separate outlet so that gases can be bubbled through a liquid (Fig. 6.4) to the more complex Boyle's vaporizing bottles which are capable of directing a varying proportion of the gases into the bottle and allowing the remainder to bypass the bottle and, furthermore, in the case of the Boyle's ether vaporizing bottle, to govern the extent to which the gases bubble through the ether by means of a cowl which can be raised or lowered over a J-shaped inlet tube (Fig. 6.5).

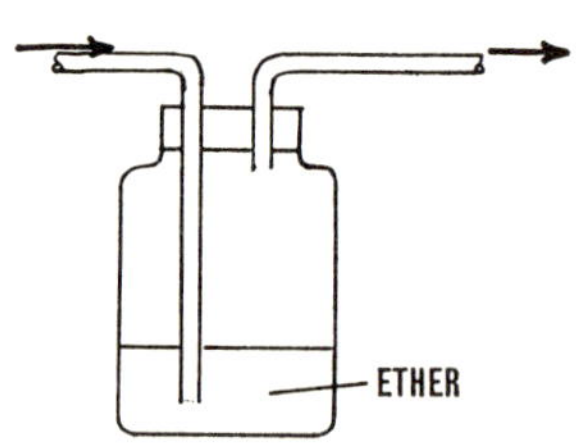

Fig. 6.4. Vaporizing bottle.

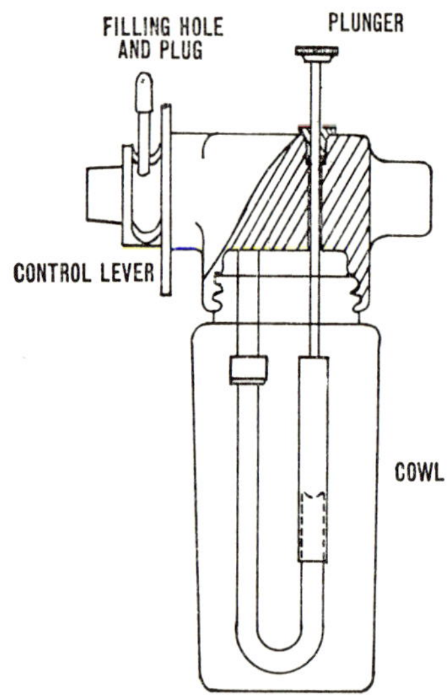

Fig. 6.5. Boyle's vaporizing bottle.

Several patterns of special vaporizers have been manufactured for halothane (Fluothane), e.g. the BOC halothane vaporizer, the Goldman vaporizer and the Fluotec.

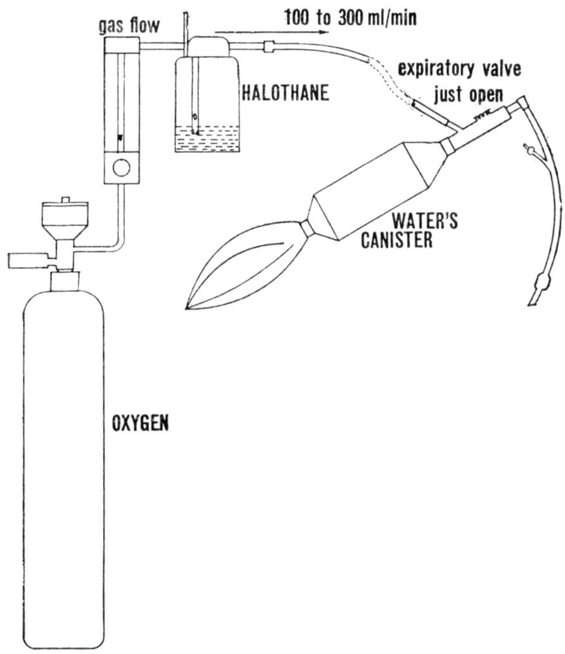

Fig. 6.6. A satisfactory method of administering halothane.

After leaving the vaporizer the gases plus anaesthetic vapour are conducted down either

(a) a narrow bore tube to an expiratory valve and *reservoir bag* (e.g. Fig. 6.6), or

(b) into a reservoir bag attached to the main part of the machine and to the patient by means of a wide corrugated (elephant) tubing to an expiratory valve (e.g. Fig. 6.7).

The expiratory valve is a spring-loaded valve sensitive to increased pressure and capable of reasonably fine adjustment.

If corrugated tubing is used from reservoir bag to expiratory valve, a connection leads directly to the *face-mask or Magill tube*. The best face-masks are made of malleable latex which mould themselves to the skull of the animal reasonably efficiently and may be secured by a strap passing behind the ears. The Magill tubes are described later (see p. 382).

If a narrow-bore tube passes from the vaporizing bottle to the expiratory valve, the latter is incorporated in a special fitting into which the gases enter by a narrow metal tube set at an angle. To one end of this fitting a connection leads to the face-mask or endotracheal tube. To the other can be fitted a rebreathing or reservoir bag (Fig. 6.6).

These bags, as other rubber parts, are usually made of anti-static rubber and are either 2 litres or 4 litres in capacity. A bag should never become distended with gas during use.

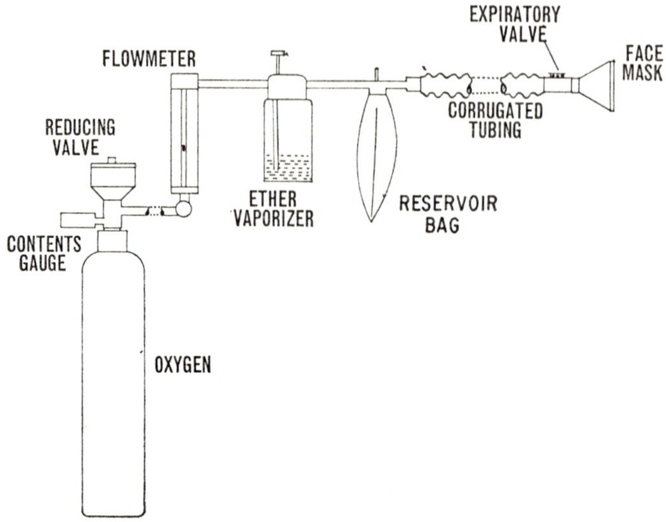

Fig. 6.7. A satisfactory method of administering ether.

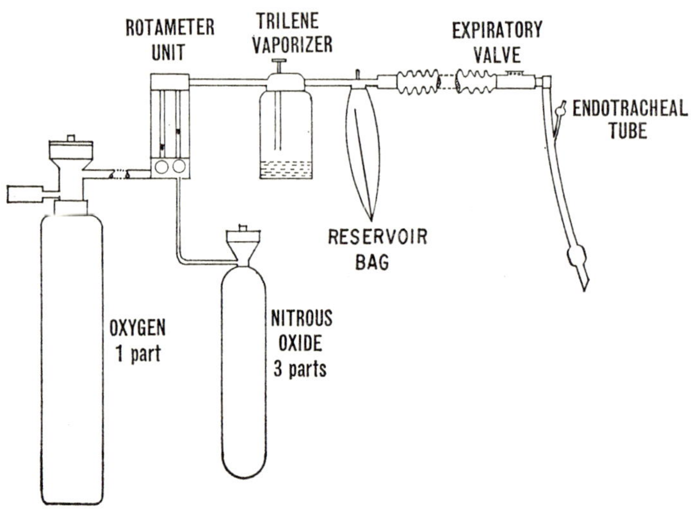

Fig. 6.8. A method for administering Trilene and nitrous oxide.

Between the expiratory valve attachment and the bag a *soda lime canister* (Water's canister) may be fitted (Fig. 6.6).

It is impossible in the scope of this book to give details of every method and system of anaesthesia, but Figs. 6.6 to 6.9 indicate a small number of methods which are in common use, but RANAs will be working under the direct supervision of a veterinary surgeon and will be required to adopt the procedures which have stood the test of time in the practice or hospital in which they are engaged.

Basic Anaesthetic Systems

OPEN METHOD

Gauze or lint is stretched over a wire frame but should not touch the animal's face so that a flow of air can be established between mask and nostril. Not all the air inspired passes through the mask, hence the term open method. Ether or chloroform is dropped on to the cloth. This is a primitive but quite effective method which may prove useful under certain difficult circumstances, for instance an emergency in an isolated area, when the bare essentials only are available.

SEMI-OPEN METHOD

Similar to above but all the inspired air passes through the gauze or lint on which ether or chloroform are vaporized. This is achieved by using two pieces of thick material, e.g. gamgee, the first having a hole just large enough to allow the nose and mouth to protrude, the other a larger hole through which the anaesthetic liquid is dropped. The mask with lint stretched across the frame is placed over the dog's nostrils as before and sandwiched between the two layers of gamgee.

CLOSED METHOD

When anaesthetic gases or vapours are inhaled by an animal they must be mixed with air or varying concentrations of oxygen. When they are exhaled they contain an increased concentration of carbon dioxide. If this exhaled mixture is passed into a closed bag the carbon dioxide must be removed if the gases are to be reinhaled. This is the basis of a closed-circuit system although, of course, in order to maintain anaesthesia small amounts of anaesthetic must be introduced into the circuit constantly together with oxygen in amounts sufficient to meet the animal's physiological requirements.

The "to and fro" system is an example of closed-circuit anaesthesia. (Fig. 6.10).

A common pattern of soda lime canister is known as a Water's canister. The exhaled gases pass over the granules of soda lime which absorb the carbon dioxide being composed of 90% calcium hydroxide, 5% sodium hydroxide and 5% silicates (to prevent powdering). Sometimes an indicator is incorporated which changes colour when the soda lime becomes exhausted. The system is closed within the animal by use of a Magill tube with an inflatable cuff which seals off the trachea from the atmosphere.

Theoretically once anaesthesia has been established and provided the anaesthetic agent, e.g. ether, is not excreted from the body except via the lung, no further agent should be needed and the animal should continue in a satisfactory state provided oxygen is fed into the circuit. In practice, however, varying amounts of the agent have to be introduced to maintain anaesthesia satisfactorily and are continually required to deepen anaesthesia. Even so this method is very economical. The chief disadvantage is the resistance to respiration created by the soda lime and therefore the method is not entirely satisfactory for very small dogs, puppies and cats. It should be remembered that when soda lime absorbs carbon dioxide, heat is produced, and if the build up within the canister is considerable, heat stroke can occur, but this only happens if anaesthesia is very prolonged.

Another method of closed-circuit anaesthesia can be achieved by the rather elaborate Circle Absorber Circuit—a satisfactory unit is made by BOC and may be studied by reference to other literature *Wright's Veterinary Anaesthesia and Analgesia*, edited by L. W. Hall).

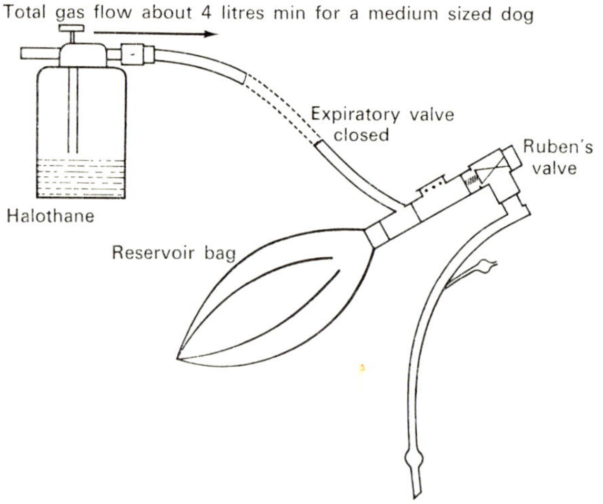

Fig. 6.9. A variation using the Ruben's non-return valve.

SEMI-CLOSED METHOD

Gases from the cylinders pass through a flowmeter which governs the rate of flow and the proportion of the gases being utilized (e.g. O_2:N_2O). These gases can then be passed over the anaesthetic liquid, which is contained in a vaporizing bottle into which is incorporated a lever mechanism to control the proportion of gas allowed to come into contact with the anaesthetic liquid. The resulting mixture then flows into a reservoir bag from which the animal inhales. Expired gases pass either partly or entirely into the atmosphere and are *not* rebreathed. To set up such a system satisfactorily a non-rebreathing valve must be incorporated into the system, examples are Weaver's valve and Ruben's valve (see Figs. 6.11 and 6.12).

It is important that air shall not be inhaled by the animal during anaesthesia. This can be prevented by delivering the anaesthetic mixture by means of a tightly fitting face-mask. Due to the wide variation of skull structure it is very difficult to devise an all-purpose mask, although malleable latex face-masks serve the purpose remarkably well, provided a full range of sizes are available.

By far the most efficient way of introducing anaesthetic gases into and out of the lungs is via an endotracheal tube. General patterns are manufactured, but perhaps the best known is the Magill endotracheal tube with an inflatable cuff in size 3 upwards

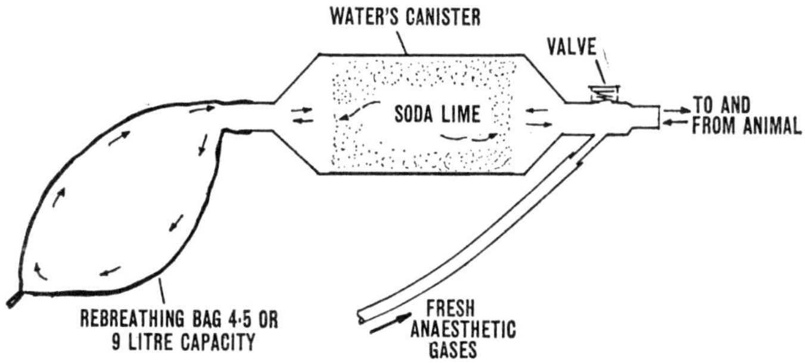

Fig. 6.10. Closed-circuit anaesthesia ("to and fro" system).

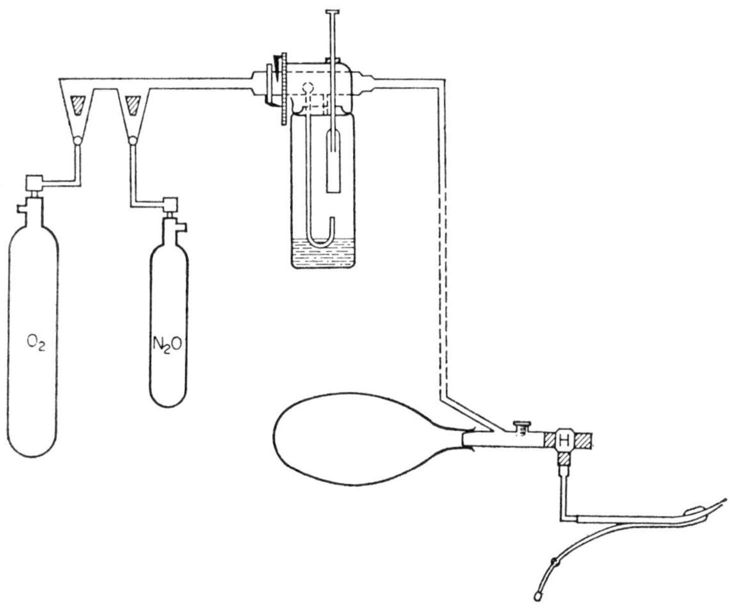

Fig. 6.11. A method of administering halothane using a vaporizing bottle and Ruben's non-return valve.

(Fig. 6.13). (Numbers 1 and 2 are very narrow, without a cuff and are used for small cats, very small dogs and puppies.)

It is important to select a size of tube which although as large as possible should pass between the vocal cords and into the trachea without undue friction.

The Magill tube is introduced when the dog is anaesthetized (usually induction and early anaesthesia is achieved by an injection of thiopeutone sodium intravenously). The tube is lubricated and the animal is either placed on its chest or on its side. Whichever position is used the mouth is opened wide and the tongue is pulled straight out between the lower canine teeth. At the base of the tongue the epiglottis will be seen. This is either depressed by means of a laryngoscope or tongue spatula or a large pair of forceps (they should not be used to grasp the epiglottis) or the end of a Magill tube is used for the same purpose. The vocal cords will be seen just within the larynx. The tube is passed between these and on into the trachea so that the tip passes a few inches down. It should never pass into the thorax as it may be diverted into one of the main bronchi and "aerate" only one lung, and in very small dogs it is possible to rupture the trachea at its bifurcation if the tube is passed down too far and with too much force. The whole procedure should be undertaken gently and easily. Once in place the cuff is inflated to a moderate degree using the pilot bulb as a guide. A special valve or a pair of old artery forceps may be used to retain air in the cuff.

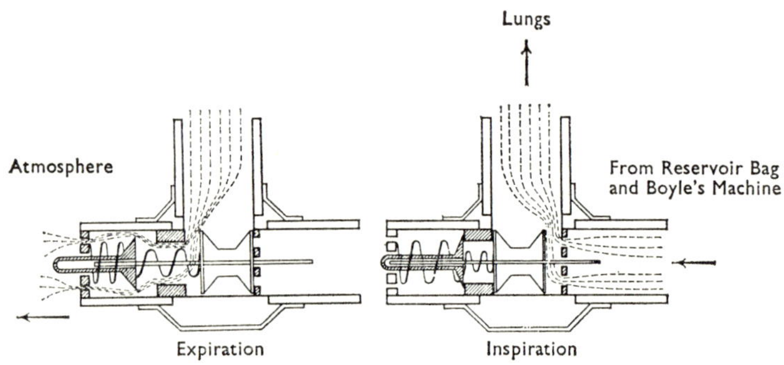

Fig. 6.12. Ruben's non-return valve.

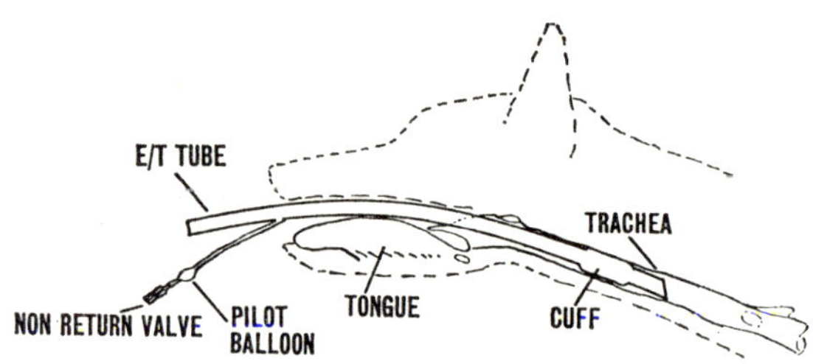

Fig. 6.13. Endotracheal tube in place.

In cats the process of passing an endotracheal tube is complicated by the fact that cats are susceptible to laryngeal spasm which can only be overcome by inducing anaesthesia deeply, or spraying the larynx with local anaesthetic or by administering a relaxant drug after the cat has been given an intravenous anaesthetic.

Note: if the animal becomes cyanosed in spite of an adequate flow of oxygen, (a) the tube may be kinked due to the head being bent down too far; (b) the tube may have passed into a main bronchus "shutting off" one lung.

Intravenous Anaesthetics

Only two drugs will be considered here, although many similar preparations exist: (a) pentobarbitone sodium—a short to medium acting anaesthetic, (b) thiopentone sodium—an ultra-short acting anaesthetic.

Pentobarbitone sodium is still used extensively as a general anaesthetic and it has undoubted value where half- to one-hour duration is required and where skilled assistance is not available. The average dosage is worked out on the basis of 29 mg/kg body weight for an 11 to 16 kg animal. Animals below this weight require slightly more and those above slightly less. Old dogs and toxic animals may take substantially less.

Induction by the intravenous route is usually smooth, but if the dog has not been premedicated recovery may be very slow and excitement and struggling may occur. Injections should always be made slowly particularly towards the point where full surgical anaesthesia is achieved, as the safety margin with pentobarbitone sodium is very small. The drug may be administered orally or intra-peritoneally although the delay in absorption and excretion makes these methods precarious and in the author's view dangerous.

Death from pentobarbitone sodium results from overdosage producing respiration failure. This is followed a few minutes later by cardiac failure. These circumstances are likely to occur about 10 to 15 minutes after administration.

Counter-action should include:

(a) The administration of oxygen via a mask accompanied by artificial respiration achieved by rhythmically pressing on the chest (the animal in lateral recumbrance) about every 3–4 seconds. Or by intubating, closing off the trachea by inflating the cuff of the tube, linking up with a reservoir bag and ventilating the lungs by gentle manipulation of the bag every 4–5 seconds.

(b) Injection of respiratory stimulants, e.g. 1 ml nikethamide BP (25% w/v solution) slowly injected intravenously or 2 ml subcutaneously (dosage assessed for 13–18 kg dog), pictrotoxin 1 mg/kg by slow intravenous injection.

Thiopentone sodium has two main uses—as an ultra-short-acting anaesthetic giving 5–15 minutes duration and as a means of induction prior to inhalation anaesthesia. The dosage rate is similar to pentobarbitone sodium, but the rate of injection is important: if injected quickly the duration of anaesthesia is short—if slowly the duration is increased. The solution must be injected intravenously, as it is an irritant to tissues and if injected in relatively large amounts subcutaneously a tissue slough may occur. The usual strength of the solution is 5%, but in small dogs it is wise to dilute to 2·5% and in toy dogs and cats to dilute further to 1·25% solution.

If prolonged anaesthesia is required, repeated injections of thiopentone sodium may be given, and some veterinary surgeons prefer to do this rather than give pentobarbitone sodium, although considerable care is still required.

MAKING AN INTRAVENOUS INJECTION

1. The area over the vein (i.e. radial or saphenous) is shaved or clipped.
2. Pressure is exerted by an assistant above the point at which the injection is to be made by the thumb or preferably by a piece of rolled 2 in. bandage.

3. The area over the vein is swabbed with spirit and allowed to dry.
4. The assistant pushes forward the leg from behind the elbow in the case of radial vein puncture and extends the stifle in the case of saphenous vein puncture.
5. A right-handed person injects the animal's right limb, grasps the limb with the left hand and runs the thumb alongside the vein—pushing it over slightly and steadying it to prevent it rolling out of place.
6. An eccentric syringe with short needle ($\frac{5}{8} \times \frac{6}{10}$ or $\frac{8}{10}$) is held in the right hand and the needle, which must be *sharp and free from barbs*, is held almost parallel to the limb but angled slightly towards the vein. It is introduced above and slightly to the opposite side of the thumb so that the vein is actually "held" between thumb and needle. It is inserted gently but quickly into the vein and blood will be seen to come back into the syringe.
7. The assistant releases pressure on the vein but still supports the limb.

Anaesthetic After-care

The patient should be kept in a warm atmosphere about 22°C (70°F). It should be placed on its side lying on a rug or blanket with a light blanket covering. If an endotracheal tube has been passed this should be left in position until the animal shows signs of mouth and tongue movement—the cuff should always be deflated as soon as anaesthesia ceases. The tube must be removed from the trachea gently to prevent the animal coughing. Once the tube has been removed the patient must be watched carefully until consciousness is regained, and until this stage is reached the tongue must be pulled well out of the mouth, particularly in short-nosed breeds.

If there is any tendency or risk of vomiting the animal must be positioned so that the body is raised above the level of the head and everything should be done to avoid inhalation of vomit.

After certain anaesthetics the animal may throw itself about rather violently during the recovery period and the RANA should hold and pacify the animal as much as possible until the stage of excitement has passed. Efficient premedication does much to prevent undue distress during recovery.

(c) THEATRE PRACTICE

W. B. SINGLETON, MRCVS

General Considerations

The success of most operations depends largely upon the thoroughness of preparation. This may take far longer than the operation itself, but operative time is vital to the patient and anything which will make the surgeon's task simpler and quicker should be part of preparation. It is a fallacy to think that animals are less susceptible to infection than humans or that their tissues heal any quicker. Even one infected operation wound in 500 is one too many. Ideally the same degree of care and preparation which precedes a human operation should be made before an operation upon an animal.

Good theatre practice should include the following duties:

1. Scrupulous cleanliness of the operating theatre.
2. Preparation and checking anaesthetic apparatus and equipment.
3. Sterilization of instruments, gloves, drapes, etc.
4. Preparation of the patient.
5. Preparation of the theatre.
6. Setting out of instruments, etc.:
   (a) in the preparation room;
   (b) in the operating theatre.
7. Preparation of the surgeon and nurses.
8. Assisting at the operations.
9. Immediate post-operative procedures.
10. Cleaning and care of instruments.

The precise order of each duty will vary slightly from practice to practice and even from one veterinary school to another. Unfortunately in practice the thoroughness with which each duty is carried out will also vary. The instructions which follow are meant to be a guide only but should fulfil the requirements of most efficiently run theatres. One point cannot be stressed too much. It is absolute folly to undertake complex preparations designed to ensure aseptic technique if one member of the team makes a careless mistake. For instance, touching the edge of an undraped operating table with scrubbed up or gloved hands, leaving on an extraction fan so that loose hair or dust is drawn into the theatre, wiping the forehead with a "sterile" hand, allowing an operation to be commenced beneath a lamp which is dusty. To twist a well-known maxim—the job is not worth doing unless it is done well.

Care of the Operating Theatre

1. As little as possible should be left on shelves—every single object should have a place and should be *replaced* immediately after use.

2. Shelves should be kept to the minimum but daily dusting or, better still, wiping with a damp wash leather of all objects on shelves, trolleys, lamps, etc., must be undertaken. A vacuum cleaner fitted with a bacterial filter is a highly satisfactory piece of equipment for cleaning shelves and other parts of the theatre.

3. The floor should be washed daily.

4. If an extraction fan is installed adjoining rooms should be kept clean and "dust free", remembering that the fan will draw dirty air into the theatre beneath doors, etc. The fan should be switched off during all operations.

5. A temperature near to 20°C (68°F) should be maintained.

Sterilization of Instruments and Materials

1. Sharp instruments, i.e. knives, needles, scissors, etc., should be kept in a sterilizing fluid (see Appendix) which contains an anti-rust compound, unless dry heat sterilization is used (see item 3).

2. Other instruments should be boiled for 30 minutes in a sterilizer and the efficiency of this procedure will be enhanced if 2% washing soda solution is used although alkaline solutions damage some materials, e.g. aluminium.

3. Or instruments may be placed in a hot air oven at 180°C (358°F) for 20 minutes.

4. Instruments may be autoclaved at 15 lb/in^2 pressure 121°C (250°F) for 15 minutes or at 20 lb/in^2 pressure 126°C (258°F) for 10 min.

An autoclave is a piece of equipment built to withstand internal pressure created by steam which is produced in a jacket around a main compartment. Into the latter, drums are placed containing the objects to be sterilized. Water within the jacket is heated by either gas or electricity. The compartment is sealed off from the jacket by a heavy lid which is usually screwed down. Pressure gauges and safety valves and thermometers are incorporated on the equipment. Three main types of autoclave are available:

1. The simplest operates by boiling-water in a closed container. A household pressure-cooker provides an example of this type and will operate at 15 lb/in^2. These cookers are very small and rarely hold sufficient items for more than one operation. Larger autoclaves operating on the same principle are available but suffer from the same major disadvantage, namely that pockets of non-sterile air may remain locked in the compartment due to the fact that steam is lighter than air and by this system not all the air is displaced from the container.
2. To overcome this point another type of autoclave is manufactured which provides for downward displacement of air—the air outlet valve being at the bottom of the apparatus and the steam inlet valve at the top. (Some autoclaves are built horizontally and some vertically but the same principle applies.) By this method the air is driven out of the container more effectively by the steam. In order to enhance the efficiency of this method and also to ensure more effective drying a further type is available.

3. This is known as the vacuum-assisted autoclave. The simple and vacuum-assisted autoclaves are available with several modifications. Perhaps the most important of these is the self-sterilizing air filter which is designed to ensure that clean air is admitted to replace steam in the final cooling stage.

The drums are packed with articles to be sterilized and a windowed cuff surrounds the outside of each drum. This can be moved so that matching windows on the drum wall can be either opened or closed. The openings may be fitted with bacterial filters in modern drums. In order to allow steam into the drums they are placed into the sterilizer with the windows open. As soon as the drums have been withdrawn from the compartment the windows are closed (unless fitted with filters) to prevent "contaminated" air being drawn into the drums as the contents cool.

The type of drum used in a vertical autoclave should have the openings at the top and bottom, for a horizontal autoclave at the sides or circumference. This will facilitate the displacement of air and the penetration of steam in each instance. In each type the contents should be packed loosely for the same reason, although when using the vacuum assisted type of autoclave the contents may be packed more tightly.

Drums are frequently replaced nowadays by bags made of nylon film. This is supplied in tubular form and a bag is produced by sealing one end with a special autoclavable tape. The instruments or other materials are placed in the bag, and after expressing as much air as possible the other end is also sealed with tape. One end can be sealed with Indicating tape on which a pattern appears after steam sterilization, and this prevents mistakes being made between sterilized and unsterilized packets. Similarly, parcels of dressings may be made up with sheets of nylon film and finally sealed with tape. The bags or parcels are placed free in the autoclave and sterilized in the usual way. The film can be obtained in various thicknesses but gauge C (0·002 in.) is the most satisfactory. Its permeability to steam is high but research has shown that the film is impervious to bacteria. After sterilization the sealed bag may be handled without danger of contaminating its contents and can be stored almost indefinitely in dust-proof boxes or cupboards. It is therefore possible to store packets of instruments, transfusion sets, drapes, syringes, ready for use at any time. This method is ideal for storing orthopaedic implants as any size of plate or screw could be available at a moment's notice. Furthermore, implants when packed individually in this way are protected from abrasion.

When the material is required for use the tape is removed from one end of the bag and its contents tipped on to a sterile towel. Similarly, a package of dressings may be opened and laid out on a trolley with Cheatle forceps.

It has been shown that the film can be re-sterilized 40–50 times. It is therefore relatively inexpensive.

The autoclave should be operated as follows:

1. The jacket should be filled with water to the indicated level (usually marked on a glass tube running vertically outside the jacket but connected with the interior by taps).

2. Taps should be closed and valves set. The escape cock (petcock) at the top of the compartment, usually on the lid, is opened.
3. Heat is applied and the petcock is not closed until steam is escaping freely.
4. The petcock is closed and pressure allowed to build up to the required pressure —it is held at this setting for the necessary time.
5. The petcock is opened, water drained off and the heat lowered but not turned off.
6. Heat is maintained for a further 10 minutes to drive off any moisture from cloths, etc. (this is not necessary with vacuum-assisted autoclaves).

   Note: damp cloths are easily contaminated. Provided they are packed in nylon bags, these can be placed into a low temperature oven to complete the drying process if the contents are not to be used immediately.

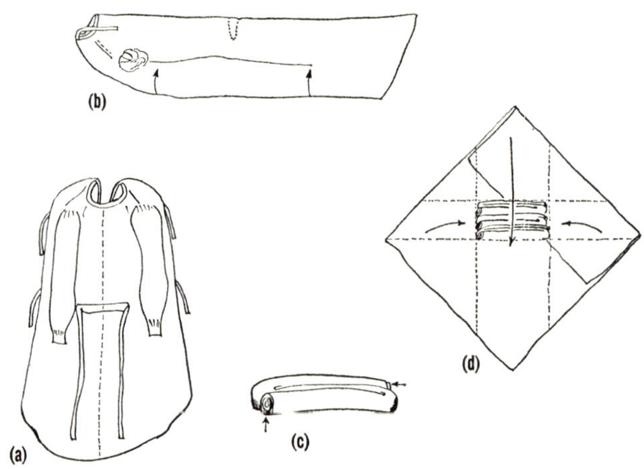

Fig. 6.14. (a)-(d) Folding and packing a surgical gown for autoclaving.

7. When the pressure has dropped the lid should be released immediately (if left until the autoclave is cool it may be very difficult to release).
8. The drums are lifted out and the windows closed immediately.

WRAPPING, PACKING AND UNWRAPPING OF CLOTHS, ETC., IN AUTOCLAVE DRUMS

(See Figs. 6.14, 6.15 and 6.16.)

STERILIZATION OF CLOTHS, DRAPES, ETC.

1. Autoclaving of 15 lb, 121°C for 30 minutes is an effective method.
2. Boiling for 45 minutes.
3. To be effective hot-air sterilization of cloths and drapes has to be carried out at

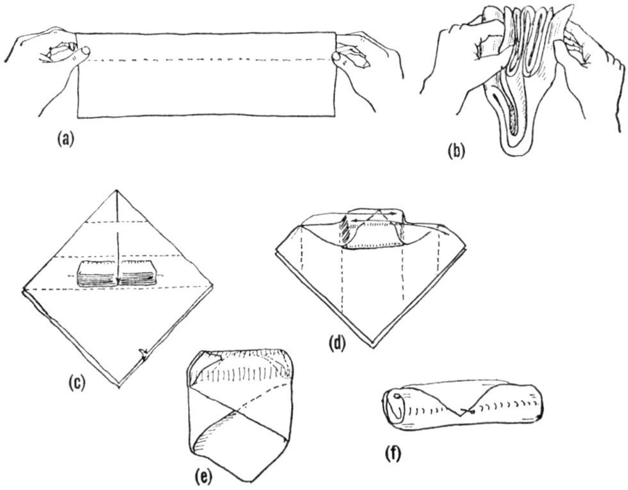

Fig. 6.15. (a)-(f) Folding and wrapping drapes into bundles of six.

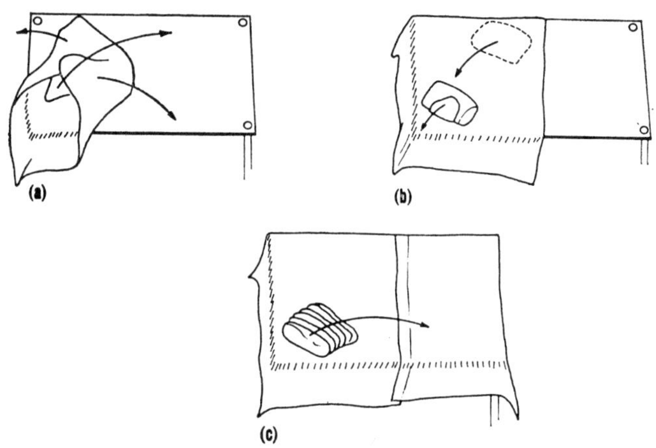

Fig. 6.16. (a)-(c) Draping the trolley.

a temperature which may cause charring if placed too close to the source of heat. Therefore they should always be placed on mesh trays.

STERILIZATION OF GLOVES

Autoclaving at 5 lb pressure for 30 minutes provided they are "clean" beforehand—if there is a possibility that the gloves are contaminated they should be boiled for $\frac{1}{2}$ hour, dried with a sterile cloth and then autoclaved. Owing to the fact that a very high percentage of gloves are punctured during a single operation, new gloves should be prepared for each operation. Cheap disposable gloves are now available.

Preparation of the Patient

Ideally the patient should be admitted 24 hours before operation so that thorough preparation may be carried out. Unfortunately, the co-operation of clients is not always possible on this point, but 4 hours prior to surgery should be looked upon as the minimum time whether the procedure is minor or major.

On admission, details of the case should be written on a record card which is fixed to the animal's cage door. Information concerning, breed, sex, age, owner's name, address and telephone number, procedure to be undertaken, whether or not the owner has agreed to a general anaesthetic being administered, time of admission, estimated time of discharge and a note of articles accompanying the animal, e.g. lead, collar, coat, basket, etc.

The owner should be asked when the animal was last fed and when the dog last passed urine and faeces. If there is doubt or the animal has not evacuated it should be walked a little and given a chance to "be clean" naturally. (Otherwise the bladder may have to be emptied immediately after induction of anaesthesia and before the wound area is scrubbed up.) If constipated a glycerine enema (1 oz glycerine to $\frac{1}{2}$ pint luke-warm water) should be administered. If a midline abdominal approach is to be undertaken the whole area should be washed with soap and water if it appears to be soiled.

The appropriate area of skin should be prepared by first, clipping the site with fine clippers and soaking with a solution of 1–2% iodine in 70% alcohol. This kills vegetative forms of bacteria in 20 seconds and is also effective against spores. The area over the radial vein, if an intravenous injection is to be given, should also be shaved. If the animal is difficult to handle the preparation may have to wait until it is tranquillized and occasionally until it is under an anaesthetic, but this type of delay should be avoided if possible.

Some veterinary surgeons like the animal to be weighed at this stage. Usually a tranquillizer is administered intramuscularly 1–2 hours prior to surgery. Many methods exist, but 1 mg of promazine per 1 lb is effective.

When the dog has been anaesthetized the area of skin should be washed well with ether soap using a soft nail-brush if necessary—several washes and rinses are necessary. Alternatively, quaternary ammonium compounds, e.g. Cetavlon 1% solution, may be used. The area is then painted again liberally with the iodine solution making quite sure that no pools of solution are left. This can occur in bitches placed on their backs on the operating table as the solution may collect between the posterior mammary glands. If this happens it might ignite if diathermy is used.

Intubation, etc., is described elsewhere, but all articles required for this procedure should be layed out as part of preparation, i.e. a range of tubes approximating to the size of the animal's trachea, lubricant ointment, forceps, if used, a gag and 1 in. adhesive tape cut into 3 × 8 in. lengths. One may be used to secure the tube to the dog's muzzle, the others may be necessary to secure drip-feed needles into the vein.

If intravenous anaesthesia is to be used the approximate amount should be placed in a syringe at the correct solution. The needle of the syringe should be protected until use by an antiseptic swab or in a sterile container.

Lighting should be checked for position in both the preparation room and the theatre. X-ray viewer, diathermy, suction pump, waste containers, etc., should all be ready to be switched on or placed into position.

SETTING OUT OF STERILIZED INSTRUMENTS

If the RANA is the surgeon's only assistant, as so often happens in veterinary practice, she will have set out instruments before the animal is prepared for surgery. Each surgeon has personal preferences about the way this should be done, but basically the following points should be observed.

1. The RANA should put on cap and mask, making sure that all hair is tucked into the cap—the operating theatre is no place to display glamorous hair styles!

2. She must discard soiled overalls and either scrub up at this stage and put on a sterile gown and gloves if used, or if she is expected to set out instruments and then do a *dirty* job, for instance helping during the initial stages of anaesthesia, she must replace the soiled overall by a freshly laundered one making certain that even this does not contact the drapes which are placed over trolley, etc. Obviously, where a high degree of asepsis is the aim, the RANA should follow the first procedure, and having set out the sterile instruments, she should wait with hands clasped together until she is asked to assist at the actual operation.

3. Having scrubbed up, etc., someone else must be asked to release autoclave drum lids, raise sterilizer lids, etc., and sterile drapes should be placed on the trolleys making certain that they *hang over the edge by at least 12 in. all round.* The instruments are then placed in groups. They may be lifted out of the sterilizer or oven by the fingers if cool enough but better still by sterile Cheatle forceps—if these are used scrubbing up at this stage need not be too rigorous. The laying out of instruments should be given careful thought so that artery forceps, Allis forceps, scissors, ligatures, etc., are grouped together in positions which relate to their actual requirement. An excellent method is to place groups of "working instruments", e.g. eight pairs of artery forceps, six pairs of Allis forceps, one straight Mayo scissor and one curved pair, one pair dissecting forceps, one pair rat-toothed forceps, two retractors, one kidney dish and swabs on to a Mayo trolley which can be swung over the patient, making the instruments readily available to surgeon and RANA. Spare instruments and those which may only be required at a certain stage of the operation may be placed on a second trolley.

Whatever method is used the laid-out instruments should be completely covered with sterile cloths until actually required.

Having done this, if there is only one RANA, she will have to become "dirty" again in order to assist with anaesthesia, etc. When this has been accomplished and the animal is happily "balanced", both surgeon and RANA will have to prepare for the operation. The ideal circumstances occur when two or more RANAs are available and one can sterilize the hands, don autoclaved clothing, set out instruments, etc., and wait for the surgeon.

Preparation of the Surgical Team

CLEANSING THE HANDS AND ARMS

The skin harbours two types of bacteria—transient and resident. The transient have been acquired by contamination, and the resident are those organisms which populate the crevices of the normal skin. Most of the latter are symbiotic. In scrubbing, bacteria are removed in two ways: by the bacteriostatic action of the soap or detergent, and by the washing of the running water, aided by the friction of the brush. Following is the procedure:

1. Put on cap and mask.
2. Trim nails short, remove nail polish, push back cuticle and clean nails.
3. Turn and regulate hot and cold water taps.
4. Wash hands, arms and elbows thoroughly with soap. Keep arms flexed so that the hands are above elbow level.
5. Rinse, removing soap and lather. Let water run off elbows.
6. Wet sterile brush, hands and arms with water and tincture of green soap, poured by assistant RANA. Scrub for 5 minutes by the clock, using soap or detergent and running water as needed.
7. Always keep hands up above elbow level. After scrubbing is begun, the hands and arms must never fall below the waist or touch the body.
8. Scrub systematically; palm, back of hand, fingers, and up the arm to 2 in. above the elbow, paying particular attention to scrubbing the nails.
9. Discard brush and rinse, letting water run off elbows.
10. Have hexachlorophene (Physohex) or similar product poured on to the palms of the hands and massage in for 1 or 2 minutes.
11. Dry with sterile towel which is accordion-folded and falls open when picked up. Dry hands in centre; dry one arm on one end, going from wrist to elbow. Dry the other arm on the other end because the towel becomes contaminated when the elbow is reached. If the operation is a major one and two people are scrubbing, the assistant RANA opens a bundle of towels. If the operation is a minor one, the surgeon and surgical RANA use the towel on top of the stack in the small bundle.
12. Ready for gown and gloves.

PUTTING ON THE STERILE GOWN

1. Pick up the gown from the opened bundle on the trolley. Grasp it firmly at the neck and let it unroll by dropping the rest of it. Be sure it does not touch anything in the room.

2. Carefully unfold the gown with back side toward the body. Do not touch the front side of the gown. With the right hand grasp the collar at the left tape and put the left arm into the sleeve and extend the hand through the wristlet.

3. With the left hand, grasp the collar of the gown at the right tape, replacing the right hand. Put the right arm into the right sleeve and extend the hand through the wristlet. Hold both arms and hands extended and up and wait for the assistant RANA to tie and adjust the gown.

4. The assistant RANA helps with the gown by standing directly behind the surgeon and surgical RANA. She must place her hands only on the shoulders and inside of the gown and may not touch the sides or front of the gown while catching the tapes.

PUTTING ON THE STERILE GLOVES

(See Fig. 6.17 (a)–(g))

1. The assistant RANA opens the glove wrap for the surgeon or surgical RANA. Each should take the powder envelope from the glove wrap and rub the powder into the surface of the hands.

2. The right glove is picked up with the left hand, grasping it by the turned-down cuff. (The outside surface of the glove is never touched by the hand because it is impossible to sterilize a hand completely.)

3. Put the right hand into the right glove about two-thirds of the way with the aid of the left hand. Care should be taken to see that the folded-down cuff is not disturbed.

4. With the right hand reach into the glove wrap and insert the gloved fingers under the cuff of the other glove.

5. Hold the left glove with the right gloved hand by means of the cuff and pull the glove over the left hand and wristlet of the gown.

6. Place the left gloved fingers under the cuff of the right glove at the palm and extend it up to the wristlet of the right sleeve. Adjust the gloves on the hands.

Assisting at Operations

Swabbing: dry autoclaved gauze swabs are the best material for swabbing; dab firmly—do not wipe as this damages fine capillaries and increases bleeding.

Passing of instruments: try to be one step ahead of the surgeon and have his next instrument ready. Learn the way he prefers the instruments to be handed to him.

Suturing: always have suture material ready with needles threaded and take the "loose" end of the material between finger and thumb or a pair of artery forceps so that the surgeon does not accidentally pull the suture end through the tissue.

Always concentrate upon the job in hand, act quickly to instructions—handle instruments firmly but with "touch" never pulling on tissues unnecessarily, remembering that the less trauma produced during an operation the quicker the healing process.

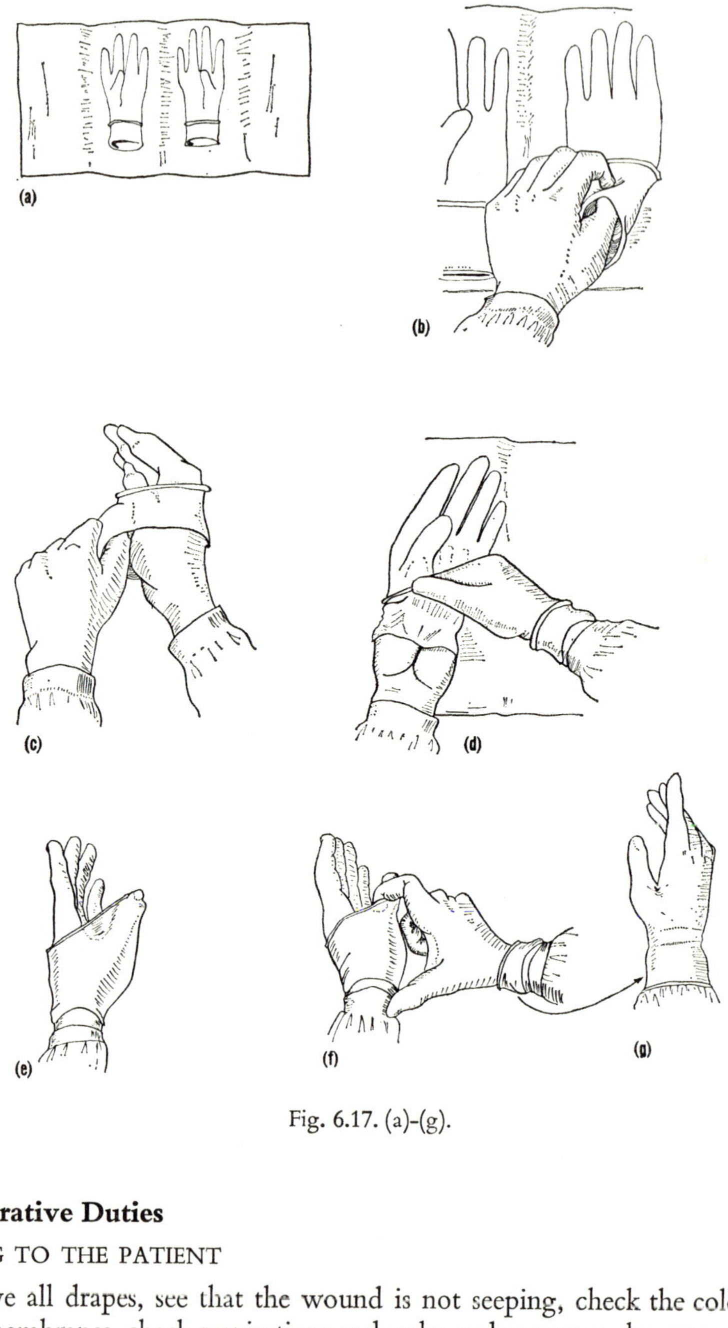

(a) (b) (c) (d) (e) (f) (g)

Fig. 6.17. (a)-(g).

Post-operative Duties

RELATING TO THE PATIENT

Remove all drapes, see that the wound is not seeping, check the colour of the mucous membranes, check respirations and pulse and report to the surgeon. Deflate the cuff, and when the dog begins to move its mouth remove the endotracheal tube when used. In short-nosed dogs the breathing should be watched carefully at this stage. It is usually wise to remove the patient to its recovery cage before removing the tube. Check repeatedly on colour, respiratory rate, pulse and for signs of haemorrhage. If post-operative haemorrhage from the wound does occur, cold compresses should be applied to the wound and secured by an elastic bandage applied with pressure. Check again in 15 minutes and if still progressing the surgeon should be informed. During the recovery period the patient should not be left, and vomiting must be watched for. If this occurs the animal's body should be raised and the mouth swabbed out thoroughly.

CARE OF INSTRUMENTS

All instruments should be washed in cold running water then rinsed in hot and dried off with a towel or placed into the dry heat sterilizer or oven. There is no doubt that dry heat sterilization and drying off preserves instruments whereas there is considerable wear and tear if they are boiled, washed and just dried off on a towel. Special instruments such as orthopaedic bone drills *must* be dried off either in an oven or over an electric fire. Delicate cutting instruments should receive a very thin covering with Vaseline or a fine mineral oil. All jointed instruments should be checked regularly for evidence of wear at the rivet and signs of rusting. Periodically they should be touched with oil (3-in-1 oil is ideal). Scissors and solid scalpels should be stood in sterilizing fluid to avoid the necessity for boiling. Again this procedure can be dispensed with if hot air sterilization is used.

A good theatre RANA must be prepared to be disciplined, must be extremely conscientious in everything she does, and therefore completely dependable. She must also treat patients with sympathy, gentleness and patience.

Appendix

Chemical agents are commonly used for their bactericidal or bacteristatic activity particularly in connection with instruments and equipment which cannot withstand high temperature sterilization.

Soaps: have a bactericidal and bacteristatic action against many bacteria but are not effective against certain pathogenic gram-positive organisms.

Alcohols: ethyl and isopropyl alcohol are useful for their fat solvent properties but bactericidal activity even in 80% solution is slow and there is virtually no action against spores. Action is delayed by the presence of organic material.

Phenols: should be avoided as they are toxic to living tissues and sporocidal activity is very limited.

Cresols are toxic to living tissues and should not be applied directly to an animal. However, 1% solutions kill vegetative organisms even in the presence of organic material and therefore cresols are useful for scrubbing floors, walls, instruments used for grooming and cleaning animals, also contaminated instruments.

Chloroxylenol (Dettol) is an effective bactericide against gram-positive organisms and the majority but not all gram-negative organisms (including a group of enteric bacteria).

Cetrimide (Cetavlon) is a quartenary ammonium compound. Gram-negative organisms, spores, fungi and acid-fact bacteria are susceptible to its bactericidal activity, therefore it is used for cleansing the skin, contaminated wounds, ointments, dishes, glassware, etc.

Benzalkenium chloride (Roccal) is similar in action to cetrimide and has similar application.

Chlorhexidine (Hibitane) is one of the most effective preparations as it has bactericidal activity against gram-negative and gram-positive organisms. It is effective in the presence of organic material including blood, mucus, pus, etc. As a 1% solution in ethylalcohol it provides a suitable solution for the sterile storage of instruments.

Hypochlorites have limited application as they damage metal and rubber. Being inexpensive solutions are useful for cleansing floors, etc.

Formaldehyde is highly effective against bacteria and bacterial spores and viruses even in the presence of organic material. A suitable solution for the chemical sterilization of instruments may be prepared as follows:

℞	Formalin	2·5 ml
	Liq. phenol	0·5 ml
	Borax	1·3 g
	Fluorescin	0·2% 0·6 g
	Water	100 ml

It should be realized that autoclaving of items which will withstand this method is preferable to any form of chemical sterilization. However, if solutions are used, several hours (usually 3 hours or more) are required for the maximum effect to be obtained. Also the presence of pus, blood, etc., on instruments may reduce the efficiency of this form of sterilization tremendously. Therefore they should be well washed and scrubbed before immersion into the solution chosen. All instruments should be rinsed well in running water before use in order to remove traces of the chemical solutions.

Using the following as examples of acceptable and efficient methods of sterilizing, a list is given of the various ways certain pieces of equipment in common use may be rendered sterile.

A = autoclaving.
B = hot air oven (dry heat).
C = chlorhexidine 1% or cetrimide 1%.
D = liq. formal.
E = Lysol 5% in water.

1. Catheters: A—stored in nylon film packs or soaked in D for 3 hours and stored in tube containing formaldehyde tablets.
2. Endoscopes: C.

3. Endotracheal tubes: D—soak for 3 hours, rinse and lay on a tray *over* solution of D in a container with well fitting lid.
4. Fluids for injection: A—timed from the moment that 121°C (250°F) is reached for 15–30 minutes depending upon volume. Containers should only be 75% full and should be allowed to cool slowly.
5. Glassware: A—flasks should be laid on their sides or with opening pointing downwards. Syringes with plungers removed from barrel may be autoclaved and later stored in nylon film.
6. Sharp instruments including scalpel blades, needles, etc.: A, B, or D.
7. Nail brushes used for scrubbing up: A, B or D—the brushes will deteriorate rapidly when frequently sterilized, but being inexpensive should be replaced frequently.
8. Nylon and other suture material, e.g. silk, linen, etc. (not catgut): A.
9. Thermometers: D.
10. Trays and large enamel or stainless steel vessels: A if size permits or E.

Note: In spite of the above recommendations it should be remembered that disposable items now available to an ever-increasing extent have distinct advantages from the point of view of asepsis and time saving. Typical examples are hypodermic syringes and needles, rubber gloves, drapes, tongue spatulae, catheters, etc.

CHAPTER 7

Obstetrical and Paediatric Nursing and the Principles of Breeding

(a) OBSTETRICAL NURSING AND THE PRINCIPLES OF BREEDING IN THE DOG

S. F. J. HODGMAN, MRCVS

Introduction

A high standard of general management should be regarded as an essential requirement for a breeding kennels. The selection of stock should be made with care, and such stock maintained in good health with adequate exercise and well balanced food. Facilities should be made for bitches in season to be kennelled and exercised separately from the stud dog, and care taken in seeing that she is not left alone in a yard or run as despite elaborate precautions in the form of high and costly fences, a dog will find some way of gaining access to her if he can; a bitch, too, will try and escape if given the chance, and it is not unknown for a bitch to have been mated through a wire-net fencing. Attention should be paid to the clothing worn by the attendants if they have to care for the stud dog as well as the bitches in season.

Oestrus

Under normal conditions a bitch first comes into season at between 7 and 12 months of age, and once every 6 months afterwards. In breeds which have a comparatively short history of domestication, the oestrus interval may easily be 12 months, as may be found in the wild dog. The actual period of oestrus lasts, on an average, for 3 weeks, but throughout this time there are only a few days during the 2nd week when she will accept a dog for mating.

The first signs of approaching oestrus are an enlargement of the vulva and a slight mucous discharge. This phase lasts for a few days and is followed by a more distinct swelling and hardening of the vulva, accompanied by a blood-stained discharge which may or may not be copious according to the individual. Ovulation begins during the first few days of the start of oestrus and this is a process by which the ova, or eggs, are liberated from the ovary and start to travel down the fallopian tube; the ova may then be fertilized if mating has taken place. By the 16th day the bitch loses her mating impulse, the normal signs of "heat" begin to wane, and by the 21st day the vulva has returned to normal size and the discharge has eased.

Anoestrus or Absence of Heat

There are cases where the normal signs of oestrus do not occur at all although the bitch may appear to be perfectly healthy in every other respect. This condition is believed to be caused by hormonal dysfunction, and as it upsets the entire oestous cycle it is naturally regarded as one of the reasons for infertility.

Silent heat is another form of abnormal oestrus whereby the external genitalia is enlarged but the bleeding is absent. This condition can cause confusion regarding the correct time for mating, it being difficult to assess the exact stage of oestrus owing to the absence of the normal blood-stained discharge. Both conditions require professional treatment as soon as possible.

There are other reasons for causing deviations of oestrus such as ovarian disease, chronic metritis, tumours or malnutrition. It is wise, however, to seek veterinary advice whenever a bitch does not appear to conform to the normal function.

The temperament of a bitch may alter when she is in season. She may become more affectionate than usual towards her handler and quite snappy and irritable with other bitches, and although the function of "heat" is a natural one, a bitch may suffer a lowered resistance at this time, therefore special attention should be paid to kennel hygiene and management.

Mating

Providing a bitch is completely ready for service this should not present difficulty, but there are many and varied occasions when a certain amount of supervision and assistance is necessary, particularly if either the dog or bitch is inexperienced.

Arrangements should be made for the mating to take place where there is enough space for the preliminary play and courtship, and yet in which dog and bitch can be controlled. It is wise to introduce them on leads but they may be released as soon as the handlers are satisfied that neither animal is going to display bad temper; maiden bitches are likely to be more hesitant than matrons, and occasionally a bitch has to be muzzled for mating, but there is no need to regard this as a routine measure.

The bitch will indicate her readiness by standing quietly, and once she has been mounted interference is not usually necessary, although if she tends to let her hindquarters sag the attendant can give some support. In the event of an unsuccessful initial attempt, the dog should be restrained from further efforts and taken away until he has quietened down; he can then be returned to her for a fresh attempt.

Once the "tie" has been established and the dogs are back to back then it is wise to keep both animals under control so as to prevent one pulling away from the other and causing injury to either or both. The "tie" may last up to half an hour or even longer, but when it has subsided they will move apart and the mating has been completed.

Many difficult or unsuccessful matings are usually the result of unreadiness on the part of the bitch. There may be other reasons, such as rough handling or fright, and in some cases *sexual frigidity* has been encountered. In such bitches the normal manifestations of oestrus and the desire for mating are present, but she will not in fact accept the dog when the time comes. Opinions vary as to how to deal with this condition, some leave dog and bitch together for long periods and some favour a forced mating, while others prefer not to breed from such bitches as the condition may be hereditary and therefore may be passed on to the progeny. Should the mating be deemed essential one can resort to artificial insemination—but if a pedigree dog, permission must be sought from the Kennel Club.

Nymphomania is another abnormal sexual condition which may give rise to trouble or even failure over mating. Some bitches display excessive desire to mate but in many cases will refuse the dog.

MISALLIANCE

Puppies born as a result of a mating between pure-bred specimens of different breeds may show evidence of the crossing at birth; on the other hand, physical appearances of such puppies may not alter until they become very much older, and sometimes not even then, but if they are later allowed to breed then evidence of their mixed parentage will invariably be obvious in the next generation. Misalliance, however, leaves no effect upon the bitch and makes no difference to her ability to produce pure-bred puppies on subsequent occasions.

Abortion

Early abortion can be carried out by a veterinary surgeon and is usually successful if performed within 48 hours of mating; natural abortion, or miscarriage, is comparatively rare in the bitch. If this does occur, it is usually as a result of an infection, violence of some kind, an endocrine abnormality or faulty nutrition.

Phantom, Pseudo of False Pregnancy (Pseudocyesis)

This may be a physiological condition but it is manifested in two ways. Some bitches display an obvious maternal instinct at a time a litter would be due had mating taken place, and the general behaviour is similar to that of a bitch with puppies—even to the extent of secreting milk. The condition may last for a week or two, or even longer, during which time plenty of exercise should be given and the diet reduced, particularly meat. The breasts should be left alone providing they do not become hard and painful, in which case a little milk may be removed. The milk, however, will usually dry up without any trouble and the bitch will return to normal.

The other type of false pregnancy is also manifested by this maternal behaviour, but the difference here can be seen in a definite enlargement of the abdomen at a time when such signs would become apparent had the bitch been mated and conceived. This condition may continue for several weeks, and many owners naturally believe the bitch must be pregnant, but the signs gradually disappear either a week or two before the whelping date or very soon after.

Pyometra is a condition sometimes associated with false pregnancy although more often encountered in elderly bitches, but the seriousness of the illness varies according to the degree of infection present in the uterus.

Pregnancy

The period between service and whelping is on the average 62–63 days; it may vary a day or two on either side of the expected date, but puppies born more than a week in advance seldom survive.

Definite signs of pregnancy vary with individuals, and in some cases it may be 6 or 7 weeks before a diagnosis can be made. While it is sometimes possible for a diagnosis to be made at the 3rd week, a lot depends on the size, nature and physical condition of the bitch.

The first visible sign will be a slight enlargement of the abdomen and a filling-out of the flanks. Owing to the better muscular tone of a maiden bitch this early fullness may become obvious sooner than in one who has had several litters. As pregnancy progresses the bitch will naturally become heavier, and at about the 6th week the mammary glands will increase in size. At this stage there may be an alteration in her behaviour, she may become quieter and less inclined for as much exercise and play as usual, and her appetite may appear to be quite insatiable. The reverse can happen and a bitch may go completely off her food, but the majority of healthy bitches eat heartily throughout pregnancy until just before parturition commences.

FEEDING THE PREGNANT BITCH

The condition of both the bitch and her pups will depend, to a great extent, on the bitch's nutrition. As her appetite increases it is as well to offer her two or three meals a day instead of the usual one, thus relieving her of too much bulk at any one time, and should consist of a plentiful supply of raw meat, biscuits, cereal, raw grated carrot, bonemeal and milk; she will, however, derive most of the nutritional benefits from the high protein value of the meat. A daily dose of cod liver oil is an important supplement to the diet, and fresh drinking water should be supplied at all times.

A watchful eye should be kept to see that the bitch does not become constipated during the latter part of pregnancy; bowel action should be regular, but if she does seem constipated a little liquid paraffin added to the food usually has the desired effect. If the condition does not improve within a day or two the matter should be reported to a veterinary surgeon.

EXERCISE

While controlled exercise is essential, too much strenuous activity, such as jumping or wild play with rough companions, is contra-indicated.

PREPARATIONS FOR PARTURITION

A whelping box should be provided for the bitch at about the 6th week so that she has plenty of time to get used to it before the puppies arrive. It should be large enough for her to lie comfortably outstretched and with plenty of room for the pups as well. The sides should be low enough for her to move in and out with ease and yet high enough to keep the puppies in and to protect them from draughts. A rail fixed around the inside of the box to prevent the puppies from being crushed by a careless mother is advisable. Plenty of newspaper is the best form of bedding, and this should be replaced frequently or whenever it has become soiled.

As the date for parturition draws nearer, a small first-aid box should be made ready containing a thermometer, scissors, cotton wool, a solution of a mild antiseptic, several squares of gauze, and a little brandy in case of need. In the event of the pups having to be removed from their mother it is as well to have a basket or box, a hot-water bottle, a blanket, and two or three towels accessible. If the weather is cold and the whelping is to take place in an unheated room or kennel, a "pig-lamp" is useful for providing both warmth and light. The amount of supervision necessary will depend largely on the temperament and general condition of the bitch, but providing the preparations have been carefully carried out and all is ready in case of emergency, it is wiser to leave the bitch, within reason, alone.

INDICATIONS OF APPROACHING LABOUR

About 24–48 hours before the start of labour the bitch's temperature usually drops, and this may continue until it is about 2°F below normal; she may seem restless and uneasy and may refuse food and, or, vomit it. The external genitalia becomes more prominent and flaccid, and a few hours before labour commences a sticky discharge will be seen. If such signs are present and labour does not start, or if, after some slight straining, the bitch settles down again, veterinary help must be obtained at once as this may be symptomatic of primary uterine inertia.

NORMAL PARTURITION

The process of parturition can be divided into two stages:

The primary stage consists of irregular and spasmodic contractions of the uterine muscles. These early contractions bring about the relaxation and dilation of the cervix, vagina and vulva through which the puppies are expelled. This stage may last for a few hours or even all day during which time the bitch may seem a little distressed and uncomfortable.

The secondary stage follows the primary stage immediately and the contractions now become powerful and perceptible. The bitch strains with each contraction in an effort to expel the puppy, but as the muscles relax she too will relax and lie resting, often panting and shivering at the same time. With the onset of the next contraction she will start straining again and this process continues until the first puppy is gradually forced through from the uterus and out through the cervix and vagina. The puppy is normally preceded by the membranes which invariably rupture from pressure as the pup is being born; if this does not happen the bitch will tear them and release the puppy herself, at the same time severing the cord. If the membranes are left behind they usually follow the next contraction. The membranes are usually eaten by the bitch. There are differences of opinion as to the advisability of allowing the bitch to eat them, but this is a perfectly natural process and many people consider that a placental hormone assists the uterus to contract and that the membranes have a high nutritional value.

If the membranes have not ruptured naturally by the time the puppy is born, and if the bitch has not dealt with it herself, then the attendant should do so immediately, as until the puppy has been released it cannot breathe. Occasionally a maiden bitch may be a little confused at the birth of her first pup and not attend to it as she should do, and in such cases assistance will have to be given. The cord can be severed in two ways—either cut or torn. In cutting, a sterile ligature should be applied first at about $1\frac{1}{2}$–2 in. from the pup's abdomen, and then cut on the distal side. If it is intended to tear the cord, great care should be taken not to put any tension on the umbilicus of the puppy as this could lead to a hernia.

Although the majority of puppies are born head first, it is not unusual for them to be presented hindlegs first. This is commonly referred to as a breech presentation and often causes some difficulty in delivery owing to the resistance caused by the hair being in the wrong direction. Many such presentations may also be lying on their backs and must be turned before delivery can take place. Such breech presentations create most difficulty in cases of brachycephalic breeds and those with very large heads, such as a Scottie. Normally such presentations should be dealt with by an expert, but in an emergency the attendant may have to act, especially if expert assistance is not readily available. Should this become necessary it must be remembered that the hindquarters presented are slippery and can be injured by undue pressure. In attempting to turn the puppy, it is best to place a piece of sterile gauze over the quarters before attempting to rotate, and while maintaining a secure but not too firm hold, the body may be slowly and gently turned; no traction should be applied until straining occurs on the part of the bitch.

The interval between births varies, but the average time is 15–30 minutes, although much longer or shorter periods are not infrequent. Pups normally commence to suckle soon after birth, but opinions differ as to whether they should be left with the mother during her labour or taken away until she has finished whelping. If she is a good mother it is better to leave the puppies with her throughout; bitches have been known to disregard the puppies when returned, but with care and patience, however, this can be overcome especially if the pups are smeared with a little of the bitch's discharge. If for any reason the puppies have to be removed then it is wiser to take them right out of her hearing so that their crying cannot cause her distress.

Apart from keeping a watchful eye on the procedure and calmly carrying out any general assistance as described above, other forms of interference in a *normal* parturition is both unnecessary and undesirable. There may be cases where labour becomes difficult and consequently a greater degree of help is required. If this appears to be likely it is as well to get in touch with a veterinary surgeon in good time, giving him as many details as possible so that he can bring with him any equipment he might need.

Malpresentations are a common cause of difficult or sometimes impossible deliveries. These cases must be attended to immediately by a veterinary surgeon who, having diagnosed the trouble and weighed up the circumstances, will act accordingly. He may be able to correct an abnormal position by manipulation and deliver the puppy with forceps through the vagina, or, on the other hand, he may decide to perform a caesarian section.

There are many other complications of parturition, amongst them being uterine inertia of which there are two types.

Primary uterine inertia can be suspected when labour starts and then ceases after only a short period, or when labour does not start at all. This condition is more often found in elderly bitches whose muscular system has become weakened either by age or having had too many litters, or even by lack of exercise during pregnancy. In some breeds it is considered to be associated with a hereditary breed incidence.

Secondary uterine inertia is similar in as much as normal contractions fail to occur, but this is caused by the exhaustion of the uterine muscle after excessive uterine activity throughout labour. Both conditions require prompt veterinary attention.

Revival of Puppies

Fortunately, most newly born puppies are surprisingly strong and healthy and they feel quite plump and warm, but there are cases where they have not had an easy passage into the world and are born blue and limp and sometimes seemingly lifeless. Such puppies need immediate attention if they are to survive, although puppies born anaemic and flaccid are usually beyond help, but it is always worth trying to resuscitate any pup which is not outwardly dead.

The first task is to ensure that the mouth and nose are free from mucus and membranes, and if not these must be removed at once and the mouth gently wiped in a downward direction with a piece of gauze. The puppy should then be placed in a warm rough towel and its body rubbed quite briskly to stimulate its circulation and respiration. The most important thing at this stage is to cause the puppy to gasp, and once air has entered the lungs normal breathing continues. Artificial respiration can be applied by *gently* compressing the ribs with forefinger and thumb in a rhythm of about twenty times a minute. Mouth-to-mouth resuscitation can also be tried, but care must be taken that the pup's lungs are not injured by too much force. A drop of brandy on the tongue is sometimes successful as is also a drop of HCN (hydrocyanic acid), but this latter treatment must only be carried out by a veterinary surgeon. Another method to be recommended is dipping the puppy alternately in hot and cold water. Once breathing has become established, however, the puppy will gradually lose its bluish colour and gain strength and should be returned to the bitch as soon as possible so that she can continue the revival process by licking.

Post-partum Care of the Bitch

It is not always easy to tell whether the last puppy has been born, but if the bitch seems to have settled down comfortably and shows no further signs of straining or panting, and if some time has elapsed since the last puppy arrived, then one can be fairly certain that all is over. It has been known, however, following such behaviour for a bitch to produce a puppy several hours later, and it is a wise precaution to have a veterinary examination to make sure that parturition has in fact ceased. The bitch can then be taken out for a short run to relieve herself; she may be very reluctant to leave her puppies and may even appear to be rather aggressive about doing so, but a little firm and kindly coaxing will soon settle her fears. While she is away the soiled newspaper in the whelping box should be replaced with fresh, and the puppies should be examined for any obvious defects such as cleft palates or hare lips, etc. On her return, the bitch may be offered a little milk and then left undisturbed for a few hours with her pups.

It takes a little time for the bitch's genital organs to return to normal after whelping, and for a week or two there may be a variable blood-stained discharge. This comes from the placental sites in the uterus and the bleeding is usually controlled by normal contraction, and unless the bleeding is excessive it should not be cause for concern; if there should be an offensive discharge, with or without pus, and an increase in temperature, veterinary help is required at once.

The bitch's stools may be rather copious and black for the first few days after parturition, particularly if she has eaten all the after-births; this is quite normal, although the condition should not be prolonged.

For the first 2 days after whelping the bitch should be given a light diet of milky preparations and nourishing meat broths. She can be given as much as she will take and as often as she wants it, and by the 3rd day she can resume her normal diet, although the supplementary milk meals should be continued. Some bitches dislike milk, and in such cases a good powdered dried milk mixed with the food is recommended. A bowl of fresh drinking water must be kept near the box at all times.

During the lactation period a bitch may suffer an acute calcium and mineral deficiency owing to the increasing demands on her milk supply. This condition is known as *eclampsia* and the symptoms are manifested by a stiffening of the legs and general body spasms, and in bad cases this can sometimes be followed by convulsions. A veterinary surgeon should be summoned at once, and after an injection of calcium the bitch usually recovers quite quickly.

Care of the bitch's breasts is an important factor during lactation. The puppies' nails may have to be trimmed to prevent them injuring the breasts, and a watch kept to see that a puppy does not suckle at an empty breast as this can make the nipple very sore. On the other hand, too much milk can cause a great deal of pain, but gentle massage and expressing a little of the milk will ease the engorged glands and make the bitch feel more comfortable. If, however, the breasts seem to be very inflamed and the bitch is still in pain after milk has been expressed, there may be an infection present. This condition is known as *mastitis* and requires immediate treatment by a veterinary surgeon, as not only is this a danger to the bitch but naturally infected milk can quickly mean death to the puppies.

As weaning time approaches the bitch should be encouraged to leave the whelping box for longer periods; most bitches are quite happy about this and will gradually return to their normal way of life and feeding and exercise.

Hand Rearing of Puppies

The best method of rearing pups is, of course, where the mother can feed and care for them herself. If this is not possible, as when, for instance, the bitch has died during whelping or is suffering from an illness or recovering from a caesarian operation, the puppies can be successfully reared by hand.

The first essential is warmth, not only in the room but also in the puppies' box or basket. This is best provided by a hot-water bottle, care being taken to see that the water is not too hot, nor that it should be allowed to get cold, and that it is well covered by a towel or blanket.

For the first 2 weeks the pups must be fed frequently; some do this every 3 hours and some every 4 hours, but puppies, like all young things, will gorge themselves and then go to sleep, and the best time to feed them is when they wake. A premature-baby's feeding bottle is commonly used, but in an emergency a 4-oz medicine bottle is perfectly adequate. The teat should be small and preferably straight as some puppies have difficulty in keeping the hard bulbous type teat in their mouths. The hole should be large enough for the milk to come through fairly freely when the bottle is shaken upside-down.

A good substitute for bitch's milk is one teaspoonful of sweetened condensed milk mixed with half a cup of cow's milk, and this should be fed at a temperature of 38·5°C (101°F). As each puppy finishes its feed it should be gently rubbed or patted to induce it to bring up its wind as in a human baby.

For the first few days of life a puppy may be unable to urinate and defecate in the absence of its mother who stimulates this process by licking, and assistance therefore must be given. This is done by gently massaging the abdomen with a small wad of moistened cotton-wool or gauze, and must be done after each feed until the puppy is old enough to relieve itself without help. A little cold cream smoothed on to the abdomen two or three times a day will prevent the skin becoming excoriated by urine.

The box and bedding must be kept clean and fresh at all times, and as bottle-reared puppies are more prone to diarrhoea and constipation than those naturally fed, these conditions must be watched for as in the very young puppy they can be serious and require prompt attention. In the event of diarrhoea, half a teaspoonful of cornflour mixed in the feed will usually improve the condition quite quickly, and for constipation two drops of liquid paraffin will help. If the puppy shows no sign of responding to these simple remedies then veterinary advice must be sought as soon as possible.

Dew claws should be removed, and tails docked if necessary, when the puppies are about 3 days old. Both these tasks should be performed by a skilled person, particularly where docking is concerned as breeds vary in the amount of tail to be removed. This is an important factor as a badly docked tail could cost a valuable dog a place in the show ring later in life; also if sufficient skin overlap is not preserved this may lead to trouble resulting from the pup biting and gnawing at the amputated stump.

Puppies should be wormed at about 5 weeks of age, although sometimes this is necessary at 3 weeks. This is an essential procedure as most puppies inherit worm larvae from their mothers before birth and the presence of worms will affect the pup's growth and development.

Weaning

A start can be made at teaching puppies to lap from a saucer at about 3 weeks of age. Not only is this the first move towards independence but it will also relieve the bitch from some of the heavy demands being made upon her system by her rapidly growing family, and most puppies will take to lapping quite readily. By the 4th week a small quantity of beef broth in which has been soaked a few finely crumbled wholemeal breadcrumbs can be introduced. At the 5th week the first real solids can be started in the form of raw minced or shredded lean meat; this can be alternated with finely flaked cooked and filleted fish, and two or three drops of cod-liver oil and a teaspoonful of egg yoke should be mixed with one of the feeds. Another very useful method in introducing meat is to nail a piece of good quality beef on to a heavy block of wood and allow the pups to suck the meat from which they will acquire a considerable amount of nourishment. The amount of food given to each puppy per feed will vary according to the size and breed of the pup, but it may be wiser at this stage to feed them separately so that the stronger and greedier ones do not deprive the others of their fair share, although sometimes a slow or disinterested feeder can be encouraged to eat more if in competitive company.

By the time they are 6 weeks old, the puppies should be having two meat meals a day and three milk meals, and fresh drinking water should always be available. They should be allowed out into the fresh air each day, providing the weather is not too cold, and be given plenty of opportunity and space for play. House training should be started during the early days of weaning and the pups either put outside or on to a sheet of newspaper or a shallow box of sawdust after each feed.

Caesarian Section

In any review of obstetrical nursing, special mention should be made of the help a RANA can give to a veterinary surgeon in the event of a caesarian operation.

In such cases it is usual for a surgeon to have an assistant who will be "scrubbed up" and will help him throughout the operation, and another attendant ready to receive and administer to the puppies as they are removed from the bitch. A box or basket should be ready in which to place the puppies, and here again warmth, both in the box and in the room, is of great importance. It is also necessary to see that the form of heating used cannot be a source of danger; hot-water bottles must be well covered and the box not placed too near a fire, and out of draughts.

As the pups are born they are handed to the attendant by the surgeon, probably still enveloped in their membranes, and the first task will be to rupture these and sever the umbilical cord; the method by which this is done has already been described. It must be remembered that a new-born puppy is very slippery and it is as well for the attendant to receive them from the surgeon with hands cupped together to avoid dropping them during the handing over, remembering also that the surgeon's gloves or hands are sterile and must not be contaminated.

Resuscitation is naturally the first consideration, and the various ways by which this may be done have also been described, with the exception of "swinging" a puppy to bring it to life. This may seem rather drastic but on occasions can be very effective. The pup should be wrapped in a clean rough towel and held firmly in both hands and swung back and forth between the attendant's legs, the greatest care being taken to see that its head does not hit anything in the process and also that the head is well supported while being swung.

Regarding the feeding of pups born by caesarian section, some people prefer them to have nothing until the bitch has recovered consciousness, some prefer them to suckle the bitch while she is still unconscious, while others prefer artificial feeding for a while. Much depends on the bitch, the amount of milk she has, her attitude towards her pups, and how she withstood the operation. There is no hard-and-fast rule, and decisions vary according to circumstances, but in normal cases, and if the bitch is a good mother, it is obviously better for her and the pups if she can feed and look after them herself.

Table 7.1
Showing when a Bitch is Due to Whelp

Served January	Whelp March	Served February	Whelp April	Served March	Whelp May	Served April	Whelp June	Served May	Whelp July	Served June	Whelp August	Served July	Whelp September	Served August	Whelp October	Served September	Whelp November	Served October	Whelp December	Served November	Whelp January	Served December	Whelp February
1	5	1	5	1	3	1	3	1	3	1	3	1	2	1	3	1	3	1	3	1	3	1	2
2	6	2	6	2	4	2	4	2	4	2	4	2	3	2	4	2	4	2	4	2	4	2	3
3	7	3	7	3	5	3	5	3	5	3	5	3	4	3	5	3	5	3	5	3	5	3	4
4	8	4	8	4	6	4	6	4	6	4	6	4	5	4	6	4	6	4	6	4	6	4	5
5	9	5	9	5	7	5	7	5	7	5	7	5	6	5	7	5	7	5	7	5	7	5	6
6	10	6	10	6	8	6	8	6	8	6	8	6	7	6	8	6	8	6	8	6	8	6	7
7	11	7	11	7	9	7	9	7	9	7	9	7	8	7	9	7	9	7	9	7	9	7	8
8	12	8	12	8	10	8	10	8	10	8	10	8	9	8	10	8	10	8	10	8	10	8	9
9	13	9	13	9	11	9	11	9	11	9	11	9	10	9	11	9	11	9	11	9	11	9	10
10	14	10	14	10	12	10	12	10	12	10	12	10	11	10	12	10	12	10	12	10	12	10	11
11	15	11	15	11	13	11	13	11	13	11	13	11	12	11	13	11	13	11	13	11	13	11	12
12	16	12	16	12	14	12	14	12	14	12	14	12	13	12	14	12	14	12	14	12	14	12	13
13	17	13	17	13	15	13	15	13	15	13	15	13	14	13	15	13	15	13	15	13	15	13	14
14	18	14	18	14	16	14	16	14	16	14	16	14	15	14	16	14	16	14	16	14	16	14	15
15	19	15	19	15	17	15	17	15	17	15	17	15	16	15	17	15	17	15	17	15	17	15	16
16	20	16	20	16	18	16	18	16	18	16	18	16	17	16	18	16	18	16	18	16	18	16	17
17	21	17	21	17	19	17	19	17	19	17	19	17	18	17	19	17	19	17	19	17	19	17	18
18	22	18	22	18	20	18	20	18	20	18	20	18	19	18	20	18	20	18	20	18	20	18	19
19	23	19	23	19	21	19	21	19	21	19	21	19	20	19	21	19	21	19	21	19	21	19	20
20	24	20	24	20	22	20	22	20	22	20	22	20	21	20	22	20	22	20	22	20	22	20	21
21	25	21	25	21	23	21	23	21	23	21	23	21	22	21	23	21	23	21	23	21	23	21	22
22	26	22	26	22	24	22	24	22	24	22	24	22	23	22	24	22	24	22	24	22	24	22	23
23	27	23	27	23	25	23	25	23	25	23	25	23	24	23	25	23	25	23	25	23	25	23	24
24	28	24	28	24	26	24	26	24	26	24	26	24	25	24	26	24	26	24	26	24	26	24	25
25	29	25	29	25	27	25	27	25	27	25	27	25	26	25	27	25	27	25	27	25	27	25	26
26	30	26	30	26	28	26	28	26	28	26	28	26	27	26	28	26	28	26	28	26	28	26	27
27	31	27		27	29	27	29	27	29	27	29	27	28	27	29	27	29	27	29	27	29	27	28
28		28		28	30	28	30	28	30	28	30	28	29	28	30	28	30	28	30	28	30	28	29
29	Apr.	29	May	29	31	29	31	29	31	29	31	29	30	29	31	29	31	29	31	29	31	29	30
30			1	30		30		30		30		30		30		30		30		30		30	
31	1		2	31	June		July	31	Aug.		Sept.	31	Oct.	31	Nov.		Dec.	31	Jan.		Feb.	31	Mar.
	2		3																				
	3				1		2		1		1		1		1		2		1		1		3
	4				2				2				2		2				2				4

General

Obstetrical nursing and the rearing of very young puppies is possibly one of the most rewarding of tasks. Continual study of routine methods, both old and new, and an understanding of the fact that every bitch is an individual and may react to the whole breeding process in an individual manner, maintains a varied interest in every case from start to finish. Conscientiousness on the part of the RANA in the keeping of correct notes and case histories combined with ability to know when to call a veterinary surgeon if everything is not as it should be, is the keynote to success.

Further Reading

FRANKLING, ELEANOR, *Popular Dog Breeding and Genetics* (Popular Dogs).

(b) OBSTETRICAL AND PAEDIATRIC NURSING IN THE CAT

G. T. Wilkinson, MVSc, MRCVS

Puberty

In the female cat or queen, sexual maturity, i.e. the ability to reproduce, is normally reached between 5 to 8 months of age, but to some extent this is dependent upon the time of the year in which the kitten was born. For instance, a kitten born in spring may not come into oestrus until the following spring when she will be around 1 year old. On the other hand, it is not unusual for a kitten to have its first oestrous cycle at 3½ months old. The male cat takes longer to reach puberty being usually about 1 year old before breeding activity occurs. Some males may not commence breeding until the second spring after their birth when they may be as much as 20 months old.

The Oestrous Cycle

The cat is polyoestrous, in contradistinction to the bitch which has a monoestrous reproductive cycle. Recurrent oestrus occurs at 14-day intervals, usually lasting for 3 to 6 days, although it may be prolonged for up to 10 days if mating does not occur. Under domesticated conditions there are two or three breeding seasons each year, the first commencing at the beginning of January and ending in May, the second extending from July to August with a possible third period in September, but this depends to some extent upon mild weather conditions. From the end of September to the end of December most queens are anoestrous. This anoestrous period can be shortened or even eliminated if desired by the provision of artificial lighting during autumn and winter.

Unlike the bitch, the cat shows little visible physical signs of oestrus, such as swelling of the vulva or vaginal discharge. The behaviour of the cat, however, presents quite striking evidence that she is in oestrus. Usually there is increased restlessness and the cat may stay out of doors for long periods, sometimes being absent for days at a time. Allied to this restlessness there is an increase in vocal activity ranging from a more frequent "talking" to a raucous shriek or howl, the latter being especially marked and distracting in the Siamese breed. This vocal activity gives rise to the lay terms of "calling" or being "on call" to denote oestrus. Some cats will become more affectionate to their owners at this time and a previously unmanageable cat will often allow itself to be groomed, evincing signs of pleasure during the procedure. Many cats indulge in constant rolling and crying and this may cause inexperienced owners to seek veterinary advice as their cat is "in agony". Other signs of oestrus are a concave curvature of the back, raising of the hindquarters, deflection of the tail to one side and treading movements with the hind feet.

The cat is a non-spontaneous ovulator, which means that ovulation does not occur automatically when the follicles ripen, but requires some stimulus to trigger it off. It is not known what constitutes the required stimulus but it has been shown that mechanical stimulation of the cervix will induce ovulation, so it may be that the act of coitus provides the trigger mechanism. This does not account for the fact that whereas the free-roaming female will almost invariably conceive, females kept in colonies with a solitary male often remain infertile although mating has apparently taken place quite normally. It is believed that a fairly prolonged period of courtship is necessary to stimulate follicle ripening to the point of rupture. This courtship period may last for up to 4 days during which the female is surrounded by several males and witnessess their frequent confrontations and battles. During this period the female will reject the advances of any of the males. This is followed by a period of about 1 day when the female will accept service from the selected male(s) several times.

During mating (coitus), the male grasps the loose skin at the back of the female's neck between his teeth and this action seems to be essential for proper mating to occur. Due to the anatomical arrangement of the external male genitalia in the cat, the full co-operation of the female is necessary for coitus to take place and forced mating of the female cannot be achieved in the cat as it can in the bitch. Following the period of acceptance, oestrous behaviour usually continues for a further 24 hours although the male is no longer accepted. Under conditions of domestication it is necessary to take the female to the male for mating as a change of surroundings has a definite inhibitory effect on the male. This appears to be bound up with the need for the male to delineate his territory by spraying with urine and scratching various objects. It may be mentioned here that by the end of the breeding season many males show a marked loss of bodily condition, with a rather "staring", hidebound coat, tucked-up abdomen, and often the enlarged kidneys of the breeding male can be seen in the flanks. Owners may think that these prominences are due to tumours in the abdomen.

Studies have indicated that ovulation occurs approximately 24 hours after mating, fertilization taking place 24 to 36 hours after mating and implantation of embryos occurring about 2 weeks thereafter.

Pregnancy

Pregnancy in the cat is usually said to average 63 days, but it would seem that this figure is on the low side. A more accurate average would be 65 days and it is unlikely that kittens born before the 56th day will survive. Some pregnant females will show signs of oestrus at about the 21st and 42nd days, which may be confusing as far as pregnancy diagnosis is concerned. Diagnosis of pregnancy can be performed by abdominal palpation at 21–35 days when the foetal units can be discerned as tense spherical swellings in the uterus, about the size of a pea in the early part of the period increasing to about 1 in. in diameter by the 35th day. After this time the uterus becomes generally enlarged and the demarcation between the foetal units is lost. About the 7th week the foetal heads and bodies become recognizably palpable and radiography during the final 2 weeks will reveal the skeletons of the kittens. Abdominal distension occurs in cats with several kittens in the litter from between the 5th and 6th weeks. In a cat pregnant for the first time the nipples become more prominent and pink after the first 2 weeks. The mammary glands become enlarged mainly during the last week of pregnancy.

The average number of kittens in a litter is four. It seems probable that more eggs are ovulated and fertilized than kittens that are born at full term. This has been shown by the examination of the uterus of a 15-day pregnant cat when twelve foetal units were present whereas the largest litter recorded by the observer was eight. Superfoetation, i.e. the presence of two or more foetuses of different ages in the same uterus, has been reported in the cat and is due to fertilization of eggs released at successive oestrous periods. This means that it is possible for kittens born in the same litter to have different sires. Superfecundation, in which two or more eggs released at the same ovulation are fertilized during successive matings at the same oestrus, is perhaps more common. Again this means that litter-mates may have two or more different sires.

The cat does not require any special management during a normal pregnancy. She should receive a balanced diet, particular attention being paid to the calcium: phosphorus ratio (Ca:P) which should be as close to 1:1 as possible, and to vitamin A, the requirement here being about 1600–2000 i.u. per day. It should be remembered that meat is very deficient in calcium. Milk contains a good supply and can provide a substantial proportion of the calcium required by the pregnant cat. Cooked fish containing the bones is another good source of the mineral. If necessary the diet can be supplemented by the addition of bone flour at a rate of up to 10% of the dry weight of the ration. The vitamin A requirement can be met by feeding a small portion of raw liver two or three times a week. Usually the actual quantity of food consumed does not increase very much until about the 6th week, from which time it increases until the cat is eating about twice her normal food intake by the 8th to 9th week. It is better to divide the daily ration into two or three smaller meals rather than one large one.

Normal exercise, jumping and climbing are allowed and, in fact, are beneficial in maintaining muscle tone. In the final week or 10 days it is advisable to provide a suitable place for the queen to have her kittens. Almost all cats like to find a spot where they are protected on at least three sides and which is in partial darkness. A cardboard box lined with several thicknessess of newspaper or wood wool and placed in the bottom of a cupboard makes an ideal nesting-place.

Abnormal Pregnancy

The vast majority of cats have a completely normal pregnancy and this applies particularly to the domestic cat which leads a fairly free existence on a good mixed diet. In the pedigree cat, especially the Siamese, however, there is quite a high incidence of abortion, foetal resorption, stillborn kittens, and weak, "fading", kittens. The reasons for these mishaps are not clear and it is probable that several causative factors are involved. Vitamin A deficiency has been shown to cause failures of implantation, abortion around the 50th day, and a high death-rate amongst the new-born kittens. Infection with bacteria, viruses, or parasites, e.g. *Eperythrozoon felis*, *Toxoplasma gondii*, may also lead to abortion, stillbirths and neonatal deaths. Finally the condition may be hormonal and of genetic origin. Pregnancy is normally maintained by progesterone, which is secreted by the corpora lutea of the ovary for the first part of pregnancy and by the placenta for the remaining period. It has been shown in the cat that ovariectomy before the 48th day of pregnancy resulted in abortion, but after this period pregnancy is maintained by the placental progesterone in the absence of the corpora lutea. Anything therefore which damages the placenta may produce abortion due to interference with the production of progesterone.

Abortion may also occur following trauma such as may result from a heavily pregnant cat being involved in a road accident or being chased and worried by a dog. This type of incident may also cause rupture of the uterus with the foetuses being liberated into the abdominal cavity. Another accident which is not uncommon in the pregnant cat is torsion of the uterus. This probably results from the cat jumping or twisting and the heavy uterus suspended by the long broad ligaments swings over itself. The torsion may involve one horn or the uterine body. The mishap usually occurs around term and parturition commences fairly shortly afterwards. If only one horn is involved then two or three kittens may be born normally after which labour ceases. Abdominal palpation reveals that there are more foetuses in the uterus which is tense and painful. Treatment is surgical and involves laparotomy and probably hysterectomy.

Parturition

As in the bitch, parturition in the cat can be divided into three stages. The first stage, when the cervix is opening, is marked by the queen becoming rather restive, occasionally crying, and making frequent trips to her box where she may indulge in some bed-making. There is often a fairly sharp drop in the rectal temperature early in this stage. Usually there is no panting as is often seen in the bitch, but this may occur during the terminal part of this stage. In most cases the first stage lasts from 12–24 hours in the cat.

In the second stage there is obvious straining and the first kitten is usually born within about 30 minutes of the onset. Quite a high proportion of the kittens are born with the hindquarters presented first and this is of little consequence, except that where it occurs with the first kitten delivery may be rather protracted. The intervals between kittens depends to some extent upon the number in the litter, being longer with fewer kittens, but are usually fairly short ranging from 10 to 60 minutes. Joshua (1965) describes an interrupted type of labour in the cat in which part of the litter is delivered normally and there is then a period of 12–24 hours when the queen behaves as if parturition was completed. Examination reveals that further kittens are present in the uterus but the cat is well and the kittens already born are apparently normal. Labour is resumed and the remainder of the litter is delivered without difficulty.

The third stage, that of expulsion of the foetal membranes, is intermingled with the second stage, the birth of each kitten being followed normally by its membranes, or the latter may precede the next kitten to be born. Sometimes two or three sets of membranes may be held up and then expelled together. The placental fluids are normally of a greenish-black colour as in the bitch.

Abnormal Parturition

In the majority of cases parturition in the cat is completely normal. Occasionally the first stage may be rather protracted in some of the pedigree breeds, especially the Siamese, the cat becoming almost hysterical and following the owner about crying. It may be necessary to administer a tranquillizer to such animals before parturition can proceed. Similarly this type of cat appears to be able to inhibit labour if the surroundings are not to her liking.

Uterine inertia is very rare in the cat and when it occurs is usually associated with a single-kitten litter. Obstruction to delivery (dystokia) may be due to healed fractures of the maternal pelvis due to road accidents, or to spontaneous fractures of the pelvis occurring in calcium-deficient animals, again more common in the Siamese. For this reason alone, all female cats sustaining fractures of the pelvis should be spayed at the earliest opportunity. Dystokia due to foetal abnormalities may result from abnormal presentations, foetal oversize (rare), or to foetal monstrosities. Due to the small size of the parts it is difficult to correct malpresentations, although it is sometimes possible to do so by manipulation of the foetus with a finger in the vagina and through the abdominal wall with the other hand. In most cases of dystokia, however, a caesarean section is necessary.

A rare complication of parturition is prolapse of the uterus in which one or both uterine horns are turned inside out and appear through the vulva. Surgical replacement is necessary, but until this can be done, the exposed organ should be covered with a clean cloth soaked in normal saline to minimize drying-out and damage.

Puerperal Abnormalities

Following parturition few complications occur in the cat. Retention of the foetal membranes is uncommon and may be unsuspected unless the owner has witnessed the birth of all the kittens and counted the membranes. Suspicion should be aroused when the queen is obviously in some abdominal discomfort, tends to neglect the kittens, runs a slight temperature, or has a brownish vaginal discharge. Abdominal palpation will usually reveal the missing membranes as a lump in the uterus. Treatment consists of administration of small doses of pituitrin combined with antibiotics.

Puerperal metritis is a more advanced stage of the previous condition and is due to infection gaining access to the uterus whilst its powers of resistance are lowered by fatigue. This may follow a protracted labour or where there have been surgical manipulations or forceps delivery. The cat has a temperature of 40·0–40·5°C (104–105°F), is off its food although it may show excessive thirst, neglects the kittens, and shows an offensive reddish-brown vaginal discharge which soils the perineum and tail. Treatment is similar to that for retained membranes. Nursing measures should include regular cleaning away of discharges, keeping the patient as comfortable as possible, tempting the appetite and caring for the kittens.

Mastitis may occur, usually in only one of the glands, and may cause rejection of the kittens. The affected gland is swollen, reddened and tender and a brownish or bloodstained fluid can be expressed through the nipple. Again there is pyrexia and anorexia. Treatment is by the use of fomentations, expressing the infected fluid from the gland and the administration of antibiotics.

Lactational tetany or eclampsia is a rare condition in the cat as few cases have been recorded in spite of the numbers of cats suckling kittens. It is more common in cats with large litters and usually the attack occurs when the kittens are between 3 to 8 weeks old, although one case has been recorded in which the condition occurred before parturition. The clinical signs vary from case to case but they are essentially nervous in character and take the form of ataxia, muscular twitching and tonic spasms of the limbs. There may be vomiting, rapid shallow breathing and hyperpyrexia; 42·7°C (109°F). There may be unusual dryness of the sclerotic of the eye and the mouth. Treatment is by injection of calcium borogluconate, removal of the kittens, and nursing the cat in a quiet, darkened room.

Management of the Newly-born Kitten

Normally the queen will free the kittens from the foetal membranes which may envelop them at birth. If she does not do this fairly promptly then the RANA must act, as delay may result in asphyxiation of the kitten. One should not be in too much of a hurry to sever the umbilical cord as there is evidence that a valuable amount of blood is expressed from the placenta and augments the kitten's blood supply in the first 2 to 3 minutes after birth. If necessary the cord should be ligated with sterile thread about $\frac{1}{2}$ in. from the kitten's abdomen and a second ligature placed nearer to the placenta; the cord is then severed between the ligatures using sterile scissors.

Occasionally apparently lifeless kittens are born but the licking action of the mother's tongue will usually revive them. If no sign of life appears within a short space of time the RANA must intervene. First ascertain whether there is a heart-beat by holding the chest lightly between the thumb and forefinger. If no beat is discernible then the kitten should be discarded. It is also as well to check for any obvious abnormalities before proceeding to revive the kitten. Clear the airway by swabbing out the mouth and pharynx with cotton-wool with the kitten held head down and compressing the chest gently a few times. Mouth to mouth resuscitation ("kiss of life") may be attempted but it is important to allow the angles of the kitten's mouth to remain open and to give very short, light puffs of breath otherwise there is a grave danger of causing over-expansion and possibly rupture of the lung alveoli. All the methods advocated in the previous chapter may be used to stimulate respiration. Other useful measures are to pinch the loose skin at the back of the neck fairly hard or to compress the chest gently in the region of the heart. Once revived, the kitten should be placed in a box on a well-padded hot-water bottle until sufficiently strong to be returned to its mother.

If the queen is very restive between the births of kittens, it is advisable to remove the kittens already born to a warm box until parturition is completed. Providing the mother is calm then the kittens should be allowed to remain and encouraged to suckle as this tends to stimulate uterine contractions.

Newly born kittens commence suckling immediately they have been washed by the mother. In the first week of life suckling occurs about every 2 hours after which the frequency falls off to around every 4 hours. If the mother's milk supply is inadequate the kittens appear hungry and nose around the mother crying continually. If there is any doubt about the supply of milk this can be checked by weighing the kittens daily. At birth a normal kitten weighs between 90–140 g (3–5 oz) depending upon the breed and the number in the litter. If the milk supply is adequate it should gain about 10 g ($\frac{1}{3}$ oz) each day doubling its birth weight in 8–9 days. A small spring balance calibrated from 0–500 g should be used for weighing with a net to hold the kitten, as the usual household scales are not sufficiently sensitive. After the first week weighing can be done weekly and a thriving kitten should gain on average between 80–100 g per week. If the mother's milk is insufficient then it must be supplemented as suggested below.

Care of the Orphaned Kitten

Orphaned kittens can be successfully reared by hand-feeding, but it is obviously much easier if a foster-mother can be found. Foster-mothers should be examined for signs of infectious or contagious disease and for the presence of ectoparasites before putting the kittens in contact with them. It is important to ensure that all the kittens are receiving sufficient milk and this is best done by daily weighing. Hand-rearing using a doll's feeding bottle necessitates feeding every 2 hours for the first week, then every 4 hours for the following week, dropping to every 6 hours in the 3rd and 4th weeks. Kittens require a high protein intake if they are to grow normally and cat's milk contains 46–49% solids as protein to supply this need. Cow's milk contains only half this amount as shown in Table 7.2.

Evaporated cow's milk contains approximately the same amount of protein as cat's milk and can be used as a substitute. Another method of increasing the protein content of cow's milk is to add 1 part of beaten egg yolk to 4 parts of milk.

Weaning

The usual period of lactation in the cat is 7 weeks and it is common practice to commence weaning at about 4 weeks after birth. Initially the kittens should be encouraged to lap evaporated or egg-yolk supplemented cow's milk to supplement the mother's milk. Once this has been accomplished then weaning foods such as

TABLE 7.2

AVERAGE PER CENT COMPOSITION BY WEIGHT OF CAT'S MILK COMPARED WITH WHOLE PASTEURIZED COW'S MILK (Scott, 1966)

	Cat	Cow
Water	82·4	87·2
Total protein	7·0	3·2
Casein	3·7	2·8
Albumin and globulin	3·3	0·4
Fat	4·8	4·0
Lactose	4·8	4·9
Ash	1·0	0·7

Farex (Glaxo), and small amounts of solids such as boiled fish, meat, etc., may be added to the milk. The amounts of solid food can be gradually increased at the expense of the milk content of the diet. It is important at weaning to accustom the kittens to as wide a variety of foods as possible as once their tastes have become established it is very difficult to make changes in the diet. Once the kittens are weaned they require three meals a day which can be reduced to two meals daily at 10–12 weeks of age. Growing kittens require a diet with a high protein content, a high calorific value and with a Ca:P ratio as near 1:1 as possible.

Common Congenital Abnormalities

Congenital abnormalities are not very common in the cat, probably due to the fact that there has not been so much human interference with breeding as there has in the dog. Cleft palate is seen occasionally but the kittens soon die as they are unable to suckle properly. A condition in which part of the brain is poorly developed, cerebellar hypoplasia, is occasionally seen and is due to infection of the mother with the virus of feline panleucopaenia. Clinical signs are a disturbed balance, ataxia and intention tremors especially when the kitten attempts to feed. Congenital heart disease is uncommon and when it occurs it is evidenced by stunting of growth, dyspnoea and ascites or hydrothorax. Extra toes (polydactylism) are quite common but have no deleterious effect on the kitten.

Some abnormalities are due to deficient feeding of the mother during pregnancy. In vitamin A deficiency kittens may be born with chests flattened dorso-ventrally, hydrocephalus, deafness, ataxia, intention tremors and spasticity of the tail and hindlegs. Where there is calcium deficiency there is malformation of the scapula, the chest and the pelvis, and growth ceases. In iodine deficiency kittens may be born with open eyes and cleft palates.

References

JOSHUA, J. O. (1965) *The Clinical Aspects of Some Diseases of Cats*, p. 123. William Heinemann Medical Books, Ltd., London.

SCOTT, P. P. (1966) in *Diseases of the Cat*, Wilkinson, G. T., p. 8. Pergamon Press, Oxford.

CHAPTER 8

Radiography

S. W. Douglas, MA, MRCVS, DVR

Introduction

When a radiographic examination is made of an animal, a beam of X-rays is passed through the patient and allowed to fall on an X-ray film. Portions of the X-ray beam will be obstructed or absorbed by the denser structures within the patient's body. This causes the beam to cast a "shadow" of the various structures penetrated, on the film.

If the part of the animal being examined is not likely to produce a distinct shadow, a dense substance, such as a barium or iodine compound, may be introduced into it in order to show the outline more distinctly on radiography. Such a substance is known as a "contrast agent".

The "shadow picture" produced on the film cannot be seen until the film is "processed" by passing it through certain chemical solutions.

The whole procedure of radiography may be divided into two main parts. The first part, which involves the necessary adjustment of the X-ray apparatus, the positioning of the machine and the patient, and the actual exposure of the film, will be undertaken by the radiographer (usually the veterinary surgeon). However, the nursing staff can be called on to assist in this; and ways in which this assistance can be given will be mentioned. Such assistance can be given more effectively if the RANA understands something of the apparatus required and its use. This cannot be explained fully in one chapter and the student is advised to study the subject more fully in *Principles of Veterinary Radiography*.

The second part of the procedure comprises the processing of the exposed film and its subsequent care and filing. These tasks may be undertaken by the nursing staff alone, and ways in which this assistance can be given will, therefore, be described in greater detail.

Assisting the Radiographer

PREPARATION OF THE PATIENT

When radiographing the abdomen of animals the presence of faeces within the alimentary tract can give rise to confusing shadows in the radiograph produced.

Therefore the patient should not be fed immediately before radiography, and, in addition, the nursing staff may be instructed to withhold all food for 24 hours or to administer an enema. In certain circumstances (e.g. when contrast agents are to be administered to be excreted through the urinary system) it may be necessary to withhold all fluids for 12 hours prior to the examination.

Any dirt, skin dressings, harness, metal fastenings or buttons, plaster casts or splints may cast a shadow on the X-ray film and, where possible, these should be removed from any part to be radiographed (obviously the veterinary surgeon should be consulted before removing splints or casts from a fracture).

POSITIONING AND RESTRAINT OF THE PATIENT

If the radiograph is to be an accurate reproduction of the area being examined, it is essential that the patient shall not move at the moment of exposure, and that the part shall be placed as close to the film as possible and centred in relation to the cassette. Suitable positions in which the patient should be placed to facilitate this are described in *Principles of Veterinary Radiography*, and the student should be familiar with most of these. In most instances two people are necessary to hold the patient, and, while owners are usually expected to undertake this, the nursing staff may be required to assist. All those taking part should wear suitable protective clothing (see subsequent section). The precise details of restraint and positioning will be explained and directed by the radiographer; and if the patient is particularly intractable he may decide that it must be sedated or anaesthetized before it can be radiographed.

The Dangers associated with Radiography

Repeated exposure of the human or animal body to X-rays can lead to injury to the body tissue. This danger is often not realized because (1) the X-ray beam is invisible, (2) the damage to the tissues may not become obvious until a considerable time after the person was exposed to X-rays.

The main effects of X-ray injury are (1) damage to the skin, (2) destruction of certain blood cells, (3) injury to the sex organs, (4) the production of malignant growths.

Injuries of this nature will occur only if the person concerned receives repeated exposure to X-rays, and, provided that the precautions which are advised are observed, there is no significant risk.

This aspect of radiography is stressed, since the nursing staff may be asked to help in restraining patients for X-ray examination, and it is essential that they should understand how exposure to X-rays can occur, and also the routine precautions to take to avoid this danger.

THE SOURCE OF EXPOSURE

X-ray apparatus will only emit X-rays at the time of making the exposure (i.e.

when the radiographer presses the exposure button). Furthermore, since the X-ray tube is surrounded with lead, the X-rays can only emerge from the tube through the aperture provided. The X-rays will emerge as a beam (known as the primary beam), and, although invisible, the size of this beam can be estimated by noting the size and angle of the lead cone which is attached to the X-ray tube or from information supplied with the set. (With some of the larger sets the extent of the primary beam is made visible by incorporating a similar sized beam of light in the apparatus.) Assistants should never place their hands, or any other portion of their body, within the primary beam while an exposure is being made.

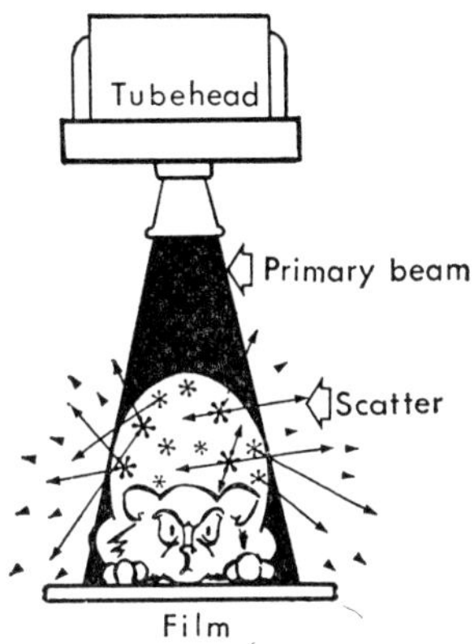

Fig. 8.1. The primary beam and "scatter".

Unfortunately, avoidance of the primary beam is not sufficient to avoid all exposure to X-rays. This is because of the phenomenon known as scatter (Fig. 8.1), whereby a small proportion of the X-rays that make up the primary beam reach the patient or the table and are then deflected in all directions and may reach those holding the animal.

The amount of X-rays received in this way is comparatively small and will become progressively less the further the assistant is from the primary beam. Adequate protection will be obtained if assistants stand as far away from the patient as possible and always wear protective clothing (lead-lined aprons and gloves).

It is usual to ask the owners of animals to hold them during radiography, so as to restrict the use of assistants for this purpose. But, since the tissues of the young are particularly susceptible to X-rays, no child under 16 or any expectant mother should be exposed to X-rays. Assistants can often help by recognizing those who come within these categories and tactfully removing them from the room before radiography is undertaken.

ROUTINE PRECAUTIONS

It is the responsibility of the radiographer to ensure that his assistants are protected from all significant irradiation during their work, and he will issue detailed instructions with regard to the particular circumstances under which he and his assistants are working. However, the following precautions apply to all situations and should be observed on all occasions when X-ray exposures are being made.

1. Always wear the protective clothing provided, even though it is heavy and uncomfortable (this will provide protection against scatter).

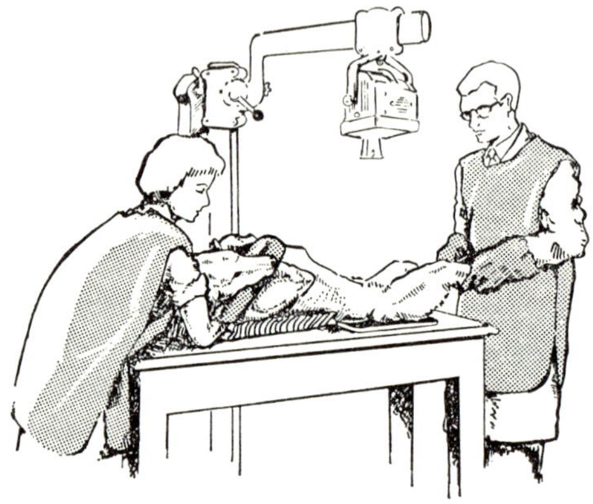

Fig. 8.2. Restraining a patient for radiography.

2. Stand as far away from the X-ray beam as is practicable. (Two people should always be available to restrain the patient since each will then be able to stand at arm's length from the animal, see Fig. 8.2.)

3. See that the task of holding animals is shared by as many persons as possible.

4. Check that protective clothing is stored or hung flat (the lead lining is easily cracked by frequent folding).

5. In particularly busy practices, monitoring badges (small films which, when processed at a special laboratory, can indicate the amount of irradiation received by the wearer) may be provided. These are pinned to one's clothing in such a way that they are not shielded by the protective clothing, and should be worn whenever radiography is undertaken.

The Code of Practice

An official document entitled "Radiation Safety in Veterinary Practice" has been issued by the Ministry of Agriculture, Fisheries and Food, for the guidance of veterinary surgeons using radiography. It is the responsibility of the Principal of the practice to ensure that the recommendations contained in the booklet are carried out. The RANA should be familiar with those sections of the document which apply to the part she is required to play in the performance of radiography. If she has any difficulty in understanding the recommendations she should ask that these should be explained to her.

Processing the Film

Processing of the exposed X-ray film is necessary before the image which has been produced on the film by the X-ray beam becomes visible and can be viewed in detail.

The production of a good radiograph requires considerable skill and experience on the part of the radiographer; but it also requires care and attention in processing. Carelessness in this procedure can waste the radiographer's efforts and render the finished radiograph useless.

Since an X-ray film is even more sensitive to light than to X-rays, it can only be handled and processed in a room from which all white light can be excluded—usually known as the dark room. The requirements and equipment of this room must be considered before the details of processing can be discussed.

THE DARK ROOM AND ITS EQUIPMENT

The type of dark room met in veterinary practices will vary very greatly, depending on the space available and the amount of use which is likely to be made of it. Some will be little more than cupboards; others are definite rooms. In all instances they must comprise a working space which can be effectively blacked out, and they are usually fitted with electrical and water supplies.

It is advisable to arrange the equipment of the dark room into two distinct sections:

1. *The dry bench.* Here the films are stored, handled dry, and loaded into and out of the cassettes.
2. *The wet bench.* This is where the processing solutions are kept and used.

It is important to keep these two sections well apart, otherwise splashes from the processing solutions will reach the dry films and the intensifying screens and produce permanent stains. Ideally the dry and wet benches should be situated on opposite sides of the dark room, but if it is necessary to arrange them side by side, then some form of partition should be erected between them (Fig. 8.3).

The equipment of the dark room will comprise:

Safelight. X-ray films can only be handled safely in a dim green or orange light. This illumination of the dark room is provided by a safelight which consists of a metal box holding a low-powered electric light bulb and fitted with a specified filter (e.g. Kodak Wratten 6B). These lights are classed as either direct, when they are placed immediately over a work point, or indirect, when they are hung from the ceiling with the light directed upwards so that it is reflected off the white ceiling. In large rooms more than one safelight may be required.

It must be realized, however, that these lights are only comparatively safe and that

X-ray films can be affected if exposed too closely or for too long a period to such illumination.

X-ray films. The type of X-ray film usually employed is known as the screen type film, because it can only be used in conjunction with intensifying screens (these will be described subsequently). The film and screens must, in turn, be encased in a film cassette to exclude light. This type of film is made in various speeds or sensitivities and each variety is marketed by different firms under different proprietary names

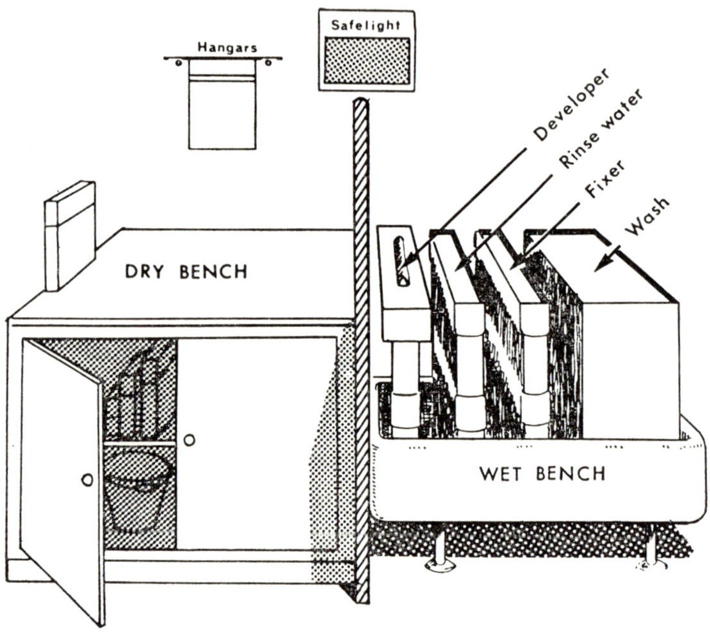

Fig. 8.3. A suitable arrangement for a small dark room.

(e.g. Kodak's Blue Brand and Royal Blue; Ilford's Red Seal and Gold Seal). These differences are of importance to the radiographer, who must adjust the controls of his apparatus to allow for variations in the film speed. Therefore, if at any time the type of film being used is changed, the radiographer must be informed of this fact.

A second type of film, known as non-screen film, is occasionally employed to show greater detail when radiographing the thinner portions of the limbs. These films are not intended for use with intensifying screens. They may be obtained in light-proof envelopes ready for use or packed in the usual way in folders in boxes and requiring to be placed in light-proof cardboard containers before use. These films, too, are sold under various proprietary names (e.g. Kodak—Kodirex; Ilford—Ilfex).

X-ray film is produced in a number of standard sizes. In most practices only a few of these sizes will be kept and used, but it is important to see that these sizes correspond with the sizes of the intensifying screens, film cassettes and film hangers employed. The sizes commonly employed are:

	(nearest metric equivalent)
$4\frac{3}{4} \times 6\frac{1}{2}$ in.	13×18 cm
$6\frac{1}{2} \times 8\frac{1}{2}$ in.	18×24 cm
8×10 in.	18×24 cm
10×12 in.	24×30 cm
12×15 in.	30×40 cm
14×14 in.	35×35 cm
14×17 in.	35×43 cm

(Other sizes can be obtained for special purposes.)

X-ray film is a particularly sensitive material which can be marked or spoilt in a number of ways, including:

1. *Exposure to X-rays.* Boxes of film or loaded cassettes must never be left near an X-ray set when it is likely to be used.
2. *Exposure to light.* Boxes of film and film cassettes must be kept closed and only opened in the dark room with safelight illumination.
3. *Dirty or greasy hands.* As far as possible film should be handled only through the paper folder which surrounds each film in the box in which it is obtained.
4. *Chemical splashes.* Hence the importance of separating the wet and dry benches.
5. *Folding or compression of film.* Boxes of X-ray film should always be stored on end and nothing heavy should be allowed to rest on these boxes.
6. *Deterioration with keeping.* Most X-ray films can be kept for a year or longer under good conditions of storage. If, however, a box of film is allowed to become damp, is exposed to any fumes, or is left at the back of a shelf and kept indefinitely, it will deteriorate. For this reason all boxes of film should be dated (in the space provided) on receipt and used in turn; and they should be stored in a clean, dry situation well away from any X-ray apparatus.
7. *Scratching during processing.* The softened emulsion of the wet film is particularly liable to be scratched and care must be taken to avoid this during processing.

Intensifying screens. These closely resemble two sheets of white cardboard, and are in fact coated with fine crystals (usually calcium tungstate). These crystals intensify the effect of the X-ray beam on the film because they fluoresce when exposed to X-rays. Thus the film is affected partly by the X-ray beam but mostly by the light produced in the screens. Because of this intensification, a smaller quantity of X-rays are required to produce the necessary changes in the film.

Intensifying screens are always used in pairs and are usually kept in film cassettes in such a way that when the film is inserted and the cassette closed, the film is tightly sandwiched between the two screens.

When inserting new screens into a cassette always follow the manufacturer's instructions with regard to fixation, and see that the front and back screens are correctly placed.

Any dirt or marks which occur on the screens will interfere with the fluorescent effect and result in similar flaws being seen on the radiograph. Precautions which can be taken to avoid the development of such screen marks include:

1. Always keep film cassettes tightly closed, except when loading or unloading.
2. Never touch the screens with the fingers.
3. Do not write (for identification purposes) on films which are still in the cassettes. (By dark room illumination it is only too easy to write on the screen instead of the film.)

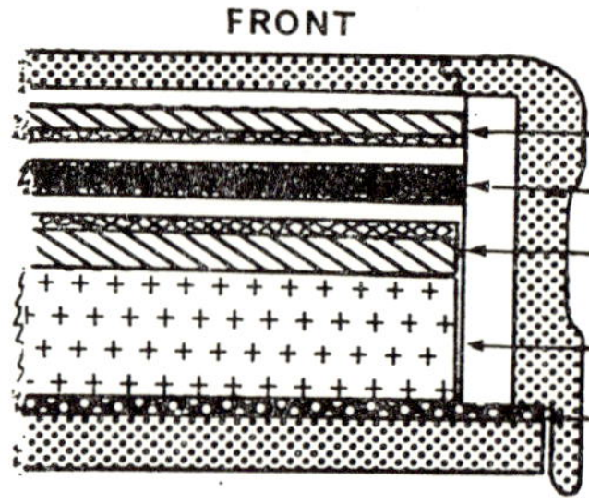

Fig. 8.4. Cross-section of a cassette.

4. Brush out dust and hairs with a fine brush. If necessary the surface of the screens can be gently washed, using damped balls of cotton wool and good quality soap. Use very little water to rinse the soap away, and see that the open cassette is allowed to dry thoroughly in a dust-free place before using again.

Film cassettes. These are light-proof metal containers (Fig. 8.4) designed to protect the film and the intensifying screens. Except when inserting or removing film, these cassettes must always be kept closed to exclude light and dirt. Furthermore, since they come into frequent contact with animals and any mark on the cassette may be reproduced on the film, they must be kept scrupulously clean.

As mentioned above, special cardboard folders are used as light-proof containers for non-screen film.

Processing frames. These are employed to hold the film while it is being passed through the tanks of solutions used in processing. There are two patterns, each with a different method of holding the film.

The channel type is easier to load but more difficult to keep clean (Fig. 8.5). The clip type hold the film more securely provided that one can avoid tearing the film during its insertion (Fig. 8.6).

Processing frames are not required if processing is carried out in dishes.

The above equipment (together with a pencil for identifying films) comprises the equipment of the dry bench.

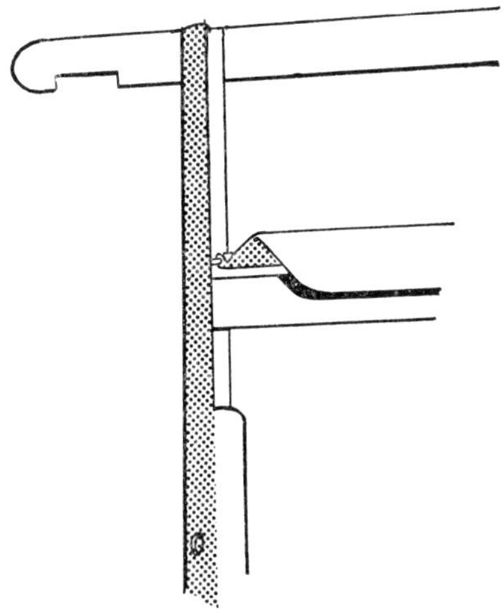

Fig. 8.5. Channel-type processing frame.

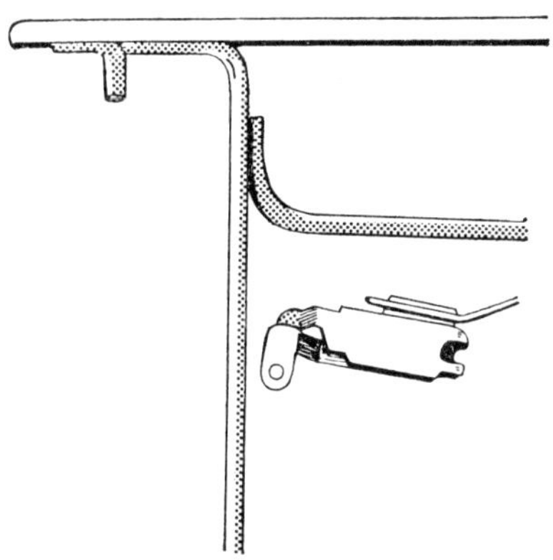

Fig. 8.6. Clip-type processing frame.

The wet bench is likely to include the following:

Processing equipment. Essentially, this will comprise four containers for (1) the developing solution, (2) water—for rinsing the film, (3) the fixing solution, (4) water—for washing the film.

Occasionally (2) and (4) are combined and only one container used, but this is not very satisfactory. If running water is not available in the dark room, the fourth container may only comprise a means of rinsing the film, and thorough washing will have to be carried out elsewhere.

The containers will either consist of a series of deep tanks into which the film is inserted vertically or else of a number of flat dishes in which the film is placed horizontally.

Processing tanks. These are more suitable for a busy unit. The tanks may be housed in a specially constructed processing unit or merely stood in a sink.

The tank intended to contain developer is fitted with a light-proof lid and also with some means of warming the solution which it contains (Fig. 8.7). The heating may be carried out by means of an immersion heater within the tank or, more frequently, by standing the tank in a larger tank of heated water (usually thermostatically controlled at 20°C (68°F)). The other processing tanks are sometimes also contained in the heated water bath, but this is not essential.

Processing dishes. These are flat dishes, similar to those used for photographic processing, but of a suitable size to take the X-ray films being used.

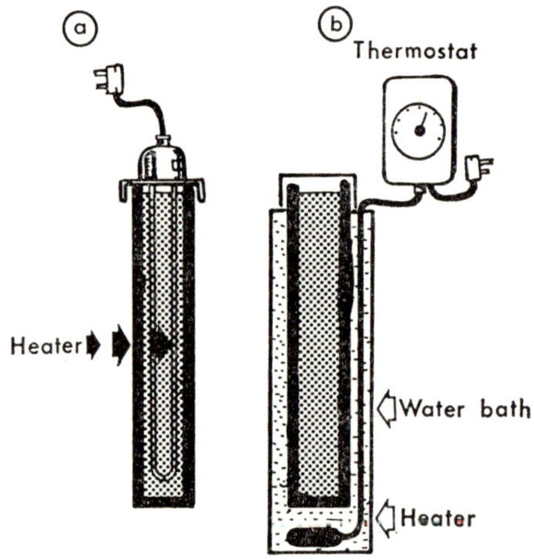

Fig. 8.7. Ways of heating the developer.

Heating of the developer is carried out by either heating the solution before it is placed in the dish or else by placing the dish on a flat low power electric heating plate.

Processing solutions. These consist of the developing solution or developer and the fixing solution or fixer. The exact composition of these solutions is not of importance since they are normally obtained in a prepared form.

The developer. This is used to develop or make visible the image produced on the film by the X-ray beam. However, the best results will only be obtained if the film is developed (immersed in the developer) for a certain time at a certain temperature (usually 3 or 5 minutes at 20°C (68°F)). The precise time and temperature will be stipulated by the manufacturers of the developer. This information is usually supplied with the developer and also some indication of how the time of development may be varied to compensate for changes in the temperature of the solution.

Developer may be purchased either in the form of a powder or as a concentrated solution, both of which are made up to a specified volume (2 or 5 gal) with water according to the capacity of the developer tanks. The liquid form can be poured directly into the tank and diluted, but the powder form should be well mixed with water in a bucket before adding to the tank.

When the developer is to be used for dish development, it is best stored in concentrated form in a dark, stoppered bottle. When required it is diluted with warm water to produce a solution of an appropriate concentration and temperature. If used in dishes the developer is particularly liable to oxygenation and should be discarded after use.

When developer is used in a tank the level of the solution will steadily drop as some of the developer is carried away with each film processed. The level of the solution should be maintained by adding a special replenisher solution prepared by the manufacturers of the developer solution. The usual practice is to make up a tank full of developer and at the same time to prepare a similar volume of replenisher. The replenisher is stored in dark, stoppered bottles and used as necessary to maintain the level of the developer. When the replenisher has been completely used, the developer is considered to be exhausted and is discarded and fresh solutions are made up. Even if the replenisher is not fully used the developer should be discarded after 3 months, as old developer produces stained, underdeveloped films.

Occasionally assistants have developed a dermatitis of the hands as a result of handling processing solutions. This is usually considered to be a form of allergic reaction to some of the chemical constituents of the developer (particularly the substance known as metol). While this is not a common occurrence, it emphasizes the need for strict cleanliness in handling all processing solutions.

Should any skin irritation be experienced, the use of gloves when handling the solutions may be of assistance. However, if the gloves are allowed to remain soiled with the chemicals, or if they contain holes, they may in fact aggravate the trouble by causing the solutions to make a more prolonged contact with the skin. Some developer solutions do not contain metol, and the substitution of these may also have to be considered.

If any marked skin trouble occurs, medical advice should always be obtained and the doctor informed that the person concerned is handling film processing chemicals.

The fixer. Film which has been passed through the developer is still sensitive to light and if exposed to white light would blacken rapidly, completely obliterating the image. This is prevented by immersing the film, after rinsing, in the fixer, which prevents any further action by light rays on the sensitive film and also hardens the film. After the film has been immersed in the fixer for some 30 seconds, it can be examined very briefly in white light, when it will be found that the film shows a whitish opaque appearance. This opacity will clear on further immersion of the film in the fixer. The time taken to achieve this is known as the clearing time, and until this has taken place the film should not be exposed to bright light for any length of time. For complete fixation and hardening of the film it should be kept in the fixer for a period at least equal to twice the clearing time.

Fixer is available both in a liquid and a powder form—to be made up to a certain volume according to the manufacturer's instructions. The temperature at which the fixer is used need not be quite so precise as is required for development, but should be kept within the range from 15·5° to 24°C (60°–75°F).

The fixer will not last as long as the developer. The time required for clearing of the film will become progressively longer with use and when the time becomes more than double the original clearing time, the fixer should be discarded and a fresh solution prepared.

Further requirements for the wet bench are:

A thermometer—to check the temperature of the developer.

A darkroom clock—to control the time of development of the film. Any clock or watch which is readable by safelight can be used for this purpose, but clocks specially made for use in dark rooms and which can be set to ring a bell after the appropriate interval have an obvious advantage.

Film clips—by which the films may be hung up to dry, either over a sink or within a heated drying cupboard.

GENERAL CARE OF THE DARK ROOM

A major requirement in the care of any dark room is to ensure that scrupulous cleanliness is observed, particularly in handling the processing solutions.

If the chemical solutions are splashed on to the surrounding walls and allowed to dry, they will produce dust which may settle on films or on screens and cause screen marks. Furthermore, the chemicals may have a corrosive action on unprotected walls and produce further dust.

Therefore the solutions should be prepared and mixed outside the dark room in clean containers made of glass, plastic, or unchipped enamel. Separate stirring rods should be employed for mixing the developer and the fixer, and containers and stirring rods should be thoroughly cleansed after use.

Splashes from the processing solutions can cause permanent stains on clothing, and plastic aprons should be worn whenever these are handled.

Clean towels for wiping the hands should be kept near the wet bench and used each time the hands are wet.

Film hangers and dishes soon become stained by chemical oxidation products and must be kept clean (when necessary, persistent stains may be removed by the use of 5% acetic acid).

DARK ROOM TECHNIQUE

Efficient processing of X-ray films requires the adoption of a definite routine at all stages of this procedure. This routine may be subdivided and summarized as follows:

1. Keep down dust by mopping the floor and dusting the walls with a damp cloth. Let in fresh air and sunshine whenever possible.

2. Note the temperature of the developer and adjust the heater if necessary.

3. Check the levels of the developing and fixing solutions. Top up the developer

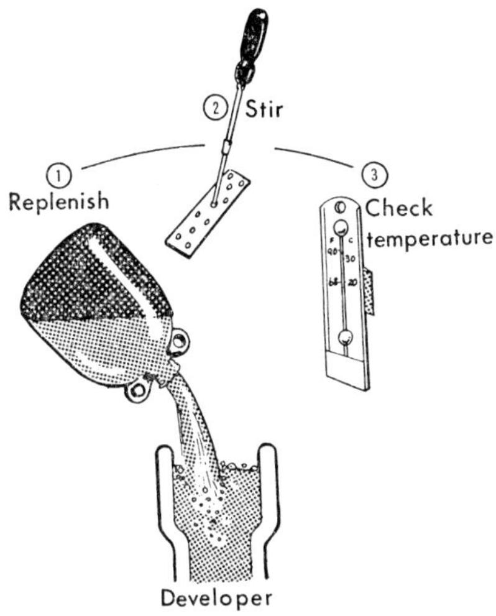

Fig. 8.8. Replenishing the developer.

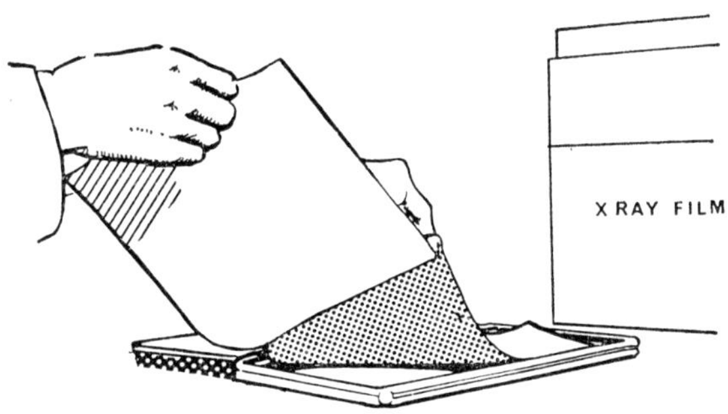

Fig. 8.9. Loading the cassette.

with the replenisher as required and see that this is well stirred in (Fig. 8.8). The level of the fixer seldom drops to any significant extent as it tends to be maintained by water carried over from the rinse. However, any marked fall might prevent complete fixation of an edge of the film, and if necessary the level can be maintained by adding further fixer.

4. See that film hangers previously used are clean and dry and ready for use.

The following procedures must, of course, only be carried out by safelight illumination.

LOADING THE FILM CASSETTE

1. Open the cassette.

2. Remove a film from the box of X-ray film, taking care to only handle the film through the paper folder which surrounds it (Fig. 8.9).

3. Pull back the top leaf of the protective paper folder and then rotate the film through 180° so that it may be dropped into the well of the cassette with the minimum of handling. Discard the folder.

4. Gently run a finger round the edge of the film to check that it is correctly placed and will not be bent when the cassette is closed.

5. Close the cassette and the box of film *before* switching on the light.

UNLOADING THE EXPOSED FILM

1. Open the cassette and gently shake out the film from the front of the cassette until it can be picked up at a corner, using the finger and thumb (Fig. 8.10).

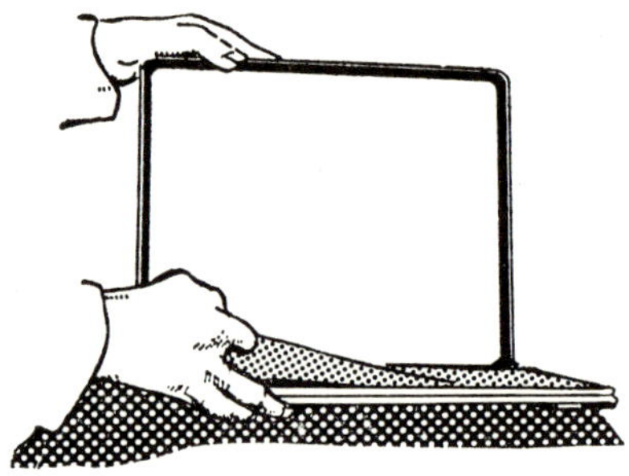

Fig. 8.10. Unloading the cassette.

2. Insert the film into a hanger with the minimum of handling. With the channel type of hanger the film is slid into the channels and the top hinge closed (Fig. 8.11). When using the clip-type hanger, fasten the lower clips first then press down the springs of the upper clips until these can be made to grasp the film and hold it taut (Fig. 8.12).

3. Identify the film by writing in pencil on the top right-hand corner (see p. 439).

4. Commence processing the film.

5. Reload and close the cassette.

PROCESSING THE FILM (TANK DEVELOPMENT) (Fig. 8.13)

1. Insert the film, supported in the hanger, gently into the developer and raise it vertically two or three times to remove air bubbles from the surface of the film. Immediately note the time or set the dark-room clock for the appropriate period.

2. Replace the lid on the developing tank and, making sure that one's hands are clean and dry, reload the film cassette. At the end of the correct period, remove the film slowly from the developer, allowing excess fluid to drain back.

3. Place the film in the rinse tank and rinse for some 10 seconds.

4. Transfer the film to the fixing tank. After it has been in this for about 30 seconds

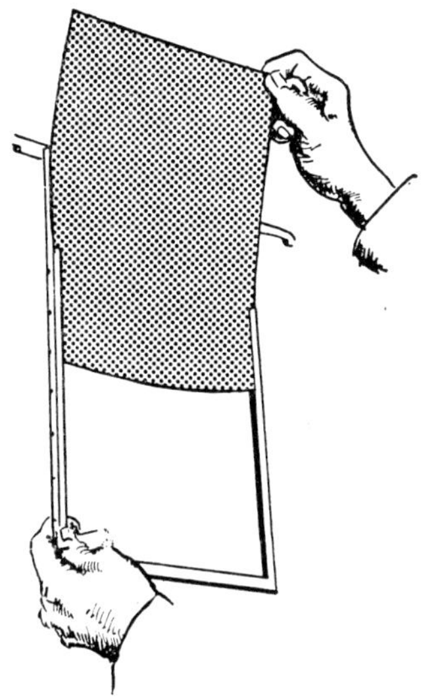

Fig. 8.11. Loading a channel-type processing frame.

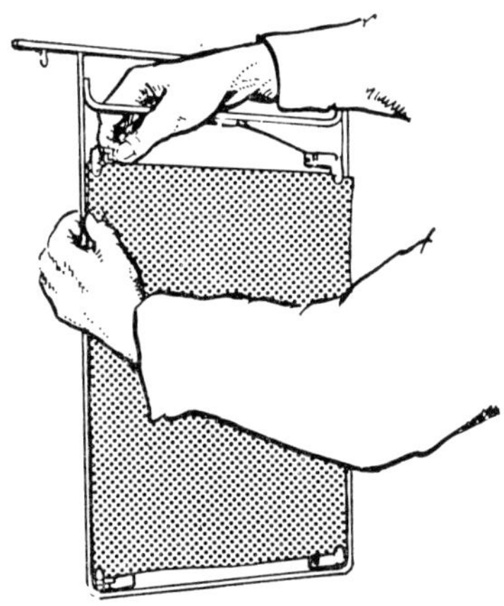

Fig. 8.12. Loading a clip-type processing frame.

the white light may be switched on, and once the film has cleared it may be examined fully in a bright light. In order that fixing may be complete the film should be left in this solution for at least 10 minutes.

5. Wash the film in running water for some 30 minutes (if running water is not available in the dark room, the film can be transferred to a suitable sink elsewhere).

6. Remove the film from the processing frame, attach a film clip and hang it up to dry in a dust free, and preferably warm, situation.

Note: If the film is left in the developer beyond the stipulated time it will be over-developed—becoming dark and losing detail.

The film should not be left in the fixer for more than an hour or the radiographic picture may lose some density.

Excessive washing (for more than a few hours) is also to be avoided, as it tends to soften the emulsion of the film and render it more liable to damage.

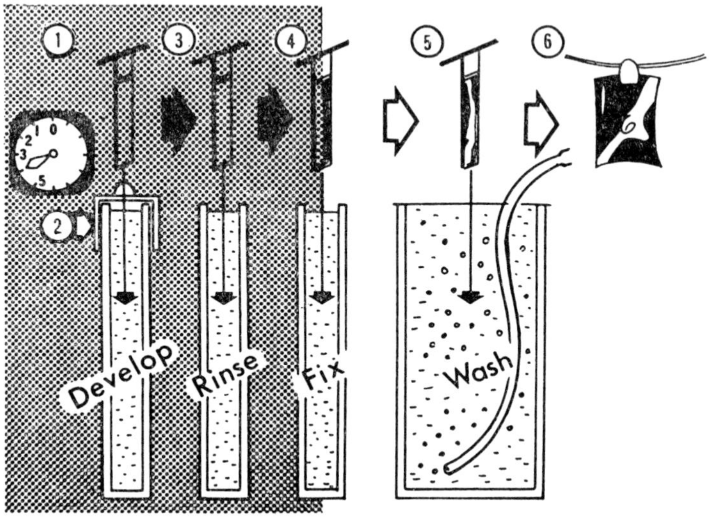

Fig. 8.13. Processing routine.

PROCESSING THE FILM (DISH DEVELOPMENT) (Fig. 8.14)

1. Check that the developer is freshly prepared, that it is at the correct temperature, and that it is of sufficient depth in the dish (about half an inch).

2. Introduce the film (no film hanger is required) by a rapid sliding action, so that the film is quickly and completely immersed.

3. Rock the dish from side to side frequently to provide movement of the developer solution and to prevent the film sticking to the bottom of the dish. Turn the film over two or three times. (The period necessary for development can be judged purely on a time basis in relation to the temperature. However, the frequent movement of the film and the developer is likely to reduce the time required for development, and it is probably more satisfactory to judge the time required by direct examination of the developing image by safelight.)

4. When adequately developed, remove the film, rinse it for 10 seconds and then immerse it in the fixer.

5. See that the film is completely covered with fixer and rock the dish frequently as the film clears.

6. After 10–30 minutes in the fixer, wash the film for at least half an hour in running water.

7. Attach a film clip and hang the radiograph up to dry in a suitable place.

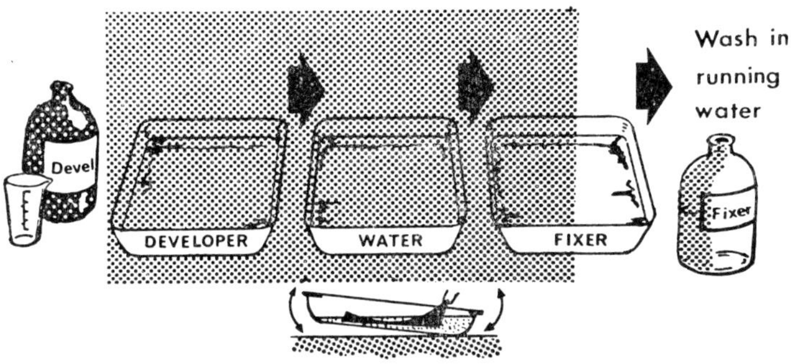

Fig. 8.14. Dish development.

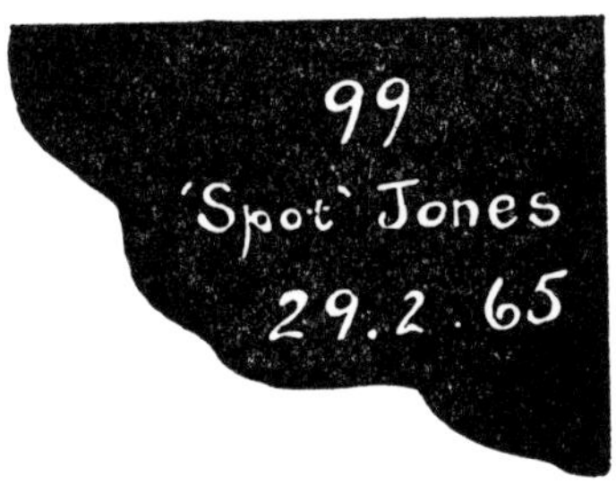

Fig. 8.15. Identification of a corner of a radiograph.

Identification and Filing of Radiographs

IDENTIFICATION

It is necessary to accurately identify each film in order to prevent the accidental muddling of the radiographs of two or more patients examined within a short time of each other, and also to permit certain reference, at a later date, to radiographs which may have been taken months or years previously.

The method of identification will vary from practice to practice, but a common practice is to write the necessary information in the top right-hand corner of the film. One suitable system is illustrated (Fig. 8.15), in which the top line represents the serial number of the radiograph, the second line gives the patient's and owner's name, and the third line indicates the date on which the radiograph was taken.

Part, or all, of the information required may be written on the X-ray film in pencil immediately before processing, in order to avoid muddling of films when washing. Ordinary pencil, however, is not suitable for permanent recording, and this identification should be rewritten in yellow chinagraph pencil or with white photographic ink when the film is dry and ready for filing.

The best permanent method of identifying radiographs is, either to place lead letters or suitably inscribed lead tape on the cassette at the time of making the exposure or to use a light contact marker in the dark room immediately prior to processing. It is essential to use one of these methods of identification if the films are to be submitted for scrutiny in connection with the hip dysplasia scheme.

FILING

In a busy practice a large number of radiographs can accumulate in the course of a year, and unless some system of filing is organized, it will not be possible to quickly locate a particular radiograph, particularly if it was taken a year or so previously.

Storage of radiographs can involve the purchase of special X-ray film envelopes and a suitable filing cabinet. However, a satisfactory method, involving no additional expense, is to replace the dry radiograph in the paper folder which protected the unexposed film, and then to store the radiographs in empty film boxes as they become available. If this system is adopted, the identification details which have been inscribed on the radiograph should be repeated on the paper folders and the radiographs placed in the boxes in chronological order. The boxes should be labelled with the date range of the radiographs which they contain. Then, provided that the date of radiography can be obtained from the patient's case history, it should be a simple matter to locate the relevant radiograph, and the owner's and patient's names will confirm the correct identification.

Before filing any radiograph it is essential to see that it is absolutely dry, otherwise it will stick to any folder or film envelope and may be ruined when any attempt is made to remove it for examination.

Further Reading

Code of Practice for the Protection of Persons Exposed to Ionising Radiation from Veterinary Uses. H.M. Stationery Office (1970).

DOUGLAS, S. W. and WILLIAMSON, H. D. (1972) *Principles of Veterinary Radiography,* Second Edition Baillière Tindall, London.

Fundamentals of Radiography, Kodak Limited, Medical Sales Division, Kingsway, W.C.2.

SMITH, R. N. (1960) *Radiography for the Veterinary Surgeon,* John Wright, Bristol.

CHAPTER 9

The Position of the RANA under the Veterinary Surgeons Act of 1966

A. R. W. PORTER, MA, Barrister-at-Law

THE Veterinary Surgeons Act of 1966 provides that "no individual shall practise or hold himself out as practising or as being prepared to practise veterinary surgery unless he is registered in the register of veterinary surgeons or the supplementary veterinary register". Since qualification as a RANA does not entitle one to be listed in either register, it follows that a RANA is no more entitled to perform any act of veterinary surgery than any other lay person.

This is not to discount the training which a RANA receives. To quote the *Guide to Professional Conduct* issued by the Royal College of Veterinary Surgeons to its members, RANAs are trained personnel "who can carry out nursing duties or assist veterinarians more competently, more expeditiously and with less explanation of what is required than untrained staff". Through their training they should, for example, be able competently to assist veterinarians in radiological examinations and the administration of anaesthetics, carry out sideroom tests and so on. This does not, however, alter the fact that RANAs are still lay persons in the context of the Veterinary Surgeons Act.

This statement of the general position still leaves two questions to be answered. First of all are there *any* acts of veterinary surgery which may be carried out by lay persons in spite of the general ruling set out above? And secondly what constitutes an act of veterinary surgery?

The answer to the first question is that the Veterinary Surgeons Act (and the subordinate legislation made thereunder) does allow certain classes of people who are not registered veterinarians to perform particular acts of veterinary surgery in certain circumstances. Doctors, dentists, physiotherapists and farmers all have special provision made for them within very closely prescribed limits. The ordinary citizen is also given the right by Schedule 3 of the Act to treat his own animals and this right is extended to the employee of the owner or any other member of the owner's household. In addition, anyone over the age of 18 years may carry out certain operations such as the docking of the tail of a dog or the amputation of its dew claws, provided that in each case this is done before the dog's eyes are open. But the general dispensation given to lay persons (and therefore to RANAs) which is of the greatest practical importance is the provision in Schedule 3 of the Act whereby it is permissible for lay persons to render first aid, in an emergency, for the purpose of saving life or relieving pain. This plainly gives a RANA the right to administer first aid to an animal when there is no veterinary surgeon available. The question is, however, often posed—"what is first aid?". To this there can be no precise answer since the first-aid measures appropriate to different cases will vary enormously. But the wording of the appropriate part of the Schedule goes some way towards providing guidance by making it plain that the treatment given to the animal must—

(a) *be given in an emergency.*
This means among other things that the RANA should not administer first aid if there is a veterinary surgeon available to treat the animal.

(b) *be given only if it is necessary to do so in order to save the animal's life or to relieve its pain.*
Thus if the animal's life is not in danger and it is not in pain, it is not permissible for a RANA to administer even first-aid treatment.

In addition one can say that the plain implication of the words "first aid" is that the treatment is given only as an interim measure until a veterinarian can take over. It is therefore not intended that this provision should be used as a cloak to enable RANAs or any other lay persons to deal completely and finally with any case.

The second question as to what is veterinary surgery is largely answered by Section 27 of the Veterinary Surgeons Act. This states that the term "veterinary surgery" includes—

(a) the diagnosis of diseases in, and injuries to, animals including tests performed on animals for diagnostic purposes;
(b) the giving of advice based upon such diagnosis;
(c) the medical or surgical treatment of animals; and
(d) the performance of surgical operations on animals.

Even although this will cover the great majority of cases in which a RANA may be wondering whether what she is going to do constitutes an act of veterinary surgery or not, this definition can be amplified a little. There are obviously some procedures which do not amount to veterinary surgery, e.g. the removal of sutures and the replacement of dressings, the cutting of nails and beaks unless performed for the relief of a pathological condition, and the scaling of teeth carried out for cosmetic or prophylactic purposes. It follows that there can be no objection to RANAs carrying out such procedures, particularly if they are carried out on the orders of a veterinary surgeon so that there can be no suggestion that there is an element of diagnosis in the RANA's actions.

At the other end of the scale there are a number of procedures which would appear to be acts of veterinary surgery and which a RANA may still be asked by a veterinary surgeon to carry out in assisting him, for example, in an operation. Although the courts alone can decide whether or not a particular act amounts to veterinary surgery, the view taken by the Royal College of Veterinary Surgeons is that in such cases it is unlikely that the RANA would be deemed to be breaking the law *provided* what was done was carried out in the form of assistance to a veterinary surgeon under his immediate and personal supervision so that the act is really the act of the veterinary surgeon and the RANA is, in a sense, his "other pair of hands".

These guidelines should enable RANAs to avoid running foul of the law relating to the practice of veterinary surgery, but in any cases of doubt the invariable rule for any RANA should be to consult the employing veterinary surgeon who can himself consult the Royal College of Veterinary Surgeons if necessary.

CHAPTER 10

The Veterinary Profession

NORMAN G. FOWLER, FRCVS, Dip Bact, DVR

The History of the Veterinary Profession

The veterinary profession is one of the oldest in the world. The "Doctor of oxen and asses" is referred to in the Laws of Hammurabi (2100 B.C.); treatises on horses were written by Simon of Athens, and by Xenophon; one of the books of Aristotle's *Historia Animalium* is devoted to veterinary medicine. In the British Isles the art was practised from the earliest times and by the fourteenth century practitioners were known as "Marshals". The "Master Marshals" of London were organized as a trade guild before 1356, in which year they were granted an ordinance by the Mayor and Alderman authorizing them to rule the craft. Later the practise of the art fell into the hands of empirics and by the end of the eighteenth century had fallen into disrepute. In 1791, however, owing mainly to the efforts of the Odiham Agricultural Society, a veterinary college was established in London, the first professor being Charles Vial de St. Bel, a French veterinary surgeon, who had been trained at the Lyons Veterinary School. In 1823 a college was established in Edinburgh by William Dick, helped by the Highland and Agricultural Society of Scotland. These two schools continued to grant certificates of competency to practise the veterinary art until 1844, by which time there were about 1000 qualified veterinary surgeons in practice.

In 1844 a Royal Charter was granted to the graduates of the two veterinary schools, forming them into a body corporate with the title of the "Royal College of Veterinary Surgeons", and declaring that the practice of Veterinary Medicine was a profession and that the members of the College "solely and exclusively of all other persons whomsoever shall be deemed and taken and recognised to be members of the said profession or professors of the said art and shall be individually known and distinguished by the name or title of Veterinary Surgeon".

Veterinary Training

The Veterinary Surgeons Act of 1948 made wide changes in the organization of veterinary education, re-enacted in the Act of 1966. Hitherto, entry to the profession had been by the candidate passing the examinations of the RCVS, for the Diploma of Member of the Royal College of Veterinary Surgeons. The Act made the veterinary degrees of certain universities admit the holders to the Register of Veterinary Surgeons provided that the said degrees have been recognized by an order of the Privy Council after consultation with the Council of the RCVS. Recognition has been given to the veterinary degrees of the Universities of Bristol, Cambridge, Edinburgh, Glasgow, Liverpool and London, and also to those of the University of Dublin and the National University of Ireland conferred on or after 1 June 1959.

Unqualified veterinary practice became illegal on the 30 July 1949, except for certain minor treatments and operations. Unqualified persons who satisfied the Council of the Royal College of Veterinary Surgeons that certain requirements contained in the Act had been met were permitted to continue the practice of veterinary surgery during their lives or until their name is removed from a new register which was called "The Supplementary Veterinary Register". A person registered in the Supplementary Veterinary Register could not take or use the title "veterinary surgeon" or anything which might lead to the belief that he was registered in the Register of Veterinary Surgeons. Such a person might call himself a "veterinary practitioner".

The course of study for a veterinary degree ranges from 5 to 6 years depending upon which university is attended. Universities lay down general requirements of entry and, in terms of the General Certificate of Education, require at least two, and in some cases three, passes at Advanced level with a background of passes at Ordinary level. In addition to satisfying a university's general entry requirements, a faculty or school may impose specific course requirements. All the university veterinary schools would wish candidates to have some knowledge of science subjects, preferably chemistry, physics and biology, although this need not preclude the possibility of entrance of candidates who have not studied all of these subjects at Advanced or Higher level. Competition for places at the universities is very keen and early application to the university of choice is advisable.

The pre-clinical part of the course is devoted to Physiology, Biochemistry, Anatomy, Histology, Animal Husbandry, Dietetics, Pharmacy, Pathology, Bacteriology, and Parasitology. The clinical years are occupied with Veterinary Surgery and Medicine. Before presenting himself for his final examination, the student must provide evidence that he has spent at least 6 months of his vacations "seeing practice" with a veterinary surgeon in general practice, and must have attended a specified number of parturition cases in the larger farm animals. Students are examined at the end of each scholastic year and progress to the next part of the course is dependent upon a good showing in these examinations. A high standard is required and up to a third of the candidates are referred for a second attempt at the examinations.

The degree awarded at the final examinations depends upon the individual university: Bristol—BVSc; Cambridge—BA, VetMB; Edinburgh—BVMS; Glasgow—BVMS; Liverpool—BVSc; London—BVetMed; Dublin—MVB(TCD); National University of Ireland—MVB(NUI). Holders of these degrees are also entitled to the letters MRCVS as their degree admits them to the Register of Veterinary Surgeons which alone allows them to practice their profession.

Post-graduate study may lead to a higher degree in Veterinary Science awarded by a university, e.g. MVSc or DVSc or PhD. The Royal College of Veterinary Surgeons also awards a Diploma of Fellowship (FRCVS) to Members who have been qualified for 5 years by examination, or by submission of a thesis or by election for meritorious contributions to learning. The Diplomas of Veterinary Radiology and Veterinary Anaesthesia may also be awarded by examination.

Other Diplomas in the field of Veterinary Science awarded by universities include those in Animal Health, Applied Parasitology and Entomology, Bacteriology, Tropical Veterinary Medicine, and Veterinary State Medicine.

Veterinary Surgery as a Career

The general public comes into contact with the veterinary surgeon mainly as the person who treats their sick animals, that is the general practitioner. It is the general practitioner, therefore, who is regarded as being the veterinary profession. In actual fact, only about two-thirds of the profession in this country is employed in general veterinary practice, the others being in research or commercial posts, veterinary education, meat and food inspection, in full-time posts with Local Government, with the Veterinary Division of the Ministry of Agriculture, or with the Royal Army Veterinary Corps. Some are employed in Commonwealth service, in British Dependencies, by the governments of foreign countries, and also by the Food and Agricultural Organisation of the United Nations.

VETERINARY PRACTICE

There are about 1500 veterinary practices in this country, just over half of which are predominantly concerned with small animals, i.e. dogs and cats. One must remember that in veterinary practice there are no public hospital services and few consultants. The veterinary surgeon in practice is dependent upon his own efforts and his own finances to provide modern hospital premises and equipment, such as X-ray plant, anaesthetic machines, instruments, etc. Such equipment and premises represent a great deal of capital invested and it is becoming increasingly difficult for individual practitioners to finance them. This is leading more and more to the group practice and the formation of animal hospitals, where the members share in providing a central hospital and administration block and all can make use of the facilities. This grouping has several advantages in that each member is encouraged to specialize in some aspect of practice, laboratory facilities can be maintained and an administration manager employed to deal with business and office organization. An obvious advantage of this type of scheme is to allow organization of leisure time and holidays.

The general practitioner may be assisted in his work by Animal Nursing Auxiliaries, the great majority of whom are employed by the veterinary surgeons in small animal practice.

The veterinary surgeon in practice must provide a 24-hour, 7 days a week, service.

It must be remembered that there is no ambulance or casualty service for animals, and it may be necessary for a surgeon to operate in some emergency outside normal working hours, a job that his colleague in medical practice passes on to the hospital service. Single-handed practitioners are thus sometimes called upon to work a very great number of hours per week. Despite long hours and the responsibility involved, financial returns may compare unfavourably with some other professions. Most practitioners, however, enter general practice because they like the direct contact with animals and their owners, because they want to practise the art as well as the science of their profession, and last but not least because they are individualists and do not like to conform to a set routine. Few would enter veterinary practice solely in anticipation of financial gain.

THE MINISTRY OF AGRICULTURE

The veterinary surgeon in the Ministry of Agriculture's Veterinary Division is a full-time civil servant concerned with the administration and application of the regulations governing animal health in this country. His job is to control and, where possible, prevent outbreaks of notifiable diseases among the farm livestock in his particular area. When a large outbreak of such a disease occurs, he may be sent to any part of the country to reinforce his colleagues in the affected area and assist in containing the spread of the disease. Examples of notifiable diseases are Foot and Mouth Disease, Fowl Pest and Swine Fever, and it is in the main due to the efforts of the Veterinary Division that this country is no longer infected by such epidemic diseases as rinderpest and bovine pleuro-pneumonia, or those communicable to man such as rabies and glanders. We are fortunate that the United Kingdom is an island and that we can regulate the entry of animals. Eternal vigilance is the price we must pay for this relative immunity. In this connection, mention should be made of the quarantine laws for animals and the danger of campaigns to get them abolished. The Veterinary Division of the Ministry through its Veterinary Investigation Service also assists the general practitioner to elucidate disease occurring on a herd or flock basis. These officers are veterinary investigation officers and have a laboratory background in addition to clinical experience.

VETERINARY RESEARCH

In the fight against animal disease, an increasing number of veterinary surgeons are employed in research establishments, by commercial organizations and pharmaceutical houses, the Ministry of Agriculture, the universities and such organisations as the Animal Health Trust. In many of these laboratories, veterinary surgeons work alongside their medical colleagues and workers in other disciplines, often in research designed to relieve human suffering. Many are engaged on pure research, that is research which has no practical value at the present time, but which has often initiated great strides forward in the advancement of knowledge.

In the clinical departments of the universities, new techniques and methods are being constantly evaluated to relieve the burden of animal ill health.

VETERINARY EDUCATION

The teaching of veterinary students is taken up by those people who have a bias towards the academic life. Most teaching posts stipulate that research must also be carried out in addition to teaching duties, so applicants should have a keen interest in research as well as teaching. Like most other university posts, salaries are lower than those obtaining in general practice, but have the attraction of a shorter working week, a more leisurely approach to life, a pensionable post, and longer holiday periods.

The Organization of the Veterinary Profession

At the present time, there are approximately 8000 members of the RCVS, which makes the veterinary profession very small in numbers compared with its sister professions of medicine and dentistry. Because of its small size and possibly the individuality of its members, the profession has not achieved much political power or even solidarity within itself. This has proved a disadvantage from the point of view of the pressure that can be brought to bear on government departments in matters of veterinary importance. It also to a certain extent effects a hindrance on the profession's striving for a greater financial reward for the services of its members.

The Royal College of Veterinary Surgeons, whose patron is Her Majesty The Queen, is the governing body of the profession, and deals with legislation affecting its members, issues the annual register, and is also concerned with various ethical considerations, such as professional conduct, veterinary education, etc. The College deals with the discipline of the profession and is empowered to remove the name of any offending veterinary surgeon from the register, i.e. withdraws his right to practise his profession. All registered veterinary surgeons must be members of the RCVS and their names are entered in the Register, an annual statutory fee being payable by the member.

The veterinary profession has a very strict code of professional ethics, mainly designed to protect the public. The veterinary surgeon must not advertise his services either openly or covertly, must not canvass for clients, must not consult with an unqualified person or usurp a case under treatment by another veterinary surgeon. These are a few of the rules governing the conduct of a veterinary surgeon and illustrate the fact that Parliament, and through it the general public, although willing to give certain preferential treatment to a profession, also imposes certain restrictions, obligations and duties on its members.

The British Veterinary Association (BVA) is a voluntary organization of veterinary surgeons established to improve the knowledge and the conditions of the veterinary profession. It publishes the only weekly veterinary journal in the world, *The*

Veterinary Record, a quarterly journal devoted to research, and handbooks dealing with recent advances in knowledge of various aspects of disease in animals. The BVA is also a political organization and brings its pressure to bear on any matter of interest to its members or to veterinary science in general. There are many local divisions of the BVA which hold regular meetings in their areas and provide a focal point for the veterinary surgeons of the area. In addition there are sectional divisions such as the British Small Animal Veterinary Association (BSAVA) and the British Equine Veterinary Association (BEVA) (each of which have their own journals), the Association of Veterinary Teachers and Research Workers and the Society of Practising Veterinary Surgeons, etc. Once a year the BVA holds a Congress for the purpose of hearing scientific papers and for social gatherings. Many world-eminent non-veterinarians have addressed plenary sessions of the Congress. Some sectional divisions also hold annual Congresses which enjoy very high repute, e.g. the BSAVA.

Future Trends

The veterinary profession has passed through some difficult phases since its inception, but it has succeeded in developing other spheres of activity in accordance with general progress. At the beginning of the century, the horse was almost the only animal of economic importance, but with the coming of the internal combustion engine and the pneumatic tyre (invented by Dunlop, a veterinarian) veterinary practice declined. Between the wars, with the decline in agriculture, the profession reached a very low ebb, but during the war years and the importance of home agriculture, the profession again flourished. Since the war, small animal practice has become increasingly important as the pet-owning public came to realize what service the profession could now offer for the health of their pets.

With the successful eradication of tuberculosis from British cattle, there was some decline in the volume of work carried out by practising veterinary surgeons acting as part-time employees (Local Veterinary Inspectors—LVIs) of the Ministry of Agriculture, but many other diseases of economic importance remain to be conquered. Work is now in hand in the eradication of contagious abortion of cattle—a disease of great economic importance to the farming industry as well as a dangerous disease communicable to man. It is possible that a nationalized veterinary service for farm animals may one day solve the problems of an effective health service to farmers coupled with adequate financial reward to the veterinary surgeon. Whatever the organization, there will always be spheres of work in which the highly trained veterinary surgeon of today may play his part in the multiple fields of animal production.

The underdeveloped countries will develop their own agricultures as their circumstances allow, and the veterinarian will be in the forefront of the battle for food production. In all matters pertaining to animal husbandry and the use of land, the wide sphere of knowledge of the veterinary profession will be increasingly called upon.

Veterinary Hospitals

In 1967 the Royal College of Veterinary Surgeons instituted a scheme for the inspection and registration of veterinary practice premises which fulfilled certain requirements. Those approved were granted the use of the title "Veterinary Hospital".

This grant by the Royal College to one of its members of the right to describe his practice premises as a veterinary hospital constitutes a guarantee that the establishment provides a very high standard of accommodation and of facilities for the diagnosis, treatment, and both post-medical and surgical care for the class of animals for which it is designed.

No member of the profession becomes entitled to describe his premises as a veterinary hospital without meeting the required standard. Authority to use this title will be granted only after a satisfactory inspection of the premises by a member of the Council of the Royal College.

In order to ensure that all veterinary hospitals continue to maintain the necessary high standards, periodic reinspections will be carried out. The first reinspection will be carried out 2 years after the original inspection and subsequent reinspections 4 years thereafter. In addition a reinspection will be carried out 6 months after change of ownership of the hospital.

A signed certificate will be issued to premises which are approved as a veterinary hospital.

The standards which must be met before an establishment may be described as a veterinary hospital are set out below:

1. The hospital must be clean and in good decorative order, creating an atmosphere of clinical cleanliness and efficiency. All parts of the premises must be kept odour-free and in an orderly condition. The buildings should be constructed of brick, stonework or other permanent materials and the internal walls and floors of such impervious materials as will permit of thorough cleansing and disinfecting. Adequate storage facilities should be provided and the area immediately surrounding the hospital must be maintained in a clean and tidy state.

2. The staff must also subscribe to this atmosphere by maintaining high standards of dress, cleanliness and personal appearance.

3. The services of the hospital must be available at all times, and a veterinary surgeon must attend daily.

4. The lay staff must be adequately trained for the efficient performance of their duties, and sufficient numbers of lay staff must be available to ensure adequate care of the animals in the hospital.

5. A waiting room or reception area of adequate size and with good fittings must be provided.

6. There must be a minimum of one examination room.

7. X-ray facilities suitable and adequate for the needs of the hospital must be provided and be readily available. Equipment should be so placed as to constitute no

risk to patients, clients or staff. Adequate safety precautions must be in operation and standards laid down by the Code of Practice observed.

8. An operating theatre must be provided, apart from the examination rooms and used only for the purpose of conducting surgical operations. The theatre must be properly equipped with a good supply of instruments and proper theatre furniture. There must be adequate facilities for sterilization, anaesthesia, and resuscitation, although not all these facilities need necessarily be provided in the theatre itself. The pre-operative preparation of surgical cases shall not be undertaken in the theatre.

9. An adequate supply of drugs used in the treatment of patients must be available. They must be properly and safely stored with accurate, well-kept stock-lists, or other efficient system which will ensure that there is no shortage of essentials.

10. Laboratory facilities for all routine diagnostic tests (such as those contained in the ANA syllabus) must be available.

11. There must be a kitchen area with suitable provision for storage and preparation of food. Feeding equipment should be sterilized or be of the disposal type.

12. Kennels and cages must be of adequate size for the type of animal housed, and made of non-permeable materials with easily disinfected fittings. Heating must be available for use as required. There should be no overcrowding and there should be suitable means of ventilation. Satisfactory arrangements for the disposal of excreta, soiled bedding and carcasses must be made. All kennels must be escape-proof, safe and comfortable. A minimum of six kennels or cages must be provided, suitable for long-term hospitalization.

13. Exercise areas must be available, adequate both in number and size for the capacity of the hospital.

14. Facilities should be provided, outside the examination or surgical areas, for the bathing and grooming of patients admitted for treatment.

15. Office facilities must be provided which will be easily accessible to the staff and to clients as required. Complete medical cards must be maintained for all patients.

16. There must be no boarding kennels at the hospital.

17. Adequate fire protection equipment must be available.

18. The display of commercially retained merchandise, or the maintenance of a trimming and clipping business within the hospital premises shall not be permissible.

Animal Nursing Auxiliaries Scheme

In 1961 the Council of the Royal College of Veterinary Surgeons introduced a scheme for the recruitment, training and registration of Animal Nursing Auxiliaries.

The scope of work open to these people may be, or may become, quite wide, but at present the great majority of them are employed by veterinary surgeons in small animal practice. It must be emphasized that the Veterinary Surgeons Act of 1966 makes it illegal for anyone other than a veterinary surgeon or veterinary practitioner to treat animals or carry out the practice of veterinary medicine and surgery, except in very limited circumstances. The work of Animal Nursing Auxiliaries both before and after qualification in no way conflicts with the terms of the Act. They are not allowed to enter into veterinary practice and must work under the direct supervision of a veterinarian. The carrying out of this work, however, entails considerable responsibility and the Auxiliary is expected to maintain a high standard of behaviour and attention to duty.

As from 1 January 1969, the entrance requirements for persons wishing to enrol in the training scheme are three passes at the Ordinary level of the GCE examination, including a pass in English Language and a pass in either a physical or biological science or mathematics, or equivalent passes in comparable examinations, including Grade 1, CSE. A trainee must be at least 17 years of age and must obtain full-time gainful employment of not less than 35 hours per week at a training centre approved under the scheme. Approved training centres comprise those veterinary practices or veterinary hospitals approved by the Royal College of Veterinary Surgeons as fulfilling certain conditions; trainees may require to attend more than one centre to gain the necessary experience. Day-release or evening courses are provided at some technical colleges.

The duties of Auxiliaries will consist mainly of nursing animals under the guidance of a veterinary surgeon or practitioner, preparations for operations, the care of instruments and assisting with anaesthesia, radiography, and side-room tests. They will also be employed in looking after, cleaning, feeding, and managing the domestic animals at the centre.

The examinations which an Auxiliary must pass to qualify as a Registered Animal Nursing Auxiliary are the Preliminary and Final examinations held by the Royal College of Veterinary Surgeons. Normally these take place annually in July; the exact time and the centres are circulated to approved training centres several months beforehand and information regarding all ANA examinations is given from time to time in the veterinary press. Each examination consists of two written papers and an oral and practical examination.

Full particulars including a detailed syllabus and specimen examination papers may be obtained on application to the Royal College of Veterinary Surgeons.

This chapter has been based on an article published in the *Journal of Small Animal Practice*, **5**, 195–200 (1964), which was prepared in conjunction with P. N. Humphreys.

INDEX